Neuropsychology of PTSD

Neuropsychology of PTSD

Biological, Cognitive, and Clinical Perspectives

Edited by

JENNIFER J. VASTERLING
CHRIS R. BREWIN

THE GUILFORD PRESS
New York   London

© 2005 The Guilford Press
A Division of Guilford Publications, Inc.
72 Spring Street, New York, NY 10012
www.guilford.com

Printed in the United States of America

This book is printed on acid-free paper.

Last digit is print number: 9   8   7   6   5   4   3

Library of Congress Cataloging-in-Publication Data

Neuropsychology of PTSD : biological, cognitive, and clinical perspectives / editors,
Jennifer J. Vasterling and Chris R. Brewin.
      p.   cm.
   Includes bibliographical references and index.
   ISBN-10: 1-59385-173-1   ISBN-13: 978-1-59385-173-6 (cloth)
   1. Post-traumatic stress disorder. 2. Neuropsychiatry. I. Vasterling, Jennifer J.
II. Brewin, Chris.
   RC552.P67N476   2005
   616.85′21—dc22

                                                                        2005001227

For Kevin and Alison
–J. J. V.

For Bernice
–C. R. B.

About the Editors

Jennifer J. Vasterling, PhD, is Associate Director for Research for the Department of Veterans Affairs South Central (VISN 16) Mental Illness Research, Education, and Clinical Center and is a clinical professor of psychiatry and neurology at Tulane University School of Medicine, New Orleans, Louisiana. Dr. Vasterling's research has focused on the application of neuropsychological assessment methods to the study of posttraumatic stress disorder in military veterans and on examination of the neuropsychological outcomes of military deployment.

Chris R. Brewin, PhD, is a professor of clinical psychology at University College London, and an honorary consultant clinical psychologist with the Camden & Islington Mental Health and Social Care Trust, London. His clinical specialization is in the treatment of posttraumatic stress disorder. Dr. Brewin is the author of *Posttraumatic Stress Disorder: Malady or Myth?* (2003).

Contributors

Amy Arnsten, MD, Department of Psychiatry, Yale University School of Medicine, New Haven, Connecticut

Jill Barron, MD, Yale University School of Medicine, New Haven, Connecticut, and VA Connecticut Healthcare System, West Haven, Connecticut

Kevin Brailey, PhD, Veterans Affairs South Central (VISN 16) Mental Illness Research, Education, and Clinical Center/Veterans Affairs Medical Center, and Department of Psychiatry and Neurology, Tulane University School of Medicine, New Orleans, Louisiana

Chris R. Brewin, PhD, Sub-Department of Clinical Health Psychology, University College London, United Kingdom

Joseph I. Constans, PhD, Mental Health Service Line, Veterans Affairs Medical Center, New Orleans, Louisiana

Michael D. De Bellis, MD, MPH, Department of Psychiatry and Behavioral Sciences and Healthy Childhood Brain Development Research Program, Duke University Medical Center, Durham, North Carolina

Lisa M. Duke, PhD, Department of Psychology, University of North Carolina–Chapel Hill, Chapel Hill, North Carolina

Matthew J. Friedman, MD, PhD, National Center for PTSD, Veterans Affairs Medical Center, White River Junction, Vermont

Mark W. Gilbertson, PhD, Department of Veterans Affairs Medical Center, Manchester, New Hampshire

Julia A. Golier, MD, Department of Psychiatry, Mount Sinai School of Medicine, Bronx Veterans Affairs, New York, New York

Allison G. Harvey, PhD, Department of Psychology, Sleep, and Psychological Disorders Lab, University of California–Berkeley, Berkeley, California

Philip D. Harvey, PhD, Department of Psychiatry, Mount Sinai School of Medicine, Bronx Veterans Affairs, New York, New York

vii

Stephen R. Hooper, PhD, Department of Psychiatry, University of North Carolina School of Medicine, Chapel Hill, North Carolina

Jennifer Sue Kleiner, PhD, Veterans Affairs Medical Center and Department of Psychiatry and Neurology, Tulane University School of Medicine, New Orleans, Louisiana

Michael D. Kopelman, PhD, Neuropsychiatry and Memory Disorders Clinic, University Department of Psychiatry and Psychology, Guy's, King's, and St. Thomas' Medical School, London, United Kingdom

Linda J. Metzger, PhD, Department of Veterans Affairs Medical Center, Manchester, New Hampshire, and Department of Psychiatry, Harvard Medical School, Boston, Massachusetts

Scott P. Orr, PhD, Department of Veterans Affairs Medical Center, Manchester, New Hampshire, and Department of Psychiatry, Harvard Medical School, Boston, Massachusetts

Roger K. Pitman, MD, Department of Psychiatry, Massachusetts General Hospital/Harvard Medical School, Boston, Massachusetts

Ann Rasmusson, MD, Department of Psychiatry, Clinical Neurosciences Division, National Center for PTSD, Yale University School of Medicine, New Haven, Connecticut, and VA Connecticut Healthcare System, West Haven, Connecticut

Scott L. Rauch, MD, Department of Psychiatry, Massachusetts General Hospital/Harvard Medical School, Boston, Massachusetts

Jennifer L. Sapia, PhD, Department of Psychiatry and Behavioral Sciences, Duke University Medical Center, Durham, North Carolina

Lisa M. Shin, PhD, Department of Psychology, Tufts University, Medford, Massachusetts

Steven M. Southwick, MD, Department of Psychiatry, Clinical Neurosciences Division, National Center for PTSD, Yale University School of Medicine, New Haven, Connecticut, and VA Connecticut Healthcare System, West Haven, Connecticut

Karina Stavitsky, BS, Department of Psychiatry, Mount Sinai School of Medicine, New York, New York

Lisa Tischler, PhD, Department of Psychiatry, Mount Sinai School of Medicine, New York, New York

Jennifer J. Vasterling, PhD, Veterans Affairs South Central (VISN 16) Mental Illness Research, Education, and Clinical Center/Veterans Affairs Medical Center, and Department of Psychiatry and Neurology, Tulane University School of Medicine, New Orleans, Louisiana

Rachel Yehuda, PhD, Department of Psychiatry, Mount Sinai School of Medicine, Bronx Veterans Affairs, New York, New York

Preface

Posttraumatic stress disorder (PTSD) first appeared as a formal diagnostic category in 1980, largely as a consequence of the Vietnam War and the large numbers of military veterans who sought assistance for stress-related symptoms. However, as described in Chapter 1, exposure to psychologically traumatic events has been part and parcel of the human experience since long before the Vietnam War and extends beyond combat experiences to such events as natural disasters, sexual assault, physical assault, life-threatening accidents, childhood neglect and abuse, domestic violence, politically motivated mass violence, and terrorist acts. Research conducted mainly in the last 20 years has highlighted the vast breadth of negative consequences that may arise and endure in response to traumatic stress exposure. It has become increasingly apparent that, in addition to emotional and behavioral symptoms, PTSD is associated with significant abnormalities in neurobiological systems and cognitive processes. As detailed in this volume, such abnormalities may have profound psychosocial consequences and direct implications for treatment.

To our knowledge, this is the first volume to provide a comprehensive examination of the neuropsychology of PTSD. We attempt to provide an integrative and balanced summary of neuropsychological research relevant to PTSD, drawing from a number of related research areas. Recent advances in functional neuroimaging have led to increased integration of biological, cognitive, and clinical approaches across neuropsychiatric disorders. Reflecting the importance of synthesizing these approaches, we adopted a broad view of neuropsychology to include relevant findings from animal research and biological challenge paradigms, electrophysiological methods, functional activation studies, experimental studies of cognition and information processing, and descriptive neuropsychological methods. This approach is reflected not only in the selection of chapter topics, but also within each chapter, leading to innovative presentations of each of these literatures.

In the past several decades researchers have gained a greater understanding of the neuropsychology of emotional disorders. PTSD presents a unique opportunity to contribute further understanding of the neuropsychological correlates of psychopathology. Specifically, PTSD differs from other neuropsychiatric disorders in that it is the only chronic mental disorder in which the experience of an environmentally induced event (i.e., the trauma) is critical to its diagnosis and development. That the development of PTSD is not genetically or biologically inevitable allows examination of the biological consequences of a psychological phenomenon.

The study of neuropsychological functioning in PTSD is an emerging area in which many questions remain. For example, does neuropsychological dysfunction represent vulnerability to, or a consequence of, PTSD? Is neuropsychological dysfunction directly attributable to PTSD, or is it better explained by iatrogenic effects or comorbidities? Are certain trauma populations or PTSD subgroups more likely to be characterized by neuropsychological impairment? How might neuropsychological features of the disorder impact assessment and treatment? Throughout the volume, chapter contributors attempt to delineate such questions and describe the degree to which these questions are addressed in the current literature.

The nature of neuropsychological impairment in PTSD has been an area of controversy, largely because of methodological challenges associated with the clinical features of the disorder. In Part I, we attempt to provide an epidemiological and methodological context in which to view the empirical literatures presented later in the volume. Part II provides a biological context with presentation of relevant findings from the animal and human neurobiological, neuroimaging, and electrophysiological literatures. Each of these chapters weaves in implications relevant to clinical neuropsychological impairments. Part III delves into cognitive and information-processing abnormalities such as biases in the way that individuals with PTSD attend to and remember emotionally relevant information and how they encode and later retrieve trauma memories. In keeping with the integrative theme of the volume, these chapters interpret such cognitive processing abnormalities within a cognitive neuroscience framework. Part IV addresses key trauma populations (children, adults, aging survivors, and victims of closed head injury) that may be expected to be associated with unique factors influencing the neuropsychological outcomes of trauma exposure, each incorporating discussion of the neurobiological context. Finally, Part V addresses clinical applications. The first of these chapters addresses clinical neuropsychological assessments in which PTSD is a central consideration. The remaining two chapters apply a neuropsychological framework to treatment issues, including psychological intervention and pharmacological approaches. This innovative approach infuses a unique perspective that we hope will spark new ways of considering the clinical management of PTSD.

We anticipate that this book will appeal to a diverse audience and provide relevant information to researchers, clinicians, and educators with backgrounds in PTSD assessment and treatment, clinical neuropsychology, or biological psychiatry. We hope that it will generate new research and clinical approaches to understanding, assessing, and treating the potentially chronic and debilitating consequences of exposure to psychological trauma.

Acknowledgments

There are a number of individuals we would like to thank. We appreciate the high quality of editorial and production support from The Guilford Press. Kelsey Oveson was helpful in formulating and editing the bibliographies of several chapters. Patricia B. Sutker was instrumental in sparking and facilitating Jennifer Vasterling's initial interest and work in the neuropsychology of PTSD. Kevin Brailey has provided extraordinary personal and professional support to Dr. Vasterling through the years as a key long-term collaborator. Finally, we would like to express our appreciation to the chapter authors. This exceptional group of experts not only generated outstanding contributions to the book, but also stimulated additional insights through their discussions with us and made the book a joy to complete.

Contents

IV. Developmental and Population-Specific Perspectives

V. Clinical Applications

PART I

Background and Context

CHAPTER 1

Epidemiological and Methodological Issues in Neuropsychological Research on PTSD

LISA M. DUKE *and* JENNIFER J. VASTERLING

Knowledge of the prevalence, clinical features, comorbidities, and natural history of any disorder is invaluable to clinicians in making informed judgments. Factors such as predisposing neurobiological vulnerabilities, comorbid psychiatric and physical problems, and trauma-related neurological insults may be particularly relevant to interpretation of neuropsychological performance data. In this chapter, we first review research concerning the epidemiology and clinical manifestations of posttraumatic stress disorder (PTSD): the prevalence of trauma exposure and of PTSD, common comorbid disorders, risk and protective factors for the development and maintenance of PTSD, and the course of the disorder. To provide an interpretive context for research findings presented in subsequent chapters, we conclude with discussion of how potentially confounding disorder-related variables are treated in the empirical literature and how other methodological issues potentially impact empirical findings.

DEFINITION AND HISTORY

PTSD is an anxiety disorder that develops in response to a traumatic experience and is characterized by the core features of reexperiencing, avoidance behaviors, numbing of responsivity, and hyperarousal (see Table 1.1 for diagnostic criteria). Although only first appearing as a formal diagnos-

4 BACKGROUND AND CONTEXT

TABLE 1.1. DSM-IV-TR Diagnostic Criteria for PTSD

A. The person has been exposed to a traumatic event in which both of the following were present:
   (1) the person experienced, witnessed, or was confronted with an event or events that involved actual or threatened death or serious injury, or a threat to the physical integrity of self or others
   (2) the person's response involved intense fear, helplessness, or horror. **Note:** In young children, this may be expressed instead by disorganized or agitated behavior

B. The traumatic event is persistently reexperienced in one (or more) of the following ways:
   (1) recurrent and intrusive distressing recollections of the event, including images, thoughts, or perceptions. **Note:** In young children, repetitive play may occur in which themes or aspects of the trauma are expressed.
   (2) recurrent distressing dreams of the event. **Note:** In children, there may be frightening dreams without recognizable content.
   (3) acting or feeling as if the traumatic event were recurring (includes a sense of reliving the experience, illusions, hallucinations, and dissociative flashback episodes, including those that occur on awakening or when intoxicated). **Note:** In young children, trauma-specific reenactment may occur.
   (4) intense psychological distress at exposure to internal or external cues that symbolize or resemble an aspect of the traumatic event
   (5) physiological reactivity on exposure to internal or external cues that symbolize or resemble an aspect of the traumatic event

C. Persistent avoidance of stimuli associated with the trauma and numbing of general responsiveness (not present before the trauma), as indicated by three (or more) of the following:
   (1) efforts to avoid thoughts, feelings, or conversations associated with the trauma
   (2) efforts to avoid activities, places, or people that arouse recollections of the trauma
   (3) inability to recall an important aspect of the event
   (4) markedly diminished interest or participation in significant activities
   (5) feelings of detachment or estrangement from others
   (6) restricted range of affect (e.g., unable to have loving feelings)
   (7) sense of foreshortened future (e.g., does not expect to have a career, marriage, children, or a normal lifespan)

D. Persistent symptoms of increased arousal (not present before the trauma), as indicated by two or more of the following:
   (1) difficulty falling or staying asleep
   (2) irritability or outbursts of anger
   (3) difficulty concentrating
   (4) hypervigilance
   (5) exaggerated startle response

E. Duration of the disturbance (symptoms in Criteria B, C, and D) is more than 1 month.

F. The disturbance causes clinically significant distress or impairment in social, occupational, or other important aspects of functioning.

(continued)

Specify if:
   Acute: if duration of symptoms is less than 3 months
   Chronic: if duration of symptom is 3 months or more
Specify if:
   With Delayed Onset: if onset of symptoms is at least 6 months after the
   stressor

tic category in the third revision of the *Diagnostic and Statistical Manual of Mental Disorders* (DSM-III; American Psychiatric Association, 1980), the psychiatric sequelae of traumatic experiences have long been reported (see Saigh & Bremner, 1999, and Trimble, 1985, for reviews). For example, in 1896, Kraepelin described a psychiatric disorder called "fright neurosis" characterized by "multiple nervous and psychic phenomena" resulting from "severe emotional upheaval or sudden fright" and observed after "serious accidents and injuries," such as fires and railway collisions (Kraepelin, 1896, as quoted in Saigh & Bremner, 1999, p. 1).

The first *Diagnostic and Statistical Manual of Mental Disorders* (DSM; American Psychiatric Association, 1952) contained a diagnostic category called "gross stress reactions." DSM-II (American Psychiatric Association, 1968) deleted the gross stress reaction category, substituting instead "transient situational disturbances." When the diagnosis of PTSD appeared in DSM-III (American Psychiatric Association, 1980), for the first time trauma-related psychological symptoms were causally attributed to the traumatic event, as opposed to individual weakness (Friedman, 2003) and acknowledged as potentially having long-lasting psychological consequences (Fairbank, Schlenger, Caddell, & Woods, 1993).

PTSD is unique among psychiatric disorders in that the symptoms of the disorder are tied directly to an etiological event, the traumatic stressor (Breslau, 2002). The core symptoms of PTSD have been largely consistent in the DSM revisions subsequent to DSM-III. In contrast, the nature of the traumatic stressor required for PTSD diagnosis has changed in the most recent DSM revisions (DSM-IV [American Psychiatric Association, 1994]; DSM-IV-TR [American Psychiatric Association, 2000]). Breslau (2002) and McNally (2003) reviewed the changing definition of the traumatic stressor since 1980. In the DSM-III, trauma was defined as "an event that is outside the range of usual human experience," meant to include events such as combat, rape, and natural disasters (American Psychiatric Association, 1980, p. 236) and exclude more usual life events, such as divorce, serious illness, and financial losses. In the DSM-IV, the definition of trauma was revised, partly in recognition of research demonstrating that traumatic events were in fact not that uncommon. DSM-IV defines the traumatic stressor as when a person "experienced, witnessed, or was confronted with an event or events that involved actual or threatened death or serious injury, or a threat to the physical integrity of self or others" and had a subjective response of "intense fear, helplessness, or horror" (American Psychiatric Association, 1994, pp. 427–428).

In a study of the effect of broadening the stressor definition in a general population survey, Breslau and Kessler (2001, pp. 701–702) found an increase from 68.1% to 89.6% in the lifetime prevalence of trauma exposure, as well as an increase in the number of reported PTSD cases, largely attributable to a single type of trauma, learning about traumatic events experienced by a close relative or friend, or about a loved one's sudden, unexpected death. The inclusion of secondary trauma exposure as a qualifying stressor remains controversial. McNally (2003, p. 231) pointed out that learning secondhand of what happened to a loved one "seems qualitatively distinct" from first-hand traumas such as those intended in the original DSM-III formulation of the PTSD diagnosis and that the inclusion of such diverse traumas may complicate attempts to identify underlying psychobiological mechanisms of PTSD. Nonetheless, DSM-IV diagnostic criteria for PTSD also contain a more stringent criterion, the requirement that the symptoms cause clinically significant functional impairment or distress, reducing the qualifying PTSD cases by 25% (Breslau, unpublished data described in Breslau, 2002).

EPIDEMIOLOGY OF TRAUMA EXPOSURE AND PTSD

Below we present a representative review of studies examining the prevalence of exposure to traumatic events and of developing PTSD upon exposure to trauma. More comprehensive reviews of the prevalence of trauma exposure and PTSD are available (Breslau, 2001a, 2002; Fairbank, Ebert, & Costello, 2002; Hidalgo & Davidson, 2000).

Prevalence of Trauma Exposure

Traumatic events appear to be relatively common experiences. Consisting of interviews of a representative national sample of 5,877 Americans, ages 15–54, the National Comorbidity Survey (NCS) found that the majority of Americans, 60.7% of men and 51.2% of women, have experienced at least one DSM-III-R (American Psychiatric Association, 1987) traumatic event in their lifetime (Kessler, Sonnega, Bromet, Hughes, & Nelson, 1995). Moreover, many trauma-exposed respondents reported having experienced two or more traumas in their lifetimes (56.3% of trauma-exposed men and 48.6% of trauma-exposed women). Traumas most frequently reported were (1) witnessing someone being badly injured or killed (35.6% of men,

14.5% of women); (2) fire, flood, natural disasters (18.9% of men, 15.2% of women); and (3) life-threatening accidents (25% of men, 13.8% of women). Men as compared to women were more frequently exposed to the above traumas, as well as to physical assaults, combat, threats with a weapon, and being kidnapped or held captive. Women reported higher rates of exposure to traumas such as rape, sexual molestation, and childhood neglect and physical abuse.

A review of recent studies concerning the prevalence of trauma exposure (Hildalgo & Davidson, 2000) found that the prevalence of trauma exposure ranged from 36.7 to 92.2% in studies conducted from 1987 to 1998. Earlier studies reported prevalence rates for trauma exposure of 40–60% (Breslau, 2002), whereas a more recent study using the DSM-IV stressor definition uncovered rates of trauma exposure of 89.6% (Breslau et al., 1998). As discussed by Breslau (2002), increased exposure rates may reflect differences in assessment strategies and differing definitions of the stressors in different DSM versions.

Risk Factors for Trauma Exposure

Traumatic events are not random (Breslau, 2002), and research has revealed a number of risk factors for trauma exposure. As described above, men have greater rates of exposure to traumatic events than do women (see Breslau et al., 1998; Gavranidou & Rosner, 2003; Kessler et al., 1995; Norris, 1992). Younger people are more likely than older individuals to be exposed to traumatic experiences (e.g., Acierno et al., 2002), with the highest rates of trauma in one study for 16- to 20-year-olds (Breslau et al., 1998). History of prior exposure to trauma increases the risk of subsequent trauma exposure in both civilian (Breslau, Davis, & Andreski, 1995) and military (Koenen et al., 2002; Orcutt, Erickson, & Wolfe, 2002) populations. Orcutt et al. (2002) noted that PTSD symptomatology, in particular reexperiencing, conferred increased risk for subsequent trauma exposure, hypothesizing that PTSD symptoms may result in impaired self-protective behavior. Finally, preexisting personal characteristics such as neuroticism and extroversion (Breslau et al., 1995), history of childhood conduct disorder (Breslau, Davis, Andreski, & Peterson, 1991; Koenen et al., 2002), pretrauma substance disorder (Koenen et al., 2002), and familial psychiatric history (Breslau et al., 1991; Koenen et al., 2002) have also been linked to subsequent trauma exposure.

Prevalence of PTSD

Earlier studies of PTSD prevalence, conducted as part of the Epidemiologic Catchment Area Survey, found estimates of lifetime PTSD prevalence of 1.0% among adults in St. Louis (Helzer, Robins, & McEvoy, 1987) and

1.3% among adults in the Piedmont area of North Carolina (Davidson, Hughes, Blazer, & George, 1991). Kessler (2000) noted that these studies did not assess the prevalence of trauma exposure, only enquiring whether respondents had experienced trauma-associated stress reactions. Higher rates of PTSD prevalence were found in subsequent studies, which included more systematic assessments of trauma exposure and resultant psychiatric symptomatology. The estimated lifetime prevalence of DSM-III-R (American Psychiatric Association, 1987) PTSD among adult Americans in the NCS was 7.8% (Kessler et al., 1995).

Lifetime prevalence of PTSD using DSM-IV criteria is higher, and prevalence rates vary depending on the method used to elicit PTSD symptomatology. Breslau et al. (1998) studied the risk of PTSD in a community-based sample of 2,181 adults in the Detroit area and found that the conditional risk of PTSD for trauma-exposed individuals was 9.2%, when estimates were derived using randomly selected traumatic events from each respondent's list. In contrast, the lifetime prevalence of PTSD associated with querying for only the worst traumatic events was 13.6% (9.5% for men and 17.7% for women).

The prevalence of PTSD is also higher in at-risk populations, such as combat veterans, inner-city children, citizens and refugees of postconflict countries, and victims of terrorist attacks, crime, and disasters. The National Vietnam Veterans Readjustment Survey (NVVRS) reported that lifetime prevalence of DSM-III-R (American Psychiatric Association, 1987) PTSD among American Vietnam veterans was 30.9% for men and 26.9% for women, with another 22.5% of men and 21.2% of women experiencing subthreshold, or partial, PTSD at some time in their lives (Kulka et al., 1990). Similarly, in a study of inner-city children and adolescents referred to a psychiatric clinic, Silva et al. (2000) found that 59% had experienced at least one qualifying traumatic stressor. Of the trauma-exposed children and adolescents, 22% met DSM-IV diagnostic criteria for PTSD and another 32% displayed symptoms consistent with subthreshold PTSD. Thus, in these two at-risk populations (Vietnam veterans and trauma-exposed inner-city children), at least half of each sample evidenced clinically significant PTSD symptoms at some point in their lives. More recently, an anonymous survey of U.S. troops assessed 3 to 4 months following return from duty in Iraq or Afghanistan combat theaters revealed high rates of PTSD in the aftermath of war-zone exposure; 12.2–12.9% of Iraq-deployed and 6.2% of Afghanistan-deployed troops met diagnostic criteria for current PTSD using a conservative checklist-based estimate (Hoge et al., 2004).

Rates of trauma exposure and PTSD vary from country to country. For example, a recent study of 3,021 German adolescents and young adults found that although 26% of young German men and 17.7% of young German women reported experiencing at least one traumatic event, rates of PTSD were only 1% among German men and 2.2% among German women (Perkonigg, Kessler, Storz, & Wittchen, 2000). In contrast, in postconflict, low-income countries, where citizens had survived prolonged traumas including war, mass violence, and torture, lifetime PTSD prevalence ranged from 15.8% (Ethiopia) to 37.4% in Algeria (DeJong et al., 2001). The authors concluded that rates of PTSD in postconflict settings vary widely and suggested that the differences in prevalence across countries may be attributable in part to differences in the cumulative number of traumas experienced in each region, noting that terrorism attacks were ongoing during the collection of Algerian study data. Similarly, refugees who have been victims of ongoing political or ethnic violence have higher rates of PTSD than do survivors of traumas characteristic of more developed countries (e.g., Eisenmann, Gelberg, Liu, & Shapiro, 2003; Kessler, 2000; Thabet & Vostanis, 1999, 2000).

Studies of the prevalence of PTSD following terrorist attacks have uncovered relatively high current rates of PTSD, with those directly affected by the attacks having higher rates of PTSD than those indirectly affected. One month after the 9/11 terrorist attacks, the prevalence of probable PTSD among Manhattan residents was 7.5%; however, 20% of respondents living in the vicinity of the World Trade Center had symptoms consistent with probable PTSD during this time period (Galea et al., 2002). Six months following the attacks, current PTSD rates for Manhattan residents dropped dramatically to 0.6% (Galea et al., 2003). Lower rates of PTSD (9.4%) were found in a representative sample of 512 Israeli adults (Bleich, Gelkopf, & Solomon, 2003) despite a relatively high prevalence of direct (16.4%) or indirect (37.4%) exposure to terrorist attacks, leading the authors to speculate that Israelis may have become somewhat habituated to the ongoing terrorist attacks in their country, as compared to the New York City residents.

PTSD also occurs at high rates among survivors of crime and disasters. In a study of 157 crime victims, 20% met criteria for DSM-III-R (American Psychiatric Association, 1987) PTSD diagnoses 6 months after the crime (Brewin, Andrews, Rose, & Kirk, 1999). In a review of studies assessing PTSD prevalence among disaster survivors, McFarlane and Potts (1999) reported PTSD prevalence to vary from 2% among tornado victims (North, Smith, McCool, & Lightcap, 1989, as cited in McFarlane & Potts, 1999) to 80% among high-stress victims of an industrial disaster (Weisaeth, 1989, as cited in McFarlane & Potts, 1999). A review of 160 samples of disaster victims from 29 countries (Norris et al., 2002) demonstrated that victims of mass violence were the most likely to report severe levels of impairment, as compared to survivors of technological or natural disasters. Of relevance to neuropsychological considerations in PTSD, Mollica, Henderson, and Tor (2002) found that among Cambodian survivors of mass violence, brain injury incurred during the traumatic event was predictive of both PTSD and depression severity.

In summary, a review of studies examining the prevalence of trauma exposure and PTSD reveals that traumatic events are relatively common. Rates of PTSD ranged from 1–9.2% in community-based studies, whereas higher rates of lifetime and current prevalence characterized at-risk populations, such as combat veterans and mass violence survivors.

Risk and Protective Factors

Despite the high prevalence of exposure to traumatic stressors, relatively few people exposed to traumas subsequently develop PTSD (McNally, 2003; Yule, 2001). On average 25% of individuals experiencing one or more traumas develop PTSD (Green, 1994). Because traumatic events trigger PTSD in only a subset of exposed individuals, the identification of risk and protective factors for developing PTSD after being exposed to a traumatic event has become of increasing interest. Knowledge concerning risk and protective factors informs treatment of PTSD, as well as prevention and early intervention strategies.

Risk factors related to PTSD development following trauma exposure can be categorized as follows: (1) factors pertaining to the trauma itself (e.g., type of trauma, severity); (2) individual characteristics (gender, age, educational level, preexisting psychiatric history, and personality); and (3) peri- and posttrauma variables. Particularly relevant to the neuropsychology of PTSD are findings that neurological soft signs (Gurvits et al., 1993; Gurvits et al., 2000), history of brain injury (Chemtob et al., 1998; Mollica et al., 2002); and lower levels of intellectual functioning moderate the relationship between stress exposure and PTSD symptomatology (Macklin et al., 1998; McNally & Shin, 1995; Silva et al., 2000; Vasterling et al., 2002).

Recent meta-analytic results have summarized and placed in context findings from the numerous PTSD risk factors studies to date. Ozer, Best, Lipsey, and Weiss (2003) included 68 studies in their meta-analysis and found significant effect sizes for seven PTSD predictors, including pretraumatic individual characteristics (i.e., history of prior trauma, previous psychological adjustment, family history of psychopathology) and peri- and posttrauma variables (i.e., perceived threat to one's life, peritraumatic emotional responses and dissociation, and posttraumatic social support). Peri- and posttraumatic variables, as compared to pretraumatic factors, were the strongest predictors of PTSD. Brewin, Andrews, and Valentine (2000) examined 77 studies and identified three pretraumatic factors that were modestly but consistently related to PTSD development: (1) history of childhood abuse, (2) psychiatric history, and (3) family psychiatric history. However, similar to results obtained by Ozer and colleagues (2003), peri- and posttraumatic factors, such as trauma severity, low levels of social support, and subsequent life stresses were stronger predictors of PTSD than pretrauma factors.

COMORBIDITIES AND COURSE OF PTSD

In this section, we review research concerning comorbid psychiatric and physical conditions in PTSD, as well as the disorder's natural history and clinical course. Our intent is to review disorder-related factors that potentially impact interpretation of neuropsychological outcome data and affect differential diagnosis.

Psychiatric Comorbidities

Individuals diagnosed with PTSD also commonly suffer from other psychiatric disorders, most commonly affective disorders, other anxiety disorders, and alcohol and substance-use disorders (see Brady, Killeen, Brewerton, & Lucerini, 2000, for review). In the NCS, 88% of men and 79% of women with lifetime PTSD met criteria for at least one other comorbid diagnosis (Kessler et al., 1995). In a study of 801 women, Breslau, Davis, Peterson, and Schultz (1997) found a similar lifetime rate (73%) of psychiatric comorbidity with PTSD.

Concurrent rates of major depression among individuals with PTSD typically range from 30 to 50% (see Shalev, 2001, for a review), with rates potentially higher in treatment-seeking populations. In a large sample of 1,127 psychiatric outpatients, 77% of PTSD patients met criteria for major depression, whereas 23% met criteria for dysthymia (Brown, Campbell, Lehman, Grisham, & Mancill, 2001). The high rate of depression comorbidity may be explained in part by shared mood and PTSD symptoms and overlap in symptom measurement. Shalev (2001) and Yule (2001) observed that PTSD and depression share 10 of 17 symptoms on the Hamilton Rating Scale for Depression (Hamilton, 1960). However, Breslau (2001b) noted that depression is comorbid with or secondary to many disorders, and the relationship between depression and anxiety is a particularly strong one, not limited to PTSD. Because the risk for major depression is elevated among trauma-exposed individuals with PTSD but not in trauma-exposed persons without PTSD, Breslau, Davis, Peterson, and Schultz (2000) theorized that traumatic events do not increase the risk for major depression independently of PTSD, but rather that the two disorders share "overlapping or common vulnerabilities" (p. 907) that represent part of the same posttraumatic syndrome, with PTSD leading to depression among trauma-exposed, vulnerable individuals.

A high-risk twin study using a subsample of the Vietnam Era Twin

Registry found that veterans with PTSD were at greater risks for lifetime major depression, dysthymia, and generalized anxiety disorder than combat-exposed veterans without PTSD or high-risk co-twins (Koenen et al., 2003). Results suggested that the comorbidity was not due to symptom overlap, but developed because both disorders were part of a syndrome of psychopathological response to combat. Results further revealed that depression was a vulnerability factor for PTSD development, as PTSD probands displayed higher rates of depression than combat controls, and high-risk co-twins displayed higher rates of depression than did low-risk co-twins.

As noted in the Koenen et al. (2003) study, anxiety disorders also frequently accompany PTSD (see Brady et al., 2000, for review). In the NCS, comorbidity of PTSD with other anxiety disorders ranged from 15.0% (generalized anxiety disorder) to 29.0% (simple phobia) in women and from 7.3% (panic disorder) to 31.4% (simple phobia) in men (Kessler et al., 1995). In the above described study of psychiatric outpatients, 23% of PTSD patients met criteria for panic disorder with agoraphobia, 38% for generalized anxiety disorder, 15% for social phobia, 31% for obsessive–compulsive disorder, and 23% for specific phobia (Brown et al., 2001).

Finally, PTSD is commonly accompanied by substance-use disorders (Breslau et al., 1991; Breslau et al., 1997; Brown et al., 2001; Kessler et al., 1995; Kulka et al., 1990), including both alcohol and nonalcohol substance-use disorders. In the NCS, for example, lifetime prevalence of alcohol abuse/dependence and drug abuse/dependence among men with histories of PTSD was 51.9% and 34.5%, respectively; rates of comorbid alcohol and drug abuse/dependence were 27.9% and 26.9%, respectively, among women with histories of PTSD (Kessler et al., 1995). McFarlane (1997) hypothesized a complex pattern of interrelationships among trauma exposure, alcohol use, and PTSD. That is, although self-medication of PTSD symptoms appears to lead to alcohol abuse, alcohol abuse also increases rates of trauma exposure and modifies PTSD symptoms in some cases.

Somatic Disorders

In addition to negatively impacting psychological well-being, PTSD appears to lead to poor physical health outcome (see Hidalgo & Davidson, 2000; Schnurr & Green, 2004, for reviews). For instance, after controlling for selection bias, socioeconomic characteristics, behavioral risk factors, and hypochondriasis among 1,399 male Vietnam veterans, Boscarino (1997) found greater rates of circulatory, digestive, musculoskeletal, nervous system, respiratory, and nonsexually transmitted infectious diseases among PTSD-diagnosed veterans as compared to combat-exposed veterans without PTSD. Similarly, in a study involving ambulatory cardiovascular monitoring, Vietnam veterans with chronic PTSD varied more in their systolic blood pressures and had a higher proportion of heart rate and systolic blood pressure readings above baseline during activity than did veterans without chronic PTSD, after controlling for demographic and other background variables and comorbid psychiatric diagnoses (Beckham et al., 2003). Of relevance to the neuropsychology of PTSD, some of the health problems associated with stress-related disorders may share neurobiological etiologies (Friedman & McEwen, 2004) and/or lead to conditions (e.g., hypertension) that increase the risk of neuropsychological compromise.

Course

Onset of PTSD typically occurs immediately following the traumatic event (see Shalev, 2000, for a review). Although a subset of PTSD-diagnosed individuals recover within a few months, many go on to develop chronic PTSD, lasting 3 months or longer. Approximately 82% of PTSD cases meet criteria for chronicity, with approximately 74% lasting 6 months or more (Breslau, 2001b). In the NCS, roughly 90% of participants retrospectively reported that PTSD symptoms persisted at 3 months, and more than 70% still experienced symptoms 1 year after the traumatic event (Kessler et al., 1995).

Unfortunately, PTSD can last for decades, or even lifetimes (see Yule, 2001, for review). Symptoms had not remitted after 10 years or more for more than one third of the NCS sample, even including those receiving treatment (Kessler et al., 1995). Similarly, 15% of veterans in the NVVRS still suffered from PTSD 19 years after combat exposure (Kulka et al., 1990). Assessment of 326 World War II and Korean War former prisoners of war (POWs) and combat veterans revealed that after 40 years or more, 88% of Korean War POWs, 76% of World War II Pacific-theater POWs, and 54% of World War II European-theater POWs met criteria for current PTSD, whereas 14% of combat veterans from both wars still suffered PTSD (Sutker & Allain, 1996). Factors predicting disorder maintenance may differ from those predicting the initial development of PTSD. In a study of Vietnam veterans, although a variety of factors spanning premilitary, military, and postmilitary time periods were related to PTSD development, variables associated with the maintenance of PTSD pertained primarily to the traumatic event itself (e.g., higher war-zone exposure, peritraumatic dissociation) and posttraumatic occurrences (e.g., lower social support during homecoming, lower current emotional sustenance and social support, and a higher number of nontraumatic stressful life events in the year prior to the interview) (Schnurr, Lunney, & Sengupta, 2004).

The pattern of symptom expression varies over time and may fluctuate in relation to ongoing life stressors and exposures to reminders of the initial traumatic event (Shalev, 2000). Port, Engdahl, and Frazier (2001) found that PTSD severity was highest among World War II and Korean War former POWs in the year after their military discharges, lower for several decades following discharge, and then higher during the 20 years prior to the most recent assessment. A study of 1991 Gulf War veterans 6 years postconflict revealed greater than chance probability of increased PTSD symptomatology and of "feeling worst" during anniversaries of trauma exposures (Morgan, Hill, Fox, Kingham, & Southwick, 1999). Finally, Osuch et al. (2001) found that symptom exacerbation was associated with varied stressful life events, leading to unique patterns of chronic PTSD within the study sample.

IMPLICATIONS FOR METHODOLOGY
IN NEUROPSYCHOLOGICAL STUDIES OF PTSD

Risk factors for trauma exposure, disorder development, and disorder maintenance; population characteristics; the comorbidity profile of PTSD; and the course of PTSD each have implications for interpretation of research relevant to neuropsychological functioning in PTSD. That is, a number of these factors (e.g., comorbid health problems, depression, neurological insult at the time of trauma, predisposing neurobiological vulnerabilities) potentially influence neuropsychological performance. In the following section, we address the treatment of these variables and other relevant methodological issues in studies examining neuropsychological functioning in PTSD.

Risk Factors and Population Characteristics

As summarized in previous sections, sociodemographic factors, familial and personal psychiatric history, and the nature and severity of the trauma exposure(s) serve as risk or protective factors for trauma exposure and the development and maintenance of PTSD. It has been suggested that such individual and population differences factor into the varied neuropsychological findings across studies (Golier & Yehuda, 2002; Vasterling, Brailey, Constans, & Sutker, 1998; see also Yehuda, Stavitsky, Tischler, Golier, & Harvey, Chapter 9, this volume). That is, it may be that PTSD-related neuropsychological deficits are more or less pronounced in certain populations in which risk factors (e.g., age, education) interact with PTSD diagnosis. For instance, PTSD-related performance deficits may be more pronounced in socioeconomically-disadvantaged populations in which academically sensitive skills are potentially more fragile. Risk factors also potentially influence findings when they are not adequately controlled within a particular study. Consider, for example, a study comparing the neuropsychological performance of PTSD-diagnosed participants to healthy controls. If age differs between the two groups, unless age-normed values are examined or age is examined statistically, it is difficult to discern whether neuropsychological performance deficits are related to PTSD specifically or instead reflect age-related performance decrements.

Given that the severity and nature of trauma exposure are related to PTSD development, it is also difficult to ferret out the relative impact of stress exposure versus PTSD on cognitive performance. The question of the relative contribution of trauma exposure to performance emphasizes the importance of including trauma-exposed, PTSD-negative comparison samples. However, even with such comparison samples, as would be expected given the typical dose–response relationship between trauma exposure and PTSD (cf. Foy, Osato, Houskamp, & Neumann, 1992), trauma exposure is often more extensive or severe in PTSD samples as compared to non-PTSD, trauma-exposed comparison samples.

Potential neurobiological and neuropsychological risk factors for PTSD present a unique interpretive question. As discussed in Vasterling and Brailey (Chapter 8, this volume), it is unclear whether cognitive functioning represents a risk–protective factor for PTSD development and maintenance, whether PTSD is associated with decline in cognition following stress exposure, or whether cognitive impairment reflects both risk for, and the sequelae of, PTSD. Most of the current body of research is cross-sectional and thus cannot address cause and effect directly. Instead, researchers have either equated groups on variables (e.g., education, IQ estimates, vocabulary) thought to be reflective of premorbid functioning (e.g., Jenkins, Langlais, Delis, & Cohen, 1998) or controlled for these variables statistically (e.g., Vasterling et al., 2002). However, in rare instances (e.g., Crowell, Kieffer, Siders, & Vanderploeg, 2002; Macklin et al., 1998), preexposure data were obtained through record review and combined with current cognitive performance data to address more directly questions related to direction of causality. In addition, in an innovative cross-sectional design, Gilbertson and his colleagues (Gilbertson et al., 2002) used twin methodology to address both neuropsychological and brain morphometric risk factors (see Shin, Rauch, & Pitman, Chapter 3, this volume; Vasterling & Brailey, Chapter 8, this volume), allowing examination of genetic versus environmental influences on cognitive performance and brain integrity. Ultimately, however, prospective data collection in populations at high risk for trauma exposure will be necessary to gain a fuller understanding of cause and effect relationships among cognitive proficiency, trauma exposure, and PTSD.

Comorbidities

As described earlier in this chapter, PTSD is associated with psychiatric comorbidities (e.g., mood disorder, substance abuse) and the development of health problems (e.g., vascular disease) potentially affecting cognitive performance either directly or indirectly (e.g., via medication). There are several ways in which the influence of comorbidities can be addressed, each associated with strengths and weaknesses regarding interpretation.

One possible method is to exclude PTSD cases with certain psychiatric or health conditions. Although this method is generally appropriate when the base rate of the comorbidity is relatively low, for disorders that are more highly comorbid with PTSD (e.g., depression), the representativeness of the remaining "cleaned" sample of PTSD-diagnosed individuals to the broader PTSD population becomes questionable. For some disorders (e.g., alcohol use disorders) with particularly high potential to impact cognitive performance adversely, researchers have adopted a compromise of excluding cases in which alcohol use is either current or relatively recent (e.g., past year) but including more remote cases. This approach eliminates the most immediate and potent effects of alcohol use; however, it does not completely eliminate subtle alcohol-related neuropsychological deficits that may be more enduring.

A second approach is to include a comparison sample that is characterized by the comorbid disorder(s) (e.g., Barrett, Green, Morris, Giles, & Croft, 1996; Crowell et al., 2002; Gil, Calev, Greenberg, Kugelmass, & Lerer, 1990; Zalewski, Thompson, & Gottesman, 1994) or, in the case of past alcohol use, to use the related approach of equating for history of use across groups (e.g., Jenkins et al., 1998). However, for some types of trauma exposure, especially when the exposure is particularly potent in terms of psychological outcome, it may be difficult to identify sufficient numbers of individuals who are trauma exposed and develop a non-PTSD psychiatric disorder but do not develop at least subthreshold manifestations of PTSD. Nonetheless, this is a viable approach in some trauma populations, especially in larger-scale studies in which access to more of the population is possible (e.g., Barrett et al., 1996). The option also remains to include disorder comparison samples comprised of individuals who were not trauma exposed; however, exposed and nonexposed samples may differ on other relevant variables associated with risk for trauma exposure.

A third approach is to examine subgroups of PTSD-diagnosed individuals with and without comorbid disorders or associated features (e.g., Beckham, Crawford, & Feldman, 1998; Vasterling, Brailey, & Sutker, 2000; Vasterling, Rogers, & Kaplan, 2000; Vasterling et al., 2002). The strength of this approach is that it takes a first step in isolating the association between the comorbidity and neuropsychological performance within the context of PTSD. The challenge in conducting such subanalyses, however, is in obtaining an adequate sample size for all subgroups.

Finally, covariance procedures that statistically control for comorbid conditions or medications are potentially informative. However, the use of covariance in quasi-experimental psychopathology research is controversial. If there is significant symptom overlap between PTSD and the comorbid condition or the comorbid condition and PTSD correlate strongly, covariance procedures may remove most of the variance associated with PTSD, leading to an overly conservative approach. Miller and Chapman (2001) argue that it may be particularly inappropriate to use covariance procedures if the diagnostic and comparison samples differ on the basis of the covariate. As articulated by Miller and Chapman, if the disorder of interest is truly associated with the covariate, removing the variance associated with the covariate would "alter the diagnostic group variable substantially."

Course of the Disorder

PTSD is often chronic (Breslau, 2001b; Kessler et al., 1995) with a fluctuating course (Shalev, 2002) in which symptoms wax and wane over the lifespan of the individual. Because most of the PTSD literature addressing neuropsychological functioning is cross-sectional, little is known about the degree to which chronicity and current symptom manifestation influence the neuropsychological profile. It could be speculated that, with increasing chronicity, neurobiological abnormalities may become more pronounced and possibly take an increasing toll on brain integrity and associated neuropsychological functioning or lead to subtle differences in the nature of the dysfunction over the course of the disorder. It may be that variance in the length of time the disorder has been endured explains some of the inconsistencies in findings across these studies. Similarly, inclusion within a single study of individuals at different stages of chronic PTSD could potentially increase interindividual variability, making it more difficult to demonstrate intergroup differences.

The question also remains whether neuropsychological performance decrements are associated with the expression of current symptoms or whether such decrements, once manifested, remain regardless of the current symptom profile. If neuropsychological deficits represent a risk factor for development of PTSD, it might be expected that symptom manifestation would not influence neuropsychological performance. However, if neuropsychological deficits are at least in part a consequence of the disorder, it is less clear whether neuropsychological impairment would be expected to exist in the absence of current symptom manifestation. Although these questions can be addressed in part through population replications, longitudinal research will more definitively address both questions regarding chronicity and symptom manifestation.

Measurement Issues

Another factor complicating comparison across neuropsychological studies of PTSD is the use of different measures to assess neuropsychological domains. Typically, multiple neuropsychological instruments, each varying slightly in instructional set, level of difficulty, and stimulus parameters, exist to measure any given neuropsychological domain. Further, neuropsychological constructs are often hierarchically organized; domains such as attention or memory may be further broken into meaningful components that tap different aspects of the construct, which may have unique brain–behavior relationships. For example, within the memory domain, performance data related to immediate recall and retention of newly learned information differ in their interpretive implications. Even when using the same instrument, if different variables are extracted, the constructs each variable measures will differ. Returning to memory as an example, if immediate recall or initial learning is taken into account when analyzing delayed recall data, the interpretation of the data would be different than if delayed recall were analyzed without taking into account initial acquisition. Thus, across studies, what may appear at first to be a failure to replicate may instead reflect inclusion of a test or a variable tapping a related, but different, neuropsychological construct.

Sample Size

In efforts to implement stringent eligibility criteria and to equate groups on key variables that could potentially confound findings, the resulting samples are often relatively small and may therefore suffer from insufficient statistical power. Only a few studies (Barrett et al., 1996; Crowell et al., 2002; Zalewski et al., 1994) have included large samples. However, these studies are all drawn from the same Centers for Disease Control database and have considerable overlap in both measures and participants, raising the question of the degree to which the findings each can be considered to be independent.

SUMMARY AND CONCLUSIONS

The epidemiology of PTSD suggests that like many other mental disorders, it is associated with a number of disorder- and population-related risk, resilience, comorbidity, and iatrogenic variables that could potentially influence neuropsychological performance. Various methodological approaches are each associated with strengths and weaknesses in addressing the relative influence of these issues, and interpretation of findings will need to be viewed in this context. Studies using longitudinal, prospective designs for assessment of at-risk populations and those using cross-sectional approaches such as twin methodology will likely help clarify many of the remaining questions in this literature.

REFERENCES

Acierno, R., Brady, K., Gray, M., Kilpatrick, D. G., Resnick, H., & Best, C. L. (2002). Psychopathology following interpersonal violence: A comparison of risk factors in older and younger adults. *Journal of Clinical Geropsychology, 8*, 13–23.

American Psychiatric Association. (1952). *Diagnostic and statistical manual of mental disorders*. Washington, DC: Author.

American Psychiatric Association. (1968). *Diagnostic and statistical manual of mental disorders* (2nd ed.). Washington, DC: Author.

American Psychiatric Association. (1980). *Diagnostic and statistical manual of mental disorders* (3rd ed.). Washington, DC: Author.

American Psychiatric Association. (1987). *Diagnostic and statistical manual of mental disorders* (3rd ed., rev.). Washington, DC: Author.

American Psychiatric Association. (1994). *Diagnostic and statistical manual of mental disorders* (4th ed.). Washington, DC: Author.

American Psychiatric Association. (2000). *Diagnostic and statistical manual of mental disorders* (4th ed., text rev.). Washington, DC: Author.

Barrett, D. H., Green, M. L., Morris, R., Giles, W. H., & Croft, J. B. (1996). Cognitive functioning and posttraumatic stress disorder. *American Journal of Psychiatry, 259*, 2701–2707.

Beckham, J. C., Crawford, A. L., & Feldman, M. E. (1998). Trail Making Test performance in Vietnam combat veterans with and without posttraumatic stress disorder. *Journal of Traumatic Stress, 11*, 811–819.

Beckham, J. C., Taft, C. T., Vrana, S. R., Feldman, M. E., Barefoot, J. C., Moore, S. D., Mozley, S. L., Butterfield, M. I., & Calhoun, P. S. (2003). Ambulatory monitoring and physical health report among Vietnam veterans with and without chronic posttraumatic stress disorder. *Journal of Traumatic Stress, 16*, 329–355.

Bleich, A., Gelkopf, M., & Solomon, Z. (2003). Exposure to terrorism, stress-related mental health symptoms, and coping behaviors among a nationally representative sample in Israel. *Journal of the American Medical Association, 290*, 612–620.

Boscarino, J. A. (1997). Diseases among men 20 years after exposure to severe stress: Implications for clinical research and medical care. *Psychosomatic Medicine, 59*, 605–614.

Brady, K. T., Killeen, T. K., Brewerton, T., & Lucerini, S. (2000). Comorbidity of psychiatric disorders and posttraumatic stress disorder. *Journal of Clinical Psychiatry, 61*(Suppl. 7), 22–32.

20   BACKGROUND AND CONTEXT

Breslau, N. (2001a). The epidemiology of posttraumatic stress disorder: What is the extent of the problem? *Journal of Clinical Psychiatry, 62*(Suppl. 17), 16–22.
Breslau, N. (2001b). Outcomes of posttraumatic stress disorder. *Journal of Clinical Psychiatry, 62(Suppl. 17)*, 55–59.
Breslau, N. (2002). Epidemiologic studies of trauma, posttraumatic stress disorder, and other psychiatric disorders. *Canadian Journal of Psychiatry, 47*, 923–929.
Breslau, N., Davis, G. C., & Andreski, P. (1995). Risk factors for PTSD related traumatic events: A prospective analysis. *American Journal of Psychiatry, 152*, 529–535.
Breslau, N., Davis, G. C., Andreski, P., & Peterson, E. (1991). Traumatic events and posttraumatic stress disorder in an urban population of young adults. *Archives of General Psychiatry, 48*, 216–222.
Breslau, N., Davis, G. C., Peterson, E., & Schultz, L. (1997). Psychiatric sequelae of posttraumatic stress disorder in women. *Archives of General Psychiatry, 54*, 81–87.
Breslau, N., Davis, G. C., Peterson, E., & Schultz, L. (2000). A second look at comorbidity in victims of trauma: The post-traumatic stress disorder–major depression connection. *Biological Psychiatry, 48*, 902–909.
Breslau, N., & Kessler, R. C. (2001). The stressor criterion in DSM-IV posttraumatic stress disorder: An empirical investigation. *Biological Psychiatry, 50*, 699–704.
Breslau, N., Kessler, R. C., Chilcoat, H. D., Schultz, L. R., Davis, G. C., & Andreski, P. (1998). Trauma and posttraumatic stress disorder in the community: The 1996 Detroit area survey of trauma. *Archives of General Psychiatry, 55*, 626–632.
Brewin, C. R., Andrews, B., Rose, S., & Kirk, M. (1999). Acute stress disorder and posttraumatic stress disorder in victims of violent crime. *American Journal of Psychiatry, 156*, 360–366.
Brewin, C. R., Andrews, B., & Valentine, J. D. (2000). Meta-analysis of risk factors for posttraumatic stress disorder in trauma-exposed adults. *Journal of Consulting and Clinical Psychology, 68*, 748–766.
Brown, T. A., Campbell, L. A., Lehman, C. L., Grisham, J. R., & Mancill, R. B. (2001). Current and lifetime comorbidity of the DSM-IV anxiety and mood disorders in a large clinical sample. *Journal of Abnormal Psychology, 110*, 585–599.
Chemtob, C. M., Muraoka, M. Y., Wu-Holt, P., Fairbank, J. A., Hamada, R. S., & Keane, T. M. (1998). Head injury and combat-related posttraumatic stress disorder. *Journal of Nervous and Mental Disease, 186*, 701–708.
Crowell, T. A., Kieffer, K. M., Siders, C. A., & Vanderploeg, R. D. (2002). Neuropsychological findings in combat-related posttraumatic stress disorder. *The Clinical Neuropsychologist, 16*, 310–321.
Davidson, J. R. T., Hughes, D., Blazer, D. G., & George, L. K. (1991). Posttraumatic stress disorder in the community: An epidemiological study. *Psychological Medicine, 21*, 713–721.
DeJong, J. T. V. M., Komproe, I. H., Van Ommeren, M. V., El Masri, M., Araya, M., Khaled, N., van de Put, W., & Somasundaram, D. (2001). Lifetime events and posttraumatic stress disorder in 4 postconflict settings. *Journal of the American Medical Association, 286*, 555–562.
Eisenmann, D. P., Gelberg, L., Liu, H., & Shapiro, M. F. (2003). Mental health and

health-related quality of life among adult Latino primary care patients living in the United States with previous exposure to political violence. *Journal of the American Medical Association, 290,* 627–634.

Fairbank, J. A., Ebert, L., & Costello, E. J. (2002). Epidemiology of traumatic events and post-traumatic stress disorder. In D. Nutt, J.R.T. Davidson, & J. Zohar (Eds.), *Post-traumatic stress disorder: Diagnosis, management, and treatment* (pp. 17–27). London: Martin Dunitz.

Fairbank, J. A., Schlenger, W. E., Caddell, J. M., & Woods, M. G. (1993). Post-traumatic stress disorder. In P. B. Sutker & H. E. Adams (Eds.), *Comprehensive handbook of psychopathology* (2nd ed., pp. 145–165). New York: Plenum Press.

Foy, D. W., Osato, S. S., Houskamp, B. M., & Neumann, D. A. (1992). Etiology of posttraumatic stress disorder. In P.A. Saigh (Ed.), *Posttraumatic stress disorder* (pp. 29–49). Boston: Allyn & Bacon.

Friedman, M. J. (2003, May 14). *Posttraumatic stress disorder: An overview.* Retrieved August 23, 2004, from *www.ncptsd.org/facts/general/fs_overview.html*

Friedman, M., & McEwen, B. S. (2004). Posttraumatic stress disorder, allostatic load, and medical illness. In P. P. Schnurr & B. L. Green (Eds.), *Trauma and health: Physical consequences of exposure to extreme stress* (pp. 157–188). Washington, DC: American Psychological Association.

Galea, S., Ahern, J., Resnick, H., Kilpatrick, D., Bucuvalas, M., Gold, J., & Vlahov, D. (2002). Psychological sequelae of the September 11 terrorist attacks in New York City. *New England Journal of Medicine, 346,* 982–987.

Galea, S., Vlahov, D., Resnick, H., Ahern, J., Sussre, E., Gold, J., Bucuvalas, M., & Kilpatrick, D. (2003). Trends of probable post-traumatic stress disorder in New York City after the September 11 terrorist attacks. *American Journal of Epidemiology, 158,* 514–524.

Gavranidou, M., & Rosner, R. (2003). The weaker sex?: Gender and posttraumatic stress disorder. *Depression and Anxiety, 17,* 130–139.

Gil, T., Calev, A., Greenberg, D., Kugelmass, S., & Lerer, B. (1990). Cognitive functioning in post-traumatic stress disorder. *Journal of Traumatic Stress, 3,* 29–45.

Gilbertson, M. W., Shenton, M. E., Ciszewski, A., Kasai, K., Lasko, N. B., Orr, S. P., & Pitman, R. K. (2002). Smaller hippocampal volume predicts pathologic vulnerability to psychological trauma. *Nature Neuroscience, 5,* 1242–1247.

Golier, J., & Yehuda, R. (2002). Neuropsychological processes in post-traumatic stress disorder. *Psychiatric Clinics of North America, 25,* 295–315.

Green, B. L. (1994). Psychological research in traumatic stress: An update. *Journal of Traumatic Stress, 7,* 343–361.

Gurvits, T. V., Gilbertson, M. W., Lasko, N. B., Tarhan, A. S., Simeon, D., Macklin, M. L., & Orr, S. P., & Pitman, R. K. (2000). Neurologic soft signs in chronic posttraumatic stress disorder. *Archives of General Psychiatry, 57,* 181–186.

Gurvits, T. V., Lasko, N. B., Schacter, S. C., Kuhne, A. A., Orr, S. P., & Pitman, R. K. (1993). Neurological status of Vietnam veterans with chronic posttraumatic stress disorder. *Journal of Neuropsychiatry and Clinical Neurosciences, 5,* 183–188.

Hamilton, M. (1960). A rating scale for depression. *Journal of Neurology, Neurosurgery, and Psychiatry, 23,* 56–61.

Helzer, J. E., Robins, L. N., & McEvoy, L. (1987). Post-traumatic stress disorder in the general population. Findings of the Epidemiologic Catchment Area Survey. *The New England Journal of Medicine, 37,* 1630–1634.

Hidalgo, R. B., & Davidson, J. R. T. (2000). Posttraumatic stress disorder: Epidemiology and health-related considerations. *Journal of Clinical Psychiatry, 61*(Suppl. 7), 5–13.

Hoge, C. W., Castro, C. A., Messer, S. C., McGurk, D., Cotting, D. I., & Koffman, R. L. (2004). Combat duty in Iraq and Afghanistan, mental health problems, and barriers to care. *New England Journal of Medicine, 351,* 13–22.

Jenkins, M. A., Langlais, P. J., Delis, D., & Cohen, R. (1998). Learning and memory in rape victims with posttraumatic stress disorder. *American Journal of Psychiatry, 155,* 278–279.

Kessler, R. C. (2000). Posttraumatic stress disorder: The burden to the individual and to society. *Journal of Clinical Psychiatry, 61*(Suppl. 5), 4–14.

Kessler, R. C., Sonnega, A., Bromet, E. Hughes, M., & Nelson, C. B. (1995). Posttraumatic stress disorder in the National Comorbidity Survey. *Archives of General Psychiatry, 52,* 1048–1060.

Koenen, K. C., Harley, R., Lyons, M. J., Wolfe, J., Simpson, J. C., Goldberg, J., Eisen, S. A., & Tsuang, M. (2002). A twin registry study of familial and individual risk factors for trauma exposure and posttraumatic stress disorder. *Journal of Nervous and Mental Disease, 190,* 209–218.

Koenen, K. C., Lyons, M. J., Goldberg, J., Simpson, J., Williams, W. M., Toomey, R., Eisen, S. A., True, W. R., Cloitre, M., Wolfe, J., & Tsuang, M. T. (2003). A high risk twin study of combat-related PTSD comorbidity. *Twin Research, 6,* 218–226.

Kulka, R. A., Schlenger, W. E., Fairbank, J. A., Hough, R. L., Jordan, B. K., Marmar, C. R., & Weiss, D. S. (1990). *Trauma and the Vietnam War generation: Report of findings from the National Vietnam Veterans Readjustment Survey.* New York: Brunner/Mazel.

Macklin, M. L., Metzger, L. J., Litz, B. T., McNally, R. J., Lasko, N. B., Orr, S. P., & Pitman, R. K. (1998). Lower precombat intelligence is a risk factor for posttraumatic stress disorder. *Journal of Consulting and Clinical Psychology, 66,* 323–326.

McFarlane, A. (1997). Epidemiological evidence about the relationship between PTSD and alcohol abuse: The nature of the association. *Addictive Behaviors, 23,* 813–825.

McFarlane, A. C., & Potts, N. (1999). Posttraumatic stress disorder: Prevalence and risk factors relative to disasters. In P. A. Saigh & J. D. Bremner (Eds.), *Posttraumatic stress disorder: A comprehensive text* (pp. 92–102). Needham Heights, MA: Allyn & Bacon.

McNally, R. J. (2003). Progress and controversy in the study of posttraumatic stress disorder. *Annual Review of Psychology, 54,* 229–252.

McNally, R. J., & Shin, L. M. (1995). Association of intelligence with severity of posttraumatic stress disorder symptoms in Vietnam combat veterans. *American Journal of Psychiatry, 152,* 936–938.

Miller, G. M., & Chapman, J. P. (2001). Misunderstanding analysis of covariance. *Journal of Abnormal Psychology, 110,* 40–48.

Mollica, R. F., Henderson, D. C., & Tor, S. (2002). Psychiatric effects of traumatic brain injury events in Cambodian survivors of mass violence. *British Journal of Psychiatry, 181*, 339–347.

Morgan, C. A., Hill, S., Fox, P., Kingham, P., & Southwick, S. M. (1999). Anniversary reactions in Gulf War veterans: A follow-up inquiry 6 years after the war. *American Journal of Psychiatry, 156*, 1075–1079.

Norris, F. N. (1992). Epidemiology of trauma: Frequency and impact of different potentially traumatic events on different demographic groups. *Journal of Consulting and Clinical Psychology, 60*, 409–418.

Norris, F. N., Friedman, M. J., Watson, P. J., Bryne, C. M., Diaz, E., & Kaniasty, K. (2002). 60,000 disaster victims speak: Part I. An empirical review of the empirical literature, 1981–2001. *Psychiatry, 65*, 207–239.

Orcutt, H. K., Erickson, D. J., & Wolfe, J. (2002). A prospective analysis of trauma exposure: The mediating role of PTSD symptomatology. *Journal of Traumatic Stress, 15*, 259–266.

Osuch, E. A., Brotman, M. A., Podell, D., Geraci, M., Touzeau, P. L., Leverich, G. S., McCann, U. D., & Post, R. M. (2001). Prospective and retrospective life charting in posttraumatic stress disorder (PTSD–LCM): A pilot study. *Journal of Traumatic Stress, 14*, 229–239.

Ozer, E., Best, S. R., Lipsey, T. L., & Weiss, D. S. (2003). Predictors of posttraumatic stress disorder and symptoms in adults: A meta-analysis. *Psychological Bulletin, 129*, 52–73.

Perkonigg, A., Kessler, R. C., Storz, S., & Wittchen, H-U. (2000). Traumatic events and post-traumatic stress disorder in the community: Prevalence, risk factors, and comorbidity. *Acta Psychiatra Scandinavica, 101*, 46–59.

Port, C. L., Engdahl, B., & Frazier, P. (2001). A longitudinal and retrospective study of PTSD among older prisoners of war. *American Journal of Psychiatry, 158*, 1474–1479.

Saigh, P. A., & Bremner, J. D. (1999). The history of posttraumatic stress disorder. In P. A. Saigh & J. D. Bremner (Eds.), *Posttraumatic stress disorder: A comprehensive text* (pp. 1–17). Needham Heights, MA: Allyn & Bacon.

Schnurr, P. P., & Green, B. L. (2004). *Trauma and health: Physical consequences of exposure to extreme stress.* Washington, DC: American Psychological Association.

Schnurr, P. P., Lunney, C. A., & Sengupta, A. (2004). Risk factors for the development versus maintenance of posttraumatic stress disorder. *Journal of Traumatic Stress, 17*, 85–95.

Shalev, A. Y. (2000). Measuring outcome in posttraumatic stress disorder. *Journal of Clinical Psychiatry, 61*(Suppl. 5), 33–42.

Shalev, A. Y. (2001). What is posttraumatic stress disorder? *Journal of Clinical Psychiatry, 62*(Suppl. 17), 4–10.

Shalev, A. Y. (2002). Post-traumatic stress disorder: Diagnosis, history, and life course. In D. Nutt, J. R. T. Davidson, & J. Zohar (Eds.), *Post-traumatic stress disorder: Diagnosis, management, and treatment* (pp. 1–15). London: Martin Dunitz.

Silva, R. R., Alpert, M., Munoz, D. M., Singh, S., Matzner, F., & Dummit, S. (2000). Stress and vulnerability to posttraumatic stress disorder in children and adolescents. *American Journal of Psychiatry, 157*, 1229–1235.

Sutker, P. B., & Allain, Jr., A. N. (1996). Assessment of PTSD and other mental disorders in World War II and Korean conflict POW survivors and combat veterans. *Psychological Assessment, 8,* 18–25.

Thabet, A. A., & Vostanis, P. (1999). Post-traumatic stress reactions in children of war. *Journal of Child Psychology and Psychiatry, 40,* 385–391.

Thabet, A. A., & Vostanis, P. (2000). Post-traumatic stress disorder reactions in children of war: A longitudinal study. *Child Abuse and Neglect, 24,* 291–298.

Trimble, M. R. (1985). Post-traumatic stress disorder: History of a concept. In C. R. Fogley (Ed.), *Trauma and its wake: The study and treatment of post-traumatic stress disorder* (pp. 5–14). New York: Brunner/Mazel.

Vasterling, J. J., Brailey, K., Constans, J. I., & Sutker, P. B. (1998). Attention and memory dysfunction in posttraumatic stress disorder. *Neuropsychology, 12,* 125–133.

Vasterling, J. J., Brailey, K., & Sutker, P. B. (2000). Olfactory identification in combat-related posttraumatic stress disorder. *Journal of Traumatic Stress, 13,* 241–253.

Vasterling, J. J., Duke, L. M., Brailey, K., Constans, J., Allain, Jr., A. N., & Sutker, P. B. (2002). Attention, learning, and memory performances and intellectual resources in Vietnam veterans: PTSD and no disorder comparisons. *Neuropsychology, 16,* 5–14.

Vasterling, J. J., Rogers, C., & Kaplan, E. (2000). Qualitative Block Design analysis in posttraumatic stress disorder. *Assessment, 7,* 217–226.

Yule, W. (2001). Posttraumatic stress disorder in the general population and in children. *Journal of Clinical Psychiatry, 62*(Suppl. 17), 23–28.

Zalewski, C., Thompson, W., & Gottesman, I. (1994). Comparison of neuropsychological test performance in PTSD, generalized anxiety disorder, and control Vietnam veterans. *Assessment, 1,* 133–142.

PART II

Biological Perspectives

CHAPTER 2

Neurobiological and Neurocognitive Alterations in PTSD

A Focus on Norepinephrine, Serotonin, and the Hypothalamic–Pituitary–Adrenal Axis

STEVEN M. SOUTHWICK, ANN RASMUSSON,
JILL BARRON, *and* AMY ARNSTEN

Over the past 20 years it has become increasingly clear that dysregulation of multiple neurobiological systems plays an important role in the pathophysiology of posttraumatic stress disorder (PTSD). During situations of threat, parallel activation of numerous brain regions and neurotransmitter systems allows the organism to assess and appropriately respond to situations of potential danger. In the short run, this process serves a protective role and facilitates fleeing from or actively confronting danger. However, for some individuals, long-standing neurobiological responses to fear and stress may prove to be maladaptive and contribute to the development of PTSD (Southwick, Yehuda, & Morgan, 1995).

In this chapter we review data on the relationship between a number of brain regions that are critically involved in the fear response (i.e., prefrontal cortex, amygdala, hippocampus, dorsal raphe nucleus, and locus coeruleus) and three neurotransmitter/neurohormone systems (i.e., noradrenergic system, serotonergic system, and hypothalamic–pituitary–adrenal [HPA] axis) known to be dysregulated in many individuals with PTSD. As such, our review is very limited and does not reflect the enormous complexity of neurobiological responses to danger or neurobiological dysregulations characteristic of PTSD. While this review is based on preclinical and clinical data, much of the discussion on clinical application is speculative in nature.

27

We begin by briefly reviewing relevant preclinical studies on the relationship between norepinephrine and arousal, sensitization and memory. We then review relevant preclinical studies related to catecholamine regulation of the prefrontal cortex (PFC), locus coeruleus (LC), and amygdala. This is followed by clinical studies on the role of norepinephrine (NE) in combat- and civilian-related PTSD. Next we briefly review preclinical and clinical studies related to the serotonin system and PTSD, with an emphasis on the orbitofrontal cortex. This is followed by a review of the HPA axis as it relates to stress, fear, PTSD, and the PFC and amygdala. Finally, we summarize the data and speculate on possible clinical relevance.

NOREPINEPHRINE

Preclinical Studies

Norepinephrine, Locus Coeruleus, Arousal, and Sensitization

Numerous preclinical studies have shown that central noradrenergic nuclei play an important role in orientation to novel stimuli, alertness, vigilance, selective attention, and cardiovascular responses to life-threatening stimuli (Aston-Jones, Rajkowski, Kubiak, & Alexinsky, 1994). For example, in rats, cats, and monkeys, drowsiness is associated with decreased rate of LC firing while alertness is associated with increased rate of LC firing. Novel sensory stimuli that interrupt ongoing vegetative behaviors (e.g., eating) are particularly likely to provoke rapid activation of the LC. As a result, the organism orients toward the novel stimulus. NE also facilitates selective attention to meaningful stimuli by enhancing excitatory or inhibitory input (signal) relative to basal activity (noise) in the same neuron. At very high rates of LC firing, selective attention is replaced by scanning and vigilance (Aston-Jones et al., 1994).

The LC contains the majority of noradrenergic cell bodies in the brain (Zigmond, Finlay, & Sved, 1995). This large cluster of noradrenergic neurons processes relevant sensory information through its diverse afferent inputs and facilitates anxiety and fear-related skeletomotor, cardiovascular, neuroendocrine, and cognitive responses through its extensive efferent network. Electrical or pharmacological stimulation of the LC elicits fear-related behaviors and increases release of NE in multiple brain regions, such as the amygdala, hippocampus, hypothalamus, and PFC. These brain regions are involved in perceiving, evaluating, remembering, and responding to potentially threatening stimuli. A marked reduction in fear-related behaviors and NE release during threatening situations has been observed secondary to bilateral lesions of the LC (Charney, Deutch, Southwick, & Krystal, 1995; Redmond, 1987).

Catecholaminergic neurons are capable of adjusting level of transmitter synthesis and release depending on current demands and past history (Abercrombie & Zigmond, 1995; Zigmond et al., 1995). For example, dopamine beta-hydroxylase activity, tyrosine hydroxylase, synaptic levels of NE, and LC responsivity to excitatory stimuli all increase when animals are exposed to repeated shock (Irwin, Ahluwalia, & Anisman, 1986; Karmarcy, Delaney, & Dunn, 1984; Melia et al., 1992; Simpson & Weiss, 1994). As a result of these and other adaptations, repeatedly stressed animals may respond to future stressors with exaggerated catecholamine, physiological, and behavioral reactivity (Southwick et al., 1995; Zigmond et al., 1995). This enhanced reactivity, often referred to as stress sensitization, is most likely to follow repeated episodes of uncontrollable, as opposed to controllable, stress. Other neurobiological factors, such as corticotropin-releasing factor (CRF) and neuropeptide Y, have also been implicated in the exaggerated noradrenergic release among animals exposed to chronic uncontrollable stress (Koob, Heinrichs, Menzaghi, Pich, & Britton, 1994; Rasmusson et al., 2000).

Norepinephrine, Amygdala, and Memory

The amygdala is a region of the brain that detects threat and controls defensive responses to these threatening situations. As such, it is involved in both the acquisition and expression of fear (Davis, 1992). The amygdala has strong connections to the hypothalamus and brainstem nuclei that mediate fear responses, including freezing behaviors, alterations in heart rate and blood pressure, sweat gland activity, and release of stress hormones. For example, threat-induced activation of the amygdala stimulates the release of catecholamines and glucocorticoids. Of note, activation of the amygdala by appropriate stimuli can change the neurochemical state of the organism, providing the amygdala with an optimal neurochemical environment for its own function.

In the amygdala, catecholamines also play a central role in the encoding and consolidation of memory for events and stimuli that are arousing, stressful, or fear-provoking. It is well known, for example, that consolidation of recently formed memories can be enhanced by posttraining administration of epinephrine or NE (Gold & Van Buskirk, 1975). These effects are dose and time dependent. The relationship between dose and degree of retention has been described as an inverted "U," where intermediate (but not low or high) doses of epinephrine enhance retention, and the memory-enhancing effects of epinephrine decrease as the time between training and epinephrine administration increases (McGaugh, 2000; Sternberg, Isaacs, Gold, & McGaugh, 1985).

While multiple other stress-induced neuromodulators, such as glucocorticoids, opioid peptides, gamma-aminobutyric acid (GABA), and glucose also affect consolidation of memory for arousing events, they appear to do so through their influence on activation or inhibition of NE in the amygdala (Introini-Collison, Nagahara, & McGaugh, 1989; McGaugh, 2000). For example, the memory enhancing effects of peripherally administered epinephrine are blocked by posttrial intra-amygdala infusion of propranolol (Liang, Juler, & McGaugh, 1990; Liang, McGaugh, & Yao, 1990), an adrenergic agent that blocks the effects of NE. Epinephrine may also enhance memory consolidation by increasing circulating levels of glucose, which readily crosses the blood–brain barrier (Gold & McCarty, 1995).

Epinephrine and NE additionally have been shown to enhance memory retrieval when administered at the time of memory testing. Stone, Rudd, and Gold (1990) found that epinephrine, amphetamine, and glucose administered 30 minutes prior to retention testing each significantly enhanced memory for a one-trial inhibitory avoidance task, and Sara (1985; Sara & Devauges, 1989) reported that yohimbine and idazoxane, both of which increase central NE, effectively alleviated forgetting. An intact central noradrenergic system appears to be necessary for effective retrieval of emotion-based learning (Sara & Devauges, 1989). It is well known that cues, which are related to the context in which the original learning took place, play an important role in the facilitation of memory retrieval (i.e., state-dependent learning).

Catecholamine Regulation of Amygdala

High levels of catecholamine and cortisol release during stress enhance the functioning of the amygdala, promoting fear conditioning and the consolidation of emotionally relevant memories. For example, fear conditioning is facilitated by dopamine projections to the amygdala (Nader & LeDoux, 1999) involving the D_1 receptor (Greba & Kokkinidis, 2000). Examination of intracellular mechanisms has shown the need for protein synthesis, and the activation of protein kinase A (PKA), protein kinase C (PKC), and mitogen-activated protein kinase (MAPK) signaling pathways (Schafe et al., 2000; Schafe, Nadel, Sullivan, Harris, & LeDoux, 1999; Weeber et al., 2000). In contrast, noradrenergic alpha$_{2A}$ receptor stimulation suppresses fear conditioning and decreases cyclic adenosine monophosphate (cAMP) response element-binding protein (pCREB) expression in the amygdala (Davies et al., 2004).

As noted above, a similar picture has emerged in neurochemical studies of the emotional enhancement of memory consolidation by the basal lateral amygdala. Numerous studies have demonstrated the critical role of NE, with special emphasis on actions at beta-adrenergic receptors (Cahill & McGaugh, 1996). Rodent studies have shown that this beta-adrenergic action is mediated by activation of cAMP/PKA signaling (Roozendaal, Quirarte, & McGaugh, 2002). The beta-adrenergic enhancement of memory is facilitated by alpha$_1$ adrenoceptor stimulation (Ferry, Roozendaal, & McGaugh, 1999) and by glucocorticoids (Roozendaal et al., 2002). Conversely alpha$_{2A}$ adrenoceptor stimulation reduces the emotional enhancement of contextual memory (Davies et al., 2004).

In summary, the amygdala potentiates the emotional control of behavior. These actions are driven by high levels of catecholamines and glucocorticoid hormones within the amygdala, and reduced by alpha$_{2A}$ adrenoceptor stimulation. The projections of the amygdala to the hypothalamus and catecholamine nuclei likely create a feedforward loop whereby the amygdala can drive its own facilitation during stress exposure. Thus, in general, catecholamines and glucocorticoids enhance amygdala function. Of note, the amygdala can also strongly influence the neurochemical environment in the PFC. Even mild psychological stressors induce high levels of catecholamine release in the PFC, as well as increased circulating corticosterone (Goldstein, Rasmusson, Bunney, & Roth, 1996). These neurochemical responses are abolished by lesions of the amygdala (Goldstein et al., 1996).

Catecholamine Regulation of Prefrontal Cortex

In contrast to their effects in the amygdala, high levels of catecholamines and glucocorticoids greatly *impair* the cognitive functioning of the PFC. The PFC regulates behavior, thought, and affect using representational knowledge (i.e., working memory) (Goldman-Rakic, 1987). The PFC plays an important role in planning, guiding, and organizing behavior. Lesions of the PFC can result in disinhibited behavior, increased motor activity, impaired attention, and diminished ability to inhibit distracting stimuli. Moderate levels of catecholamines are essential to PFC working memory function, but high levels of catecholamines and glucocorticoids impair the working memory functions of the PFC (Arnsten, 2000b). In both rats and monkeys, exposure to mild, uncontrollable stress impairs performance of a working memory task, while having little effect on control tasks with similar motor and motivational demands (Arnsten, 1998b; Murphy, Arnsten, Goldman-Rakic, & Roth, 1996). Dopamine has an important role in this response. For example, stress-induced impairments can be prevented by dopamine D$_1$ receptor blockade (Arnsten, 1998b; Murphy et al., 1996), and mimicked by infusion of a D$_1$ agonist into the PFC (Zahrt, Taylor, Mathew, & Arnsten, 1997). Dopamine D$_2$/D$_4$ receptors likely contribute as well (Arnsten, 2000a; Druzin, Kurzina, Malinina, & Kozlov, 2000), although this family of receptors has not been studied as thoroughly.

In addition to dopamine, NE plays a critical role in stress-induced PFC dysfunction. Noradrenergic projections from the LC modulate PFC functioning through postsynaptic alpha$_1$ and alpha$_2$ receptors. Preclinical research in rodents and primates suggests that moderate basal release of NE improves PFC cognitive functioning through preferential binding to post-synaptic alpha$_{2A}$ receptors. Arnsten (Arnsten, 1998a) has proposed that postsynaptic alpha$_{2A}$ receptor stimulation inhibits irrelevant and distracting sensory processing through effects on pyramidal cells that project to sensory association cortices. Inhibition or gating of irrelevant sensory stimuli allows the organism to concentrate on the contents of working memory. However, under stressful conditions (especially uncontrollable stress) when NE release is increased above basal levels in the PFC, postsynaptic alpha$_1$ receptors become activated causing a decline in PFC functioning. It has been proposed that this inhibition of PFC functioning during stressful or dangerous situations has value for survival by allowing the organism to employ rapid habitual subcortical modes of responding (Arnsten, 1998a; Birnbaum, Gobeske, Auerbach, Taylor, & Arnsten, 1999).

Thus, stress-induced PFC dysfunction can be prevented by alpha$_1$ adrenoceptor antagonists such as urapidil and prazosin (Arnsten & Jentsch, 1997; Birnbaum et al., 1999), and mimicked by alpha$_1$ agonist infusion into the PFC in rats (Arnsten, Mathew, Ubriani, Taylor, & Li, 1999) and monkeys (Li, Mao, Wang, & Mei, 1999). More recent research suggests that activation of beta$_1$ adrenoceptors in PFC may also impair working memory (Ramos & Arnsten, unpublished), although the mixed beta$_1$/beta$_2$ antagonist, propranolol, has little effect on working memory under non-stress conditions (Arnsten & Goldman-Rakic, 1985; Aston-Jones et al., 1994). The intracellular cascades initiated by high levels of catecholamines in PFC have just begun to be examined. Evidence to date indicates that activation of both cAMP/PKA (Arnsten et al., 1999) and PKC (Birnbaum et al., 2004) intracellular signaling cascades contribute to PFC cognitive impairment during stress.

In contrast to noradrenergic actions at alpha$_1$ and beta$_1$ receptors, stimulation of alpha$_2$ adrenoceptors protects PFC cognitive function during stress. The alpha$_2$ agonist, guanfacine, was more potent than clonidine in protecting against stress-induced PFC dysfunction (Birnbaum, Podell, & Arnsten, 2000). As clonidine is more potent than guanfacine at presynaptic alpha$_2$ receptors, these results suggest that postsynaptic alpha$_2$ receptors play an important protective role. Studies of genetically altered mice have confirmed that working memory enhancement results from actions at alpha$_{2A}$ adrenoceptors (Franowicz et al., 2002), and infusion of the alpha$_{2A}$ agonist, guanfacine, directly into monkey PFC produces a delay-related enhancement of working memory (Li et al., 1999). Alpha$_{2A}$ adrenoceptor stimulation likely strengthens PFC function by reducing cAMP/PKA signaling (Ramos & Arnsten, unpublished).

The strengthening of PFC function by alpha$_{2A}$ receptor stimulation has been observed at the cellular level as well. PFC neurons can fire during the delay interval, representing information in the absence of environmental stimulation (Funahashi, Bruce, & Goldman-Rakic, 1989; Fuster, 1973) and despite the presence of distractors (Miller, Li, & Desimone, 1993). Delay-related firing also contributes to behavioral inhibition such as the ability to suppress a prepotent response (Funahashi, Chafee, & Goldman-Rakic, 1993). Thus, it is of great interest that alpha$_2$ adrenoceptor stimulation increases the delay-related firing of PFC cells (Anderson, Bechara, Damasio, Tranel, & Damasio, 1999). Conversely, yohimbine, an alpha$_2$ adrenergic receptor antagonist that increases the release of NE, impairs working memory (Aston-Jones et al., 1994) and reduces delay-related firing (Anderson et al., 1999; Sawaguchi, 1998). In sum, alpha$_{2A}$ adrenoceptor stimulation strengthens PFC function, while alpha$_1$, beta$_1$, and high levels of D$_1$ receptor stimulation impair PFC function.

In this context, it is important to note that NE has higher affinity for alpha$_{2A}$ receptors (O'Rourke, Blaxall, Iversen, & Bylund, 1994) than for alpha$_1$ receptors (Mohell, Svartengren, & Cannon, 1983) or beta receptors (Pepperl & Regan, 1994). Therefore, conditions of modest NE release (i.e., during alert but nonstressful wakefulness) would predominantly engage alpha$_{2A}$ adrenoceptors, facilitating PFC regulation of behavior, and suppressing the role of the amygdala. In contrast, high levels of NE release during stress would engage alpha$_1$ and beta adrenoceptors, impairing PFC function and promoting amygdala regulation of behavior. In this way NE can act as a chemical switch, determining which brain structures have control over our behavior.

In summary, during uncontrollable stress, the amygdala induces the release of high levels of catecholamines and cortisol, thus optimizing its own neurochemical environment while impairing PFC regulation of behavior, thought, and affect. It is important to note that the PFC has extensive projections to the amygdala (Ghashghaei & Barbas, 2002), and can potently inhibit amygdala function (Quirk, Likhtik, Pelletier, & Pare, 2003). Thus, when the amygdala floods the PFC with catecholamines and takes the PFC "off-line," it also releases PFC inhibition of the amygdala and sensorimotor cortex, diminishing rational influences on behavior and thought.

Clinical Studies

General

A large body of clinical physiological, neuroendocrine, receptor binding, pharmacological challenge, brain imaging, and pharmacological treatment studies have provided compelling evidence for exaggerated noradrenergic activity in traumatized humans with PTSD (Friedman & Southwick, 1995; Southwick et al., 1999a). This exaggerated activity is generally observed in response to a variety of stressors but not under baseline or resting conditions. It has been suggested that altered reactivity of noradrenergic neurons is associated with a variety of hyperarousal and reexperiencing symptoms characteristic of PTSD (Southwick et al., 1999a).

Baseline Norepinephrine

Most studies measuring baseline or resting indices of catecholamine activity have found insignificant differences between subjects with PTSD and control groups. This includes psychophysiology studies, which compare indices of resting heart rate, blood pressure and galvanic skin conductance as well as neuroendocrine studies measuring plasma NE and epinephrine. (Southwick et al., 1999a, 1999b). For example, in a large multicenter psychophysiology study, Keane et al. (1998) reported no differences between baseline heart rate, blood pressure, and galvanic skin response between Vietnam combat veterans with PTSD, Vietnam combat veterans without PTSD, and healthy controls. Similarly, at least three studies of combat veterans with PTSD have reported resting plasma levels of NE that did not differ from levels in healthy controls (reviewed in Southwick, 1999a).

24-Hour Urine Catecholamines and Platelet Adrenergic Receptors

Unlike baseline psychophysiology and neuroendocrine data, studies of 24-hour plasma NE levels, 24-hour urine hormone excretion, and platelet adrenergic receptor number have found significant differences between subjects with PTSD and controls (Southwick et al., 1999a). Under resting or unstimulated conditions, Yehuda et al. (1998) sampled plasma 3-methoxy-4-hydroxyphenylglycol (MHPG) and NE over a period of 24 hours in subjects with PTSD compared to healthy controls and found significantly higher mean NE levels in combat veterans with PTSD compared to combat veterans with PTSD and comorbid depression, patients with MDD alone, and healthy controls. There were no differences in MHPG between groups.

Most studies of combat veterans and civilians (e.g., residents living near the Three Mile Island Nuclear Power Plant accident) (Davidson & Baum, 1996); and of women with histories of child abuse (Limieux & Coe, 1995) have found elevated 24-hour urine excretion of NE in subjects with PTSD compared to controls. It is possible that 24-hour catecholamine levels reflect the summation of both phasic physiological changes in response to meaningful stimuli and tonic resting levels of catecholamines, while single plasma samples reflect only tonic activity (Southwick et al., 1999a, 1999b).

Reduced platelet alpha$_2$-adrenergic receptor number has been reported in combat veterans and traumatized children with PTSD compared to healthy controls (Perry, 1994). It has been hypothesized that downregulation of alpha$_2$-adrenergic receptors serves as an adaptive response to chronic elevation of circulating catecholamines. This hypothesis is consistent with the finding that patients with congestive heart failure and hypertension (conditions characterized by chronic elevated levels of plasma catecholamines) also have reduced numbers of platelet alpha$_2$ receptors.

Catecholamine Challenge Paradigms

Studies that challenge catecholamine systems have been designed to evaluate catecholamine activity under controlled conditions where the subject is intentionally exposed to provocative auditory or visual stimuli or exogenously administered biological substances, such as lactate or yohimbine. Challenge paradigms using platelets and lymphocytes have also been used to assess adrenergic receptor reactivity.

A review of the scientific literature suggests that trauma survivors with PTSD experience greater physiological reactivity (particularly heart rate) in response to trauma-relevant stimuli than do trauma survivors without PTSD and nontraumatized healthy controls. Trauma-relevant stimuli have included sights and sounds of combat as well as scripts of personally experienced traumas. In all published studies approximately two thirds of PTSD subjects have demonstrated exaggerated reactivity to trauma-associated cues. The percentage appears to be even higher in subjects with severe PTSD (Keane et al., 1998; Orr, 1997a; Orr et al., 1997b). On the other hand, most studies have found that subjects with PTSD do not experience exaggerated physiological reactivity in response to generic non-trauma-related stimuli (Orr, 1997a). Of note, a relationship between physiological reactivity to traumatic cues and elevation in endogenous catecholamines has been supported by McFall, Murburg, Ko, and Veith (1990), who found parallel increases in subjective distress, blood pressure, heart rate, and plasma epinephrine among combat veterans with PTSD in response to viewing a combat film. Similar findings have been reported by Blanchard, Kolb, Prins, Gates, and McCoy (1991) with respect to heart rate and plasma NE.

In a study designed to assess dynamic functioning of alpha$_2$ receptors, Perry (1994) incubated intact platelets with high levels of epinephrine and found a greater and more rapid loss in receptor number among subjects with PTSD compared to controls, suggesting that alpha$_2$ adrenergic receptors in subjects with PTSD were particularly sensitive to stimulation by the agonist epinephrine. Challenge studies assessing epinephrine on forskolin-stimulated adenylate cyclase activity and the lymphocyte beta-adrenergic receptor-mediated cyclic adenosine 3'5'-monophosphate system in subjects with PTSD have been mixed (Southwick et al., 1999a).

While a number of pharmacological challenges have been used in the study of PTSD, investigations employing yohimbine have been most relevant to understanding catecholamine systems. Yohimbine is an alpha$_2$-adrenergic receptor antagonist that increases presynaptic release of NE by blocking the alpha$_2$-adrenergic autoreceptor. When administered to healthy subjects, yohimbine has few effects. However, subjects diagnosed with panic disorder experience marked yohimbine-induced increases in subjective anxiety, heart rate, and biochemical indices of noradrenergic activity. Additionally, approximately 60% experience yohimbine-induced panic attacks. Similarly, in subjects with PTSD, yohimbine causes significant increases in subjective anxiety, heart rate, and plasma MHPG, a metabolite of NE. In one study (Southwick et al., 1993), 70% of combat veterans with PTSD experienced yohimbine-induced panic attacks. However, unlike panic disorder patients, subjects with PTSD also experienced marked increases in yohimbine-induced PTSD symptoms such as hypervigilance and intrusive memories. In fact, nearly 80% of combat veterans with PTSD, when administered yohimbine, experience vivid intrusive memories of combat traumas and 40% experienced yohimbine-induced flashbacks.

In the above cited study, it is possible that yohimbine-induced increases in NE impaired PFC functioning, which contributed to intrusive memories among individuals with PTSD. These intrusive memories and flashbacks were accompanied by increased heart rate and catecholamine activity (i.e., increased plasma MHPG). The retrieval of traumatic memories secondary to yohimbine infusion is consistent with animal studies demonstrating enhanced retrieval of aversive memories through adrenergic and noradrenergic stimulation (Conway, Anderson, & Larsen, 1994). Creating a biological context (yohimbine-induced increase in catecholamine activity) that resembles the biological state at the time of encoding (fear-enhanced increase in catecholamine activity) may have served to facilitate the retrieval of frightening memories (state-dependent recall).

Forty percent of PTSD subjects who received IV yohimbine also experienced full-blown flashbacks. It is possible that impaired PFC functioning (secondary to exaggerated release of NE and engagement of postsynaptic alpha$_1$ receptors) may have compromised a number of executive functions, such as simulation and reality testing, that are needed to differentiate past experiences from experiences occurring in the present. Simulation involves the generation of internal models of reality while reality testing includes the monitoring of information sources. Thus, elevated NE in the amygdala and hippocampus may have facilitated retrieval of past memories but deficits in simulation and reality testing may have made it difficult to discriminate between the current external world and the internally generated memory of the past. The result may have been a flashback where the past memory was experienced as if it were occurring in the present.

This model is consistent with results from a recent positron emission tomography (PET) study where healthy controls had increased yohimbine-induced metabolism and PTSD subjects decreased yohimbine-induced metabolism in neocortical brain regions (orbitofrontal cortex, temporal cortex, PFC, parietal cortex). It is possible that yohimbine-induced release of NE (which was greater in PTSD subjects compared to controls) in the PFC resulted in exaggerated alpha$_1$ adrenergic receptor occupancy with a subsequent decrease in regional metabolism.

Of course, genetic factors clearly play a role in sympathetic nervous system (SNS) reactivity to stress. Recent evidence suggests that alpha$_2$ adrenoreceptor gene polymorphisms may play a role in baseline catecholamine levels, intensity of stress-induced SNS activation, and rate of catecholamine return to baseline after stress. In a study of healthy subjects, homozygous carriers for the alpha$_2$cDel322-325-AR polymorphism had exaggerated total body noradrenergic spillover at baseline, exaggerated yohimbine-induced increases in anxiety and total body noradrenergic spillover, and a slower than normal return of total body noradrenergic spillover to baseline after yohimbine infusion (Neumeister et al., in press). Such individuals may be more vulnerable to stress-related psychiatric disorders such as PTSD and depression.

SEROTONIN
General Characteristics and Relevant Brain Regions

Serotonin is a monoamine that is synthesized from tryptophan in serotonergic neurons within the brain and gastrointestinal tract. Neurons that synthesize and release serotonin are found almost exclusively in the raphe nuclei of the brainstem (Nestler, Hyman, & Malenka, 2001). Serotonergic neurons project to many brain regions including limbic structures and all areas of the cerebral cortex (Nestler et al., 2001). Serotonin receptors (14 receptor subtypes) can be found in multiple brain regions including the PFC, amygdala, LC, hippocampus, dorsal raphe nucleus, nucleus accumbens, and hypothalamus. The serotonergic system is a complex system that has both inhibitory and excitatory actions.

Serotonin is specifically known to play an important role in regulation of the PFC, the amygdala, and the hippocampus, each of which has been implicated in the pathophysiology of PTSD. These three brain regions have intricate neuroanatomical connections with one another and with other structures, such as the LC, which appear to be involved in the pathophysiology of PTSD. The hippocampus receives projections from brainstem regions (LC, raphe nucleus, ventral tegmental area), the amygdala, and the cortex. Major hippocampal efferents project to the amygdala, hypothalamus, and septum (Clark & Boutros, 1999). The amygdala is divided into three nuclei, and receives inputs from various areas including the PFC, cingulate gyrus, and ventral striatum. All three nuclei have connections with the hypothalamus for expression of emotion by way of the autonomic and endocrine systems (Clark & Boutros, 1999).

Relationship to Orbitofrontal Cortex

The effects of serotonin on prefrontal cortical function are still under investigation, and likely very complex given the large number of serotonin receptors. Mounting evidence suggests that serotonin may play an important role in orbitofrontal cortical functioning. The orbitofrontal cortex is known for its role in filtering, processing, and evaluating social and emotional information. It assists in evaluating cues within a social context and in interpreting the emotional properties of stimuli. It also plays a role in the emotional processing of affective memories. These functions are believed to be important for social and emotional decision making. Patients with damage to the orbitofrontal cortex tend to have deficits in social decision making and difficulty inhibiting inappropriate social responses, including aggressive impulses. They often demonstrate behaviors marked by impulsivity and aggression (Blair, Morris, Frith, Perrett, & Dolan, 1999). In addition, orbitofrontal damage can result in impaired recognition of emotions in others. Accurate recognition of emotional stimuli and drawing on emotional memory is important for the appropriate modulation of behavioral responses to a host of everyday situations.

The effects of serotonin on orbitofrontal function have been examined in a series of tryptophan-depletion studies. Tryptophan depletion involves the oral administration of a drink mixture of 15 large neutral amino acids without tryptophan. Ingestion of a tryptophan depleting drink mixture, followed by a low-tryptophan diet, has been shown to reduce plasma tryptophan in humans by over 80%, which subsequently causes a transient depletion of 5-HT stores by approximately 50% (Young, Smith, Phil, & Ervin, 1985). Tryptophan-depletion studies have demonstrated that low serotonin levels are associated with impairment in a number of psychological tasks, including reversal learning (Park et al., 1994; Young et al., 1985). Reversal tasks measure an individual's ability to evaluate, integrate, and act on environmental cues. More specifically, reversal tasks require an individual to stop responding to a stimulus that previously has been reinforced and begin responding to a previously non-reinforced stimulus in order to receive a reward (Robbins & Everitt, 1995).

Optimal performance on reversal-learning tasks requires intact serotonergic innervation of an intact orbitofrontal cortex. Performance on these tasks is impaired in animals with lesions of the orbitofrontal cortex (Dias, Roberts, & Robbins, 1996a), in humans with damage to the orbitofrontal cortex, and in humans whose serotonin has been depleted (Rolls, Hornak, Wade, & McGrath, 1994). While the effects of serotonin are probably not specific to the orbitofrontal cortex, the orbitofrontal cortex (compared to the dorsolateral cortex) may be especially sensitive to the effects of serotonin (Park et al., 1994).

Studies in individuals with PTSD have demonstrated alterations in both serotonergic function and in orbitofrontal cortex-mediated tasks, as reflected by impaired ability to perform object-alteration and reversal tests. Regarding the orbitofrontal cortex, Koenen et al. (2001) reported impaired performance on object alteration and reversal learning in combat veterans with PTSD. Among women with PTSD, Bremner et al. (2003) found decreased regional cerebral blood flow (rCBF) in areas of the PFC (including the orbitofrontal cortex) during retrieval of emotionally balanced word pairs. Additionally, a number of symptoms that are commonly observed in patients with PTSD, including misinterpretation of emotionally laden cues, impulsivity, aggression, and enhanced emotional memory have been described in patients with orbitofrontal cortex lesions. Receptor, challenge, and pharmacological treatment studies have all implicated altered serotonin function in the pathophysiology of PTSD. The above findings suggest that deficits in object alteration and reversal learning among individuals with PTSD might, in part, reflect altered serotonin modulation of the orbitofrontal cortex.

Relationship to the Amygdala and Locus Coeruleus

Serotonin also affects the amygdala. Reduced levels of serotonin in the amygdala have been associated with a decrease in threshold of amygdala firing (i.e., increased activation of the amygdala) through effects on GABAergic interneurons, which modulate glutamatergic input (Morgan, Krystal, & Southwick, 2003). Furthermore, the ability of 5-HT to modulate glutamatergic activity is dependent on the presence of corticosterone (Stutzmann & LeDoux, 1999; Stutzmann, McEwen, & LeDoux, 1998). On the other hand, increased 5-HT has been found to increase the threshold of amygdala firing with a resultant decrease in vigilance and fear-related behaviors. Efficacy of selective serotonin reuptake inhibitors (SSRIs) in patients with PTSD may be related, in part, to an increased threshold of amygdala firing.

Serotonin also has important effects on the LC. An inhibitory role of 5-HT on LC and NE neurons has been demonstrated in lesion, electrophysiological, and biochemical studies (Aston-Jones et al., 1991; Bobker & Williams, 1989). For example, lesions of the raphe nuclei as well as pretreatment with 5-HT synthesis inhibitors (which effectively release inhibitory control of the LC by 5-HT) have been shown to increase tyrosine hydroxylase activity and firing rate of LC/NE neurons in the LC. More specifically, in rats with lesions of 5-HT neurons, firing activity of NE neurons is approximately 50% greater than that recorded in intact animals (Blier, 2001). In a related study, prolonged administration of the SSRI citalopram (14 and 21 days) led to a progressive decrease in the firing activity of NE neurons (Blier, 2001).

The interaction between serotonin and NE has also been studied in healthy humans. In order to assess the modulating effects of 5-HT on NE, 11 healthy human subjects were depleted of tryptophan and then administered yohimbine, an alpha$_2$-adrenergic antagonist (Goddard et al., 1995). In separate studies, tryptophan depletion has been shown to cause mild decreases in mood and concentration among healthy subjects while a clinically significant worsening of depressive symptoms has been observed in remitted patients on antidepressants (Delgado et al., 1990; Young et al., 1985). Yohimbine administration has produced modest or no increase in subjective nervousness among healthy subjects, but in patients with panic disorder, yohimbine has caused marked increases in symptoms consistent with anxiety and panic as well as elevations on physiological and neuroendocrine measures associated with heightened arousal and anxiety (Charney, Woods, Krystal, Nagy, & Heninger, 1992). In Goddard's tryptophan–yohimbine study, healthy subjects who underwent tryptophan depletion and then received yohimbine experienced a synergistic increase in subjective nervousness compared to administration of either yohimbine alone or a placebo (Goddard et al., 1995). Tryptophan depletion caused a marked reduction in 5-HT, which in turn left the noradrenergic response to yohimbine partially unchecked.

Relationship to Clinical Symptoms

Alterations in serotonin have been implicated in PTSD as well as in disorders of mood, impulsivity, and aggression. It is likely that the effects of altered serotonergic function among subjects with PTSD are mediated by multiple brain regions known to be involved in central fear circuitry. Preclinical and clinical data have shown that alterations in serotonin affect orbitofrontal cortex functioning, orbitofrontal cortex inhibition of the amygdala, threshold of amygdala firing, and the firing rate of the LC. It is possible that these alterations contribute to a number of symptoms commonly described in PTSD. For example, serotonin's effect on orbitofrontal cortex might contribute to misinterpretation of emotion-laden stimuli including accurate recognition of emotions in others, impulsivity and aggression, and socially inappropriate decision making. Alterations in serotonin also contribute to exaggerated alerting and fear-related behaviors through release of orbitofrontal cortex inhibitory control of the amygdala, effects on GABAergic interneurons within the amygdala, and diminished tonic inhibition of LC/NE firing.

Despite the above evidence, which implicates serotonin in the pathophysiology of multiple symptoms commonly seen in trauma victims with PTSD (i.e., aggression, impulsivity, depression), relatively little research to date has actually investigated serotonergic function in subjects with PTSD per se. Several reports of baseline serotonergic function in PTSD have reported decreased platelet uptake in subjects with PTSD (Arora, Fichtner, O'Connor, & Crayton, 1993; Bremner, Southwick, & Charney, 1999). A number of studies have also used challenge paradigms to assess serotonergic activity in trauma victims with PTSD. Davis, Clark, Kramer, Moeller, and Petty (1999) in a study of combat veterans with PTSD, reported a blunted prolactin response to the serotonin-releasing and uptake inhibitor D-fenfluramine. In a study comparing the effects of the noradrenergic probe yohimbine to the serotonergic probe MCPP, 40% of combat veterans with PTSD experienced a panic attack in response to yohimbine and 30% in response to MCPP (Southwick, Bremner, Rasmusson, Morgan, Arnsten, & Charney, 1999a). This study provided preliminary evidence for possible neurobiological subgroups of patients with PTSD, one showing increased reactivity of the noradrenergic system and the other increased reactivity of the serotonergic system.

Further evidence that indirectly supports a role for serotonin in the pathophysiology of PTSD comes from studies in subjects with aggression, impulsivity, and depression. These include reduced cerebrospinal fluid (CSF) 5-HIAA in aggressive psychiatric patients, impulsive violent men, and suicide victims who have killed themselves through violent means (Davidson, Putnam, & Larson, 2000). Genetic evidence includes the relationship between a polymorphism in the gene that codes for tryptophan hydroxylase and individual differences in aggressive behavior (Manuck et al., 1999; Nielsen et al., 1994). The link between genetic predisposition for altered serotonergic function and life traumas has been further demonstrated in a recent study by Caspi et al. (2003) who found that one or two copies of the short allele of the 5-HT transporter promoter polymorphism, in association with a life stress, significantly increased the risk for developing depression, a disorder that frequently accompanies PTSD.

Perhaps the strongest clinical evidence speaking to serotonin's role in PTSD comes from pharmacological treatment studies. Currently only two medications have been approved by the U.S. Food and Drug Administration (FDA) for the treatment of PTSD. Both agents, sertraline and paroxetine, are SSRIs. In large multicenter treatment trials, these agents have been shown to significantly improve all three PTSD symptom clusters (reexperiencing, avoidance, arousal), when compared to placebo. Additionally monoamine oxidase inhibitors, which increase serotonin by inhibiting its degradation, have shown promise in treating trauma victims with PTSD (Foa, Keane, & Friedman, 2000).

THE HYPOTHALAMIC-PITUITARY-ADRENAL AXIS

General Characteristics

Alterations in HPA-axis functioning have been reported in patients diagnosed with PTSD. In response to acute and chronic stress, the paraventricular nucleus of the hypothalamus secretes corticotropin-releasing factor (CRF), which, in turn, stimulates the anterior pituitary gland to synthesize and release adrenocorticotropin (ACTH). ACTH then stimulates the synthesis and release of adrenal cortical glucocorticoids. Cortisol mobilizes and replenishes energy stores, inhibits growth and reproductive systems, contains the immune response, and affects behavior through actions on multiple neurotransmitter systems and brain regions.

Relationship to Amygdala and Prefrontal Cortex

As previously noted, threat activates the amygdala. The amygdala, in turn, projects to the hypothalamus, which activates the pituitary and adrenal glands. Glucocorticoids (cortisol in humans and corticosterone in many animals) that are released by the adrenal gland then cross the blood–brain barrier and exert effects on the amygdala and PFC. While high levels of glucocorticoids facilitate functioning of the amygdala, they impair functioning of the PFC. For example, systematic administration of glucocorticoids or local glucocorticoid infusion into the PFC has been shown to impair working memory (Roozendaal, McReynolds, & McGaugh, 2004). Further, high levels of glucocorticoids in the PFC are known to augment synaptic catecholamine levels via blockade of catecholamine reuptake (Grundemann, Schechinger, Rappold, & Schomig, 1998). The result is impaired working memory and decreased cortical inhibition of limbic activity. The combination of glucocorticoid-mediated enhancement of amygdala functioning (e.g., fear conditioning and consolidation of emotional memory) and glucocorticoid-mediated impairment in PFC functioning can leave the organism in a physiological state dominated by poorly inhibited limbic reactivity.

Cortisol and PTSD

The above preclinical findings suggest that abnormal CNS cortisol levels among individuals with PTSD may contribute to some of the deficits in cognitive functioning that have been observed in this patient population.

However, the HPA axis is complex and findings to date in subjects with PTSD have been both inconsistent and, at times, difficult to interpret. Thus, a clear association between abnormalities in the HPA axis and cognitive dysfunction in PTSD has not yet been clearly established.

Although a number of studies have found decreased 24-hour urine cortisol levels, others have reported elevated levels. For example, studies of HPA-axis function in male veterans have produced mixed findings with some showing low, some similar, and some high 24-hour urine cortisol levels in veterans with PTSD compared to combat veterans and healthy controls without PTSD (reviewed in Rasmusson et al., 2003). Similarly, studies of premenopausal women and children with PTSD have reported increased 24-hour urinary cortisol output, apparently related to increased pituitary adrenocorticotropic hormone and adrenal cortisol reactivity. In contrast, a study performed in postmenopausal female survivors of the Holocaust showed decreased 24-hour urinary cortisol output, as did a study in male Holocaust survivors. Insufficient control for nicotine, psychotropics, and alcohol use by PTSD subjects may have contributed to inconsistent findings across studies (reviewed in Rasmusson et al., 2003). In addition, it is possible that genetic factors may have contributed to variable findings. For instance, functional mutations in the 21-hydroxylase gene, frequently present in some ethnic groups, are associated with diminished cortisol synthesis (Witchel, Lee, Suda-Hartman, Trucco, & Hoffman, 1997).

Of note, however, Baker and colleagues (1999) found that CSF cortisol levels in male veterans with chronic PTSD were high even when their urinary cortisol levels were not different from healthy controls. These data suggest that urinary cortisol levels may not always adequately reflect the level of glucocorticoid exposure experienced in the central nervous system. Other evidence of hyperactive or sensitized HPA activity in individuals with PTSD is reviewed by Yehuda (2002).

Dehydroepiandrosterone and Frontal Cortex

Cortisol is not the only adrenal neuroactive steroid of potential relevance to functioning of the frontal cortex. Dehydroepiandrosterone (DHEA) is another steroid that is secreted from the adrenal gland episodically and synchronously with cortisol in response to fluctuating ACTH levels (Rosenfeld et al., 1971). Indeed, DHEA derived from the periphery is thought to be the primary source of DHEA in the brain (Compagnone & Mellon, 2000). DHEA and its sulfated metabolite, DHEAS, have antiglucocorticoid effects and positively modulate N-methyl-D-aspartate (NMDA) receptor function and antagonize $GABAA_A$ receptor-mediated chloride ion flux (Baulieu & Robel, 1998). As a result, DHEA would be expected to enhance monoaminergic responses during initial traumatic stress exposure or during reexposure to cues previously associated with traumatic experiences.

It is of interest that higher DHEA and/or DHEAS levels have been observed in Israeli combat veterans with PTSD compared to Israeli veterans without PTSD (Spivak et al., 2000) while DHEAS levels have been found to rise over several months in association with the development of PTSD among Kosovo refugees (Sondergaard, Hansson, & Theorell, 2002). In addition, Rasmusson and colleagues (2004) found that DHEA responses to maximum stimulation of the adrenal gland during an ACTH stimulation test were significantly increased in premenopausal women with PTSD. Interestingly, the magnitude of the DHEA response to ACTH was inversely related to PTSD symptoms as measured by the Clinician Administered PTSD Scale (CAPS). This relationship was explained primarily by a negative relationship between DHEA reactivity and avoidance or hyperarousal symptoms of PTSD.

The study by Rasmusson et al. (2004) showing a negative relationship between the adrenal capacity for DHEA release and PTSD symptoms suggested that DHEA may confer resistance to some of the disabling effects of traumatic stress exposure, perhaps in part by enhancing frontal lobe functioning. This possibility is supported by the work of Morgan et al. (2004) showing a negative relationship between the ratio of plasma DHEAS/cortisol levels and dissociation as well as a positive relationship between the DHEAS/cortisol ratio and behavioral performance during severe acute stress in apparently healthy military personnel undergoing survival training. In contrast, low levels of DHEA(S) alone or in relation to cortisol have been repeatedly associated with depressed mood and reduced feelings of vigor and well-being, while DHEA itself has been found to effectively treat at least a subpopulation of patients with refractory major depression, a condition known to be associated with deficiencies in frontal lobe processing. And finally, a recent study by Strous et al. (2003) found that DHEA reduced negative symptoms of schizophrenia without worsening positive symptoms when administered in addition to the subjects' usual medication regimens.

DHEA(S) may directly affect frontal lobe function through modulation of GABAergic and NMDA receptor function as well as indirectly through secondary effects on monoamine release. In addition, DHEA may indirectly promote optimum frontal lobe function through effects in the amygdala. Activation of NMDA receptors in the amygdala has been found to facilitate extinction as well as formation of conditioned fear-based memories (Walker & Davis, 2002). Thus, heightened DHEA release in the period following trauma exposure when natural extinction occurs in some individuals or during exposure-based therapy may promote extinction and prevent future disruption of frontal lobe function by catecholamine fluxes induced by trauma-related cue exposure. It is also possible that "antiglucocorticoid" effects exerted by DHEA in many tissues including brain may be found to pertain specifically to the frontal cortex. Thus far, however, research has focused on the hippocampus where hydroxylated metabolites of DHEA have been shown to interfere with the nuclear uptake of activated glucocorticoid receptors (Morfin & Starka, 2001).

Neuroactive Steroids and Activation of the Hypothalamic–Pituitary-Adrenal Axis

Adrenally derived neuroactive steroids that positively modulate $GABA_A$ receptors and enhance chloride flux into neurons also deserve mention, with allotetrahydro-deoxycorticosterone and allopregnanolone being the most potent of these (Compagnone & Mellon, 2000). Recent data show allopregnanolone levels in the CSF of premenopausal women in the follicular phase of the menstrual cycle to be about 50% lower than in healthy nontraumatized women (Rasmusson, Pinna, Weisman, Gottschalk, Charney, Krystal, et al., 2005). Allopregnanolone is released by the adrenal gland in response to stress and is thought to provide delayed negative feedback inhibition of the HPA axis as well as exert anxiolytic and anesthetic effects. Thus, reductions in this neuroactive steroid may prolong activation of the HPA axis and promote the enhancement of monoamine effects in the frontal lobe and amygdala by DHEA and cortisol. As noted above, under such conditions, amygdala-mediated defense responses and sensory processing would be expected to hold sway over cognitive and behavioral functions subserved by frontal-lobe-mediated working memory.

Gene Polymorphisms and Responses to Trauma

There are many points at which variations in genetic endowment or stress-induced alterations in gene regulation could affect biosynthesis or degradation of adrenally derived neuroactive steroids. Indeed, there are more than 65 different functional mutations of the 21-hydroxylase gene already known to affect cortisol production. Other HPA-axis-related genes with polymorphisms known to enhance either ACTH or cortisol responses to stress include the catechol-O-methyltransferase (COMT) gene (Hernandez-Avila, Wand, Luo, Gelernter, & Kranzler, 2003; Oswald, McCaul, Choi, Yang, & Wand, 2004), angiotensin I-converting enzyme (ACE-I) gene (Baghai et al., 2002), the glucocorticoid receptor gene (Wust et al., 2004), the ACTH gene (Slawik et al., 2004) and the CRF or CRF receptor gene (Challis et al., 2004; Gonzalez-Gay et al., 2003; Kyllo et al., 1996; Smoller et al., 2003). No doubt others will be identified in the near future. Assessment of the effects of functional mutations of such genes on other

neuroactive steroids including DHEA, allopregnanolone, and allotetrahy-
drocorticosterone in addition to ACTH and cortisol will likely be important in understanding individual variability in acute cognitive reactions to
traumatic stress and cognitive dysfunction subsequent to trauma. In addition, it will be important to understand epigenetic factors that regulate the
function of such genes. Hopefully, this line of research will promote our
understanding of HPA-axis-related risk factors that predispose to stress-
induced dysregulation of frontal lobe function and also lead to the development of novel strategies for the prevention or treatment of PTSD and
PTSD-related disabilities.

CONCLUSIONS AND IMPLICATIONS

In summary, we have briefly reviewed preclinical and clinical data related
to three neurotransmitter/neuroendocrine systems that are known to be involved in the pathophysiology of PTSD and that may contribute to some of
the symptoms and neurocognitive deficits that have been reported in this
patient population. These neurotransmitters appear to exert their stress-
related effects through actions in multiple brain regions including the PFC,
amygdala, hippocampus, dorsal raphe nucleus, and the LC.

As noted earlier, stress sensitization of noradrenergic systems results in
increased synthesis and release of NE. When stress-sensitized organisms are
subsequently stressed, the amygdala and the PFC become flooded with NE.
In the PFC, high levels of NE preferentially engage postsynaptic alpha$_1$ receptors, which in essence take the PFC "off-line." In humans with PTSD,
impairment in PFC functioning would likely compromise executive functioning and decrease inhibitory control of the amygdala with a resultant increase in fear-related behavior (Davis, 1999).

It is possible that PFC functioning might also be affected by alterations
in serotonin, cortisol, and DHEA among subjects with PTSD. For example,
decreased serotonergic stimulation of the orbitofrontal cortex would be expected to impair reversal learning. Behavioral effects might include misinterpretation of social and emotional information, faulty interpretation of
emotion in others, impaired emotional processing of affective memories,
and difficulty inhibiting inappropriate social responses (e.g., aggressive impulses). Similarly, high levels of stress-induced glucocorticoids are likely to
impair working memory and to augment synaptic catecholamine levels,
which likely would lead to a further engagement of postsynaptic alpha$_1$ receptors. On the other hand, stress-induced release of DHEA might enhance
PFC functioning by direct effects on GABAergic and NMDA receptor function as well as indirect effects on monoamine release.

In this chapter, we have also reviewed data showing that NE, serotonin, and cortisol have important effects on the amygdala. For example, high levels of stress-induced catecholamines and cortisol enhance functioning of the amygdala (e.g., enhanced fear conditioning and consolidation of emotional memories) while low levels of serotonin reduce the threshold of amygdala firing through effects on GABA. In addition to orchestrating the fear response, the amygdala also modulates the neurochemical environment of the PFC.

Taken together, findings from preclinical and clinical studies suggest that alterations in NE, 5-HT, and adrenal hormones may contribute to psychological symptoms and neuropsychological deficits described in patients with PTSD through effects on multiple brain regions including the PFC and amygdala. Reduced serotonin (through effects on the orbitofrontal cortex), elevated NE (through actions at the postsynaptic $alpha_1$-adrenergic receptor) and cortisol (through interactions with catecholamines) may all contribute to impaired PFC functioning, including reduced inhibition of the amygdala. Decreased inhibition by the PFC, in combination with excitation secondary to elevated levels of catecholamines and cortisol, and reduced levels of 5-HT, would leave the amygdala in an activated and "unleashed" state. Activation of the amygdala, in the presence of impaired PFC executive functioning, might activate release of NE (LC), dopamine (ventral tegmental area) and acetylcholine (dorso lateral tegmental nucleus); diminish capacity for rational problem solving and rational influence on behavior and thought; exaggerate the startle response; increase fear conditioning; enhance consolidation of emotional memory; and increase vigilance, insomnia, impulsivity, intrusive memories, flashbacks, and other fear-related behaviors.

We have also focused in this chapter on the PFC and amygdala. Clearly, other brain regions such as the anterior cingulate cortex and the hippocampus play an important role in mediating stress-induced effects of neurotransmitters/neurohormones. For example, preclinical and clinical studies have clearly demonstrated a relationship between chronic stress and hippocampal function. In animals, inescapable stress has been associated with hippocampal damage and inhibition of neurogenesis. Some human studies have reported reduced hippocampal volume and deficits in hippocampal-based declarative verbal memory among subjects with PTSD. Further, in a recent study of women with PTSD, Vermetten and colleagues found a significant increase in hippocampal volume and verbal memory after long-term treatment with the SSRI paroxetine (Vermetten, Vythilingam, Southwick, Charney, & Bremner, 2003). Finally, pretreatment with an SSRI has been shown to prevent the development of many fear-induced behaviors in animals. This effect is probably mediated through activation of postsynaptic 5-HT 1A receptors (reviewed in Bonne, Grillon, Vythilingam, Neumeister, & Charney, 2004).

The discussion in this chapter has potential clinical implications (see Friedman, Chapter 13, this volume). For example, alpha$_2$-adrenergic receptor agonists (e.g., clonidine, guanfacine) might be helpful through effects on presynaptic alpha$_2$ receptors in the LC (reduced NE release and reduced NE stimulation of the amygdala) as well as increased occupancy of prefrontal cortical alpha$_2$-adrenergic receptors (enhanced PFC function and inhibition of the amygdala). Alpha$_1$-adrenergic-receptor antagonists (e.g., prazosin) might help by reducing NE occupancy of alpha$_1$-adrenergic receptors (decreased impairment of PFC functioning and improved inhibition of the amygdala). SSRIs might exert positive effects by increasing orbitofrontal cortex inhibition of the amygdala and by increasing threshold of amygdala firing through effects on GABA. CRF antagonists might also reduce trauma-related symptoms and cognitive deficits through effects on multiple brain regions, neurotransmitter and neuropeptide systems, and the HPA axis.

It is important to note that the above discussion is speculative in nature since direct evidence for these ideas is largely lacking in clinical populations. It is also important to remember that the relationship between neurobiology and behavior is exceptionally complex. In discussing only three neurotransmitters/neurohormones, we have presented an incomplete and extremely simplistic model. Much research remains to be conducted on the interface between trauma-related neurotransmitter/neurohormone alterations, regional brain function, psychological symptoms, and neuropsychological deficits in trauma survivors with PTSD.

REFERENCES

Abercrombie, E. D., & Zigmond, M. J. (1995). Modification of central catecholaminergic systems by stress and injury. In F. E. Bloom & D. J. Kupfer (Eds.), *Psychopharmacology: The fourth generation of progress* (pp. 355–361). New York: Raven Press.

Anderson, S. W., Bechara, A., Damasio, H., Tranel, D., & Damasio, A. R. (1999). Impairment of social and moral behavior related to early damage in human prefrontal cortex. *Nature Neuroscience, 2*(11), 1032–1037.

Arnsten, A. F. T. (1998a). Catecholamine modulation of prefrontal cortical cognitive function. *Trends in Cognitive Sciences, 2*(11), 436–447.

Arnsten, A. F. (1998b). The biology of being frazzled. *Science, 280*(5370), 1711–1712.

Arnsten, A. F. (2000a). Stress impairs prefrontal cortical function in rats and monkeys: Role of dopamine D1 and norepinephrine alpha$_1$ receptor mechanisms. *Progress in Brain Research, 126*, 183–192.

Arnsten, A. F. (2000b). Through the looking glass: Differential noradrenergic modulation of prefrontal cortical function. *Neural Plasticity, 7*(1–2), 133–146.

Arnsten, A. F., & Goldman-Rakic, P. S. (1985). Alpha$_2$-adrenergic mechanisms in prefrontal cortex associated with cognitive decline in aged nonhuman primates. *Science, 230*(4731), 1273–1276.

Arnsten, A. F., & Jentsch, J. D. (1997). The alpha$_1$ adrenergic agonist, cirazoline, impairs spatial working memory performance in aged monkeys. *Pharmacology, Biochemistry, and Behavior, 58*(1), 55–59.

Arnsten, A. F., Mathew, R., Ubriani, R., Taylor, J. R., & Li, B. M. (1999). Alpha-1 noradrenergic receptor stimulation impairs prefrontal cortical cognitive function. *Biological Psychiatry, 45*(1), 26–31.

Arora, R. C., Fichtner, C. G., O'Connor, F., & Crayton, J. W. (1993). Paroxetine binding in the blood platelets of post-traumatic stress disorder patients. *Life Sciences, 53*(11), 919–928.

Aston-Jones, G., Rajkowski, J., Kubiak, P., & Alexinsky, T. (1994). Locus coeruleus neurons in monkeys are selectively activated by attended cues in a vigilance task. *Journal of Neuroscience, 14*(7), 4467–4480.

Aston-Jones, G., Shipley, M. T., Chouvet, G., Ennis, M., van Bockstaele, E., Pieribone, V., et al. (1991). Afferent regulation of locus coeruleus neurons: Anatomy, physiology and pharmacology. *Progress in Brain Research, 88*, 47–75.

Baghai, T. C., Schule, C., Zwanzger, P., Minov, C., Zill, P., Ella, R., et al. (2002). Hypothalamic–pituitary–adrenocortical axis dysregulation in patients with major depression is influenced by the insertion/deletion polymorphism in the angiotensin I-converting enzyme gene. *Neuroscience Letters, 328*(3), 299–303.

Baker, D. G., West, S. A., Nicholson, W. E., Ekhator, N. N., Kasckow, J. W., Hill, K. K., et al. (1999). Serial CSF corticotropin-releasing hormone levels and adrenocortical activity in combat veterans with posttraumatic stress disorder. *American Journal of Psychiatry, 156*, 585–588.

Baulieu, E. E., & Robel, P. (1998). Dehydroepiandrosterone (DHEA) and dehydroepiandrosterone sulfate (DHEAS) as neuroactive neurosteroids. *Proceedings of the National Academy of Sciences of the United States of America, 95*(8), 4089–4091.

Birnbaum, S., Gobeske, K. T., Auerbach, J., Taylor, J. R., & Arnsten, A. F. (1999). A role for norepinephrine in stress-induced cognitive deficits: Alpha$_1$-adrenoceptor mediation in the prefrontal cortex. *Biological Psychiatry, 46*(9), 1266–1274.

Birnbaum, S. G., Podell, D. M., & Arnsten, A. F. (2000). Noradrenergic alpha-2 receptor agonists reverse working memory deficits induced by the anxiogenic drug, FG7142, in rats. *Pharmacology, Biochemistry, and Behavior, 67*(3), 397–403.

Birnbaum, S. B., Yuan, P., Bloom, A., Davis, D., Gobeske, K., Sweatt, D., et al. (2004). *Protein kinase C overactivity impairs prefrontal cortical regulation of behavior.* Manuscript under review.

Blair, R. J., Morris, J. S., Frith, C. D., Perrett, D. I., & Dolan, R. J. (1999). Dissociable neural responses to facial expressions of sadness and anger. *Brain, 122*(Pt 5), 883–893.

Blanchard, E. B., Kolb, L. C., Prins, A., Gates, S., & McCoy, G. C. (1991). Changes in plasma norepinephrine to combat-related stimuli among Vietnam veterans with posttraumatic stress disorder. *Journal of Nervous and Mental Disease, 179*(6), 371–373.

Blier, P. (2001). Crosstalk between the norepinephrine and serotonin systems and its role in the antidepressant response. *Journal of Psychiatry and Neuroscience, 26,* S3–10.

Bobker, D. H., & Williams, J. T. (1989). Serotonin agonists inhibit synaptic potentials in the rat locus coeruleus *in vitro* via 5-HT 1A and 5 HT1B receptors. *Journal of Pharmacology and Experimental Therapeutics, 250,* 37–43.

Bonne, O., Grillon, C., Vythilingam, M., Neumeister, A., & Charney, D. S. (2004). Adaptive and maladaptive psychobiological responses to severe psychological stress: Implications for the discovery of novel pharmacotherapy. *Neuroscience and Biobehavioral Reviews, 28*(1), 65–94.

Bremner, J., Southwick, S., & Charney, D. (1999). The neurobiology of posttraumatic stress disorder: An integration of animal and human research. In P. A. Saigh & J. D. Bremner (Eds.), *Posttraumatic stress disorder: A comprehensive text* (pp. 103–143). Boston: Allyn & Bacon.

Bremner, J. D., Vythilingam, M., Vermetten, E., Southwick, S. M., McGlashan, T., Staib, L. H., et al. (2003). Neural correlates of declarative memory for emotionally valenced words in women with posttraumatic stress disorder related to early childhood sexual abuse. *Biological Psychiatry, 53*(10), 879–889.

Cahill, L., & McGaugh, J. L. (1996). Modulation of memory storage. *Current Opinion in Neurobiology, 6*(2), 237–242.

Caspi, A., Sugden, K., Moffitt, T. E., Taylor, A., Craig, I. W., Harrington, H., et al. (2003). Influence of life stress on depression: Moderation by a polymorphism in the 5-HTT gene. *Science, 301*(5631), 386–389.

Challis, B. G., Luan, J., Keogh, J., Wareham, N. J., Farooqi, I. S., & O'Rahilly, S. (2004). Genetic variation in the corticotropin-releasing factor receptors: Identification of single-nucleotide polymorphisms and association studies with obesity in UK Caucasians. *International Journal of Obesity and Related Metabolic Disorders, 28*(3), 442–446.

Charney, D. S., Deutch, A. Y., Southwick, S. M., & Krystal, J. H. (1995). Neural circuits and mechanisms of post-traumatic stress disorder. In M. J. Friedman, D. S. Charney, & A. Y. Deutch (Eds.), *Neurobiological and clinical consequences of stress: From normal adaptation to post traumatic stress disorder* (pp. 271–287). Philadelphia: Lippincott-Raven.

Charney, D. S., Heninger, G. R., & Breier, A. (1984). Noradrenergic function in panic anxiety. Effects of yohimbine in healthy subjects and patients with agoraphobia and panic disorder. *Archives of General Psychiatry, 41*(8), 751–763.

Charney, D. S., Woods, S. W., Krystal, J. H., Nagy, L. M., & Heninger, G. R. (1992). Noradrenergic neuronal dysregulation in panic disorder: The effects of intravenous yohimbine and clonidine in panic disorder patients. *Acta Psychiatrica Scandinavica, 86*(4), 273–282.

Clark, D. L., & Boutros, N. N. (1999). *The brain and behavior: An introduction to behavioral neuroanatomy* (Vol. 1). Oxford, UK: Blackwell.

Compagnone, N. A., & Mellon, S. H. (2000). Biosynthesis and function of these novel neuromodulators. *Neuroendocrinology, 21,* 1–56.

Conway, M. A., Anderson, S. J., & Larsen, S. F. (1994). The formation of flashbulb memories. *Memory and Cognition, 22,* 326–343.

Davidson, L. M., & Baum, A. (1996). Chronic stress and posttraumatic stress disorder. *Journal of Clinical Psychology, 54,* 303–308.

Davidson, R. J., Putnam, K. M., & Larson, C. L. (2000). Dysfunction in the neural circuitry of emotion regulation—A possible prelude to violence. *Science, 289*(5479), 591–594.

Davies, M. F., Tsui, J., Flannery, J. A., Li, X., DeLorey, T. M., & Hoffman, B. B. (2004). Activation of alpha2 adrenergic receptors suppresses fear conditioning: Expression of c-Fos and phosphorylated CREB in mouse amygdala. *Neuropsychopharmacology, 29*(2), 229–239.

Davis, L. L., Clark, D. M., Kramer, G. L., Moeller, F. G., & Petty, F. (1999). D-fenfluramine challenge in posttraumatic stress disorder. *Biological Psychiatry, 45*(7), 928–930.

Davis, M. (1992). The role of the amygdala in fear and anxiety. *Annual Review of Neuroscience, 15,* 353–375.

Davis, M. (1999). Functional Neuroanatomy of anxiety and fear: A focus on the amygdala. In D. S. Charney, E. J. Nestler, & B. S. Bunney. (Eds.), *Neurobiology of mental illness* (pp. 463–474). New York: Oxford Press.

Delgado, P. L., Charney, D. S., Price, L. H., Aghajanian, G. K., Landis, H., & Heninger, G. R. (1990). Serotonin function and the mechanism of antidepressant action. Reversal of antidepressant-induced remission by rapid depletion of plasma tryptophan. *Archives of General Psychiatry, 47*(5), 411–418.

Dias, R., Roberts, A., & Robbins, T. W. (1996a). Dissociation in prefrontal cortex of affective and attentional shifts. *Nature, 380,* 69–72.

Druzin, M. Y., Kurzina, N. P., Malinina, E. P., & Kozlov, A. P. (2000). The effects of local application of D2 selective dopaminergic drugs into the medial prefrontal cortex of rats in a delayed spatial choice task. *Behavioral Brain Research, 109*(1), 99–111.

Ferry, B., Roozendaal, B., & McGaugh, J. L. (1999). Involvement of alpha1-adrenoceptors in the basolateral amygdala in modulation of memory storage. *European Journal of Pharmacology, 372*(1), 9–16.

Foa, E. B., Keane, T. M., & Friedman, M. J. (Eds.). (2000). *Effective treatments for PTSD: Practice guidelines from the International Society for Traumatic Stress Studies.* New York: Guilford Press.

Franowicz, J. S., Kessler, L. E., Borja, C. M., Kobilka, B. K., Limbird, L. E., & Arnsten, A. F. (2002). Mutation of the alpha2A-adrenoceptor impairs working memory performance and annuls cognitive enhancement by guanfacine. *Journal of Neuroscience, 22*(19), 8771–8777.

Friedman, M. J., & Southwick, S. M. (1995). Towards pharmacotherapy for posttraumatic stress disorder. In M. J. Friedman, D. S. Charney, & A. Y. Deutch (Eds.), *Neurobiological and clinical consequences of stress* (pp. 465–482). Philadelphia: Lippincott-Raven.

Funahashi, S., Bruce, C. J., & Goldman-Rakic, P. S. (1989). Mnemonic coding of visual space in the monkey's dorsolateral prefrontal cortex. *Journal of Neurophysiology, 61*(2), 331–349.

Funahashi, S., Chafee, M. V., & Goldman-Rakic, P. S. (1993). Prefrontal neuronal activity in rhesus monkeys performing a delayed anti-saccade task. *Nature, 365*(6448), 753–756.

Fuster, J. M. (1973). Unit activity in prefrontal cortex during delayed-response performance: Neuronal correlates of transient memory. *Journal of Neurophysiology,* 36(1), 61–78.

Ghashghaei, H. T., & Barbas, H. (2002). Pathways for emotion: Interactions of prefrontal and anterior temporal pathways in the amygdala of the rhesus monkey. *Neuroscience, 115*(4), 1261–1279.

Goddard, A. W., Charney, D. S., Germine, M., Woods, S. W., Heninger, G. R., Krystal, J. H., et al. (1995). Effects of tryptophan depletion on responses to yohimbine in healthy human subjects. *Biological Psychiatry, 38*(2), 74–85.

Gold, P. E., & McCarty, R. C. (1995). Stress regulation of memory processes: Role of peripheral catecholamines. In M. J. Friedman, D. S. Charney, & A. Y. Deutch (Eds.), *Neurobiological and clinical consequences of stress: From normal adaptation to post traumatic stress disorder* (pp. 151–162). Philadelphia: Lippincott-Raven.

Gold, P. E., & Van Buskirk, R. B. (1975). Facilitation of time-dependent memory processes with posttrial epinephrine injections. *Behavioral Biology, 13*(2), 145–153.

Goldman-Rakic, P. S. (1987). Circuitry of the primate prefrontal cortex and the regulation of behavior by representational memory. In F. Plum (Ed.), *Handbook of physiology, The nervous system, higher functions of the brain* (pp. 373–417). Bethesda: American Physiological Society.

Goldstein, L. E., Rasmusson, A. M., Bunney, B. S., & Roth, R. H. (1996). Role of the amygdala in the coordination of behavioral, neuroendocrine, and prefrontal cortical monoamine responses to psychological stress in the rat. *Journal of Neuroscience, 16*(15), 4787–4798.

Gonzalez-Gay, M. A., Hajeer, A. H., Garcia-Porrua, C., Dababneh, A., Amoli, M. M., Botana, M. A., et al. (2003). Corticotropin-releasing hormone promoter polymorphisms in patients with rheumatoid arthritis from northwest Spain. *Journal of Rheumatology, 30*(5), 913–917.

Greba, Q., & Kokkinidis, L. (2000). Peripheral and intraamygdalar administration of the dopamine D1 receptor antagonist SCH 23390 blocks fear-potentiated startle but not shock reactivity or the shock sensitization of acoustic startle. *Behavioral Neuroscience, 114*(2), 262–272.

Grundemann, D., Schechinger, B., Rappold, G. A., & Schomig, E. (1998). Molecular identification of the corticosterone-sensitive extraneuronal catecholamine transporter. *Nature Neuroscience, 1*(5), 349–351.

Hernandez-Avila, C. A., Wand, G., Luo, X., Gelernter, J., & Kranzler, H. R. (2003). Association between the cortisol response to opioid blockade and the Asn40Asp polymorphism at the mu-opioid receptor locus (OPRM1). *American Journal of Medical Genetics, 118B*(1), 60–65.

Introini-Collison, I. B., Nagahara, A. H., & McGaugh, J. L. (1989). Memory enhancement with intra-amygdala post-training naloxone is blocked by concurrent administration of propranolol. *Brain Research, 476*(1), 94–101.

Irwin, J., Ahluwalia, P., & Anisman, H. (1986). Sensitization of norepinephrine activity following acute and chronic footshock. *Brain Research, 379*(1), 98–103.

Karmarcy, N. R., Delaney, R. L., & Dunn, A. L. (1984). Footshock treatment activates catecholamine synthesis in slices of mouse brain regions. *Brain Research, 290,* 311–319.

Keane, T. M., Kolb, L. C., Kaloupek, D. G., Orr, S. P., Blanchard, E. B., Thomas, R. G., et al. (1998). Utility of psychophysiological measurement in the diagnosis of posttraumatic stress disorder: Results from a Department of Veterans Affairs Cooperative Study. *Journal of Consulting and Clinical Psychology, 66*(6), 914–923.

Koenen, K. C., Driver, K. L., Oscar-Berman, M., Wolfe, J., Folsom, S., Huang, M. T., et al. (2001). Measures of prefrontal system dysfunction in posttraumatic stress disorder. *Brain and Cognition, 45*(1), 64–78.

Koob, G., Heinrichs, S., Menzaghi, F., Pich, E., & Britton, K. (1994). Corticotropin releasing factor, stress and behavior. *Seminars in Neuroscience, 6,* 221–229.

Kyllo, J. H., Collins, M. M., Vetter, K. L., Cuttler, L., Rosenfield, R. L., & Donohoue, P. A. (1996). Linkage of congenital isolated adrenocorticotropic hormone deficiency to the corticotropin releasing hormone locus using simple sequence repeat polymorphisms. *American Journal of Medical Genetics, 62*(3), 262–267.

Li, B. M., Mao, Z. M., Wang, M., & Mei, Z. T. (1999). Alpha-2 adrenergic modulation of prefrontal cortical neuronal activity related to spatial working memory in monkeys. *Neuropsychopharmacology, 21*(5), 601–610.

Liang, K. C., Juler, R. G., & McGaugh, J. L. (1990). Modulating effects of posttraining epinephrine on memory: Involvement of the amygdala noradrenergic system. *Brain Research, 31,* 247–260.

Liang, K. C., McGaugh, J. L., & Yao, H. Y. (1990). Involvement of amygdala pathways in the influence of post-training intra-amygdala norepinephrine and peripheral epinephrine on memory storage. *Brain Research, 508*(2), 225–233.

Limieux, A. M., & Coe, C. L. (1995). Abuse-related posttraumatic stress disorder: Evidence for chronic neuroendocrine activation in women. *Psychomatic Medicine, 57,* 105–115.

Manuck, S. B., Flory, J. D., Ferrell, R. E., Dent, K. M., Mann, J. J., & Muldoon, M. F. (1999). Aggression and anger-related traits associated with a polymorphism of the tryptophan hydroxylase gene. *Biological Psychiatry, 45*(5), 603–614.

McFall, M. E., Murburg, M. M., Ko, G. N., & Veith, R. C. (1990). Autonomic responses to stress in Vietnam combat veterans with posttraumatic stress disorder. *Biological Psychiatry, 27*(10), 1165–1175.

McGaugh, J. L. (2000). Memory—A century of consolidation. *Science, 287*(5451), 248–251.

Melia, K. R., Rasmussen, K., Terwilliger, R. Z., Haycock, J. W., Nestler, E. J., & Duman, R. S. (1992). Coordinate regulation of the cyclic AMP system with firing rate and expression of tyrosine hydroxylase in the rat locus coeruleus: Effects of chronic stress and drug treatments. *Journal of Neurochemistry, 58*(2), 494–502.

Miller, E. K., Li, L., & Desimone, R. (1993). Activity of neurons in anterior inferior temporal cortex during a short-term memory task. *Journal of Neuroscience, 13*(4), 1460–1478.

Mohell, N., Svartengren, J., & Cannon, B. (1983). Identification of [3H]prazosin binding sites in crude membranes and isolated cells of brown adipose tissue as alpha 1-adrenergic receptors. *European Journal of Pharmacology, 92*(1–2), 15–25.

Morfin, R., & Starka, L. (2001). Neurosteroid 7-hydroxylation products in the brain. *International Review of Neurobiology, 46,* 79–95.

Morgan, C. A., III, Krystal, J. H., & Southwick, S. M. (2003). Toward early pharmacological posttraumatic stress intervention. *Biological Psychiatry, 53*(9), 834–
843.

Morgan, C. A., III, Southwick, S., Hazlett, G., Rasmusson, A., Hoyt, G., Zimolo, Z.,
et al. (2004). Relationships among plasma dehydroepiandrosterone sulfate and
cortisol levels, symptoms of dissociation, and objective performance in humans
exposed to acute stress. *Archive of General Psychiatry, 61*(8), 819–825.

Murphy, B. L., Arnsten, A. F., Goldman-Rakic, P. S., & Roth, R. H. (1996). Increased
dopamine turnover in the prefrontal cortex impairs spatial working memory
performance in rats and monkeys. *Proceedings of the National Academy of Sciences of the United States of America, 93*(3), 1325–1329.

Nader, K., & LeDoux, J. E. (1999). Inhibition of the mesoamygdala dopaminergic
pathway impairs the retrieval of conditioned fear associations. *Behavioral Neuroscience, 113*(5), 891–901.

Nestler, E. J., Hyman, S. E., & Malenka, R. C. (2001). *Molecular neuropharmacology: A foundation for clinical neuroscience.* New York: McGraw-Hill.

Neumeister, A., Charney, D. S., Belfer, I., Geraci, M., Holmes, C., Sherabi, Y., et al. (in
press). Sympathoneural and adrenomedullary functional effects of A2c-
adrenoreceptor gene polymorphism in healthy humans. *Pharmacogenetics.*

Nielsen, D. A., Goldman, D., Virkkunen, M., Tokola, R., Rawlings, R., & Linnoila,
M. (1994). Suicidality and 5-hydroxyindoleacetic acid concentration associated
with a tryptophan hydroxylase polymorphism. *Archives of General Psychiatry,
51*(1), 34–38.

O'Rourke, M. F., Blaxall, H. S., Iversen, L. J., & Bylund, D. B. (1994). Characterization of [3H]RX821002 binding to alpha-2 adrenergic receptor subtypes. *Journal
of Pharmacology and Experimental Therapeutics, 268*(3), 1362–1367.

Orr, S. P. (1997a). Psychophysiologic reactivity to trauma-related imagery in PTSD.
Diagnostic and theoretical implication of recent findings. In R. Yehuda & A. C.
McFarlane (Eds.), *Psychobiology of posttraumatic stress disorder. Annals of the
New York Academy of Sciences* (pp. 114–124). New York: New York Academy
of Sciences.

Orr, S. P., Lasko, N. B., Metzger, L. J., Berry, N. J., Ahern, C. E., & Pitman, R. K.
(1997b). Psychophysiologic assessment of PTSD in adult females sexually
abused during childhood. In R. Yehuda & A. C. McFarlane (Eds.), *Psychobiology of posttraumatic stress disorder. Annals of the New York Academy of
Sciences* (pp. 491–493). New York: New York Academy of Sciences.

Oswald, L. M., McCaul, M., Choi, L., Yang, X., & Wand, G. S. (2004). Catechol-O-
methyltransferase polymorphism alters hypothalamic–pituitary–adrenal axis
responses to naloxone: A preliminary report. *Biological Psychiatry, 55*(1), 102–
105.

Park, S. B., Coull, J. T., McShane, R. H., Young, A. H., Sahakian, B. J., Robbins, T. W.,
et al. (1994). Tryptophan depletion in normal volunteers produces selective impairments in learning and memory. *Neuropharmacology, 33,* 575–588.

Pepperl, D. J., & Regan, J. W. (1994). Adrenergic receptors. In S. Peroutka (Ed.), *G
protein-coupled receptors* (pp. 45–78). Boca Raton, FL: CRC Press.

Perry, B. D. (1994). Neurobiological sequelae of childhood trauma: PTSD in children.

In M. Murburg (Ed.), *Catecholamine function in post-traumatic stress disorders: Emerging concepts, progress in psychiatry* (pp. 233–255). Washington, DC: American Psychiatric Press.

Quirk, G. J., Likhtik, E., Pelletier, J. G., & Pare, D. (2003). Stimulation of medial prefrontal cortex decreases the responsiveness of central amygdala output neurons. *Journal of Neuroscience, 23*(25), 8800–8807.

Ramos, B., Colgan, L., Nou, E., Ovadia, S., Wilson, S., & Arnsten, A. (in press). The beta-1 antagonist, betaxolol, improves working memory performance in rats and monkeys. *Biological Psychiatry.*

Rasmusson, A., Pinna, G., Weisman, D., Gottschalk, C., Charney, D., Krystal, J., et al. (2005, May). *Decreases in CSF allopregnanolone levels in women with PTSD correlate negatively with reexperiencing symptoms.* Paper presented at Society of Biological Psychiatry Annual Meeting, Atlanta, GA.

Rasmusson, A. M., Hauger, R. L., Morgan, C. A., Bremner, J. D., Charney, D. S., & Southwick, S. M. (2000). Low baseline and yohimbine-stimulated plasma neuropeptide Y (NPY) levels in combat-related PTSD. *Biological Psychiatry, 47*(6), 526–539.

Rasmusson, A. M., Vasek, J., Lipschitz, D. S., Vojvoda, D., Mustone, M. E., Shi, Q., et al. (2004). An increased capacity for adrenal DHEA release is associated with decreased avoidance and negative mood symptoms in women with PTSD. *Neuropsychopharmacology, 29*(8), 1546–1557.

Rasmusson, A. M., Vythilingham, M., & Morgan, C. A., III. (2003). The neuroendocrinolgy of posttraumatic stress disorder: New directions. *CNS Spec, 8*(9), 651–656, 665–667.

Redmond, D. E. J. (1987). Studies of the nucleus locus-coeruleus in monkeys and hypotheses for neuropsychopharmacology. In H. Y. Meltzer (Ed.), *Psychopharmacology: The third generation of progress* (pp. 967–975). New York: Raven Press.

Robbins, T., & Everitt, B. J. (1995). Central norepinephrine neurons and behavior. In F. E. Bloom & D. J. Kupfer (Eds.), *Psychopharmacology: The fourth generation of progress* (pp. 363–372). New York: Raven Press.

Rolls, E. T., Hornak, J., Wade, D., & McGrath, J. (1994). Emotion-related learning in patients with social and emotional changes associated with frontal lobe damage. *Journal of Neurology, Neurosurgery and Psychiatry, 57*, 1518–1524.

Roozendaal, B., McReynolds, J. R., & McGaugh, J. L. (2004). The basolateral amygdala interacts with the medial prefrontal cortex in regulating glucocorticoid effects on working memory impairment. *Journal of Neuroscience, 24*(6), 1385–1392.

Roozendaal, B., Quirarte, G. L., & McGaugh, J. L. (2002). Glucocorticoids interact with the basolateral amygdala beta-adrenoceptor—cAMP/cAMP/PKA system in influencing memory consolidation. *European Journal of Neuroscience, 15*(3), 553–560.

Rosenfeld, R. S., Hellman, L., Roffwarg, H., Weitzman, E. D., Fukushima, D. K., & Gallagher, T. F. (1971). Dehydroisoandrosterone is secreted episodically and synchronously with cortisol by normal man. *Journal of Clinical Endocrinology and Metabolism, 33*(1), 87–92.

Sara, S. J. (1985). The locus-coeruleus and cognitive function: Attempts to relate noradrenergic enhancement of signal/noise in the brain. *Physiological Psychology, 13*, 151–162.

Sara, S. J., & Devauges, V. (1989). Idazoxan, an alpha-2 antagonist, facilitates memory retrieval in the rat. *Behavioral and Neural Biology, 51*(3), 401–411.

Sawaguchi, T. (1998). Attenuation of delay-period activity of monkey prefrontal neurons by an alpha2-adrenergic antagonist during an oculomotor delayed-response task. *Journal of Neurophysiology, 80*(4), 2200–2205.

Schafe, G. E., Atkins, C. M., Swank, M. W., Bauer, E. P., Sweatt, J. D., & LeDoux, J. E. (2000). Activation of ERK/MAP kinase in the amygdala is required for memory consolidation of pavlovian fear conditioning. *Journal of Neuroscience, 20*(21), 8177–8187.

Schafe, G. E., Nadel, N. V., Sullivan, G. M., Harris, A., & LeDoux, J. E. (1999). Memory consolidation for contextual and auditory fear conditioning is dependent on protein synthesis, PKA, and MAP kinase. *Learning and Memory, 6*(2), 97–110.

Simpson, P. E., & Weiss, J. M. (1994). Altered electrophysiology of the locus coeruleus following uncontrollable stress. In M. Murburg (Ed.), *Catecholamine function in post-traumatic stress disorder: Emerging concepts* (pp. 63–86). Washington, DC: American Psychiatric Press.

Slawik, M., Reisch, N., Zwermann, O., Maser-Gluth, C., Stahl, M., Klink, A., et al. (2004). Characterization of an adrenocorticotropin (ACTH) receptor promoter polymorphism leading to decreased adrenal responsiveness to ACTH. *Journal of Clinical Endocrinology and Metabolism, 89*(7), 3131–3137.

Smoller, J. W., Rosenbaum, J. F., Biederman, J., Kennedy, J., Dai, D., Racette, S. R., et al. (2003). Association of a genetic marker at the corticotropin-releasing hormone locus with behavioral inhibition. *Biological Psychiatry, 54*(12), 1376–1381.

Sondergaard, H. P., Hansson, L. O., & Theorell, T. (2002). Elevated blood levels of dehydroepiandrosterone sulphate vary with symptom load in posttraumatic stress disorder: Findings from a longitudinal study of refugees in Sweden. *Psychotherapy and Psychosomatics, 71*(5), 298–303.

Southwick, S. M., Bremner, J. D., Rasmusson, A., Morgan, C. A., III, Arnsten, A., & Charney, D. S. (1999a). Role of norepinephrine in the pathophysiology and treatment of posttraumatic stress disorder. *Biological Psychiatry, 46*(9), 1192–1204.

Southwick, S. M., Krystal, J. H., Morgan, C. A., Johnson, D., Nagy, L. M., Nicolaou, A., et al. (1993). Abnormal noradrenergic function in posttraumatic stress disorder. *Archives in General Psychiatry, 50*(4), 266–274.

Southwick, S. M., Paige, S., Morgan, C. A., III, Bremner, J. D., Krystal, J. H., & Charney, D. S. (1999b). Neurotransmitter alterations in PTSD: Catecholamines and serotonin. *Seminars in Clinical Neuropsychiatry, 4*(4), 242–248.

Southwick, S. M., Yehuda, R., & Morgan, C. A. I. (1995). Clinical studies of neurotransmitter alterations in post-traumatic stress disorder. In M. J. Friedman, D. Charney, & A. Y. Deutch (Eds.), *Neurobiological and clinical consequences of stress: From normal adaptation to post traumatic stress disorder* (pp. 335–350). Philadelphia: Lippincott-Raven.

Spivak, B., Maayan, R., Kotler, M., Mester, R., Gil-Ad, I., Shtaif, B., et al. (2000). Elevated circulatory level of GABA(A)—antagonistic neurosteroids in patients with combat-related post-traumatic stress disorder. *Psychological Medicine, 30*(5), 1227–1231.

Sternberg, D. B., Isaacs, K. R., Gold, P. E., & McGaugh, J. L. (1985). Epinephrine facilitation of appetitive learning: Attenuation with adrenergic receptor antagonists. *Behavioral and Neural Biology, 44*(3), 447–453.

Stone, W. S., Rudd, R. J., & Gold, P. E. (1990). Amphetamine, epinephrine and glucose enhancement of memory retrieval. *Psychobiology, 18*, 227–230.

Strous, R. D., Maayan, R., Lapidus, R., Stryjer, R., Lustig, M., Kotler, M., et al. (2003). Dehydroepiandrosterone augmentation in the management of negative, depressive, and anxiety symptoms in schizophrenia. *Archives in General Psychiatry, 60*(2), 133–141.

Stutzmann, G. E., & LeDoux, J. E. (1999). GABAergic antagonists block the inhibitory effects of serotonin in the lateral amygdala: A mechanism for modulation of sensory inputs related to fear conditioning. *Journal of Neuroscience, 19*(11), RC8.

Stutzmann, G. E., McEwen, B. S., & LeDoux, J. E. (1998). Serotonin modulation of sensory inputs to the lateral amygdala: Dependency on corticosterone. *Journal of Neuroscience, 18*(22), 9529–9538.

Vermetten, E., Vythilingam, M., Southwick, S. M., Charney, D. S., & Bremner, J. D. (2003). Long-term treatment with paroxetine increases verbal declarative memory and hippocampal volume in posttraumatic stress disorder. *Biological Psychiatry, 54*(7), 693–702.

Walker, D. L., & Davis, M. (2002). The role of amygdala glutamate receptors in fear learning, fear-potentiated startle, and extinction. *Pharmacology, Biochemistry, and Behavior, 71*(3), 379–392.

Weeber, E. J., Atkins, C. M., Selcher, J. C., Varga, A. W., Mirnikjoo, B., Paylor, R., et al. (2000). A role for the beta isoform of protein kinase C in fear conditioning. *Journal of Neuroscience, 20*(16), 5906–5914.

Witchel, S. F., Lee, P. A., Suda-Hartman, M., Trucco, M., & Hoffman, E. P. (1997). Evidence for a heterozygote advantage in congenital adrenal hyperplasia due to 21-hydroxylase deficiency. *Journal of Clinical Endocrinology and Metabolism, 82*(7), 2097–2101.

Wust, S., Van Rossum, E. F., Federenko, I. S., Koper, J. W., Kumsta, R., & Hellhammer, D. H. (2004). Common polymorphisms in the glucocorticoid receptor gene are associated with adrenocortical responses to psychosocial stress. *Journal of Clinical Endocrinology and Metabolism, 89*(2), 565–573.

Yehuda, R. (2002). Current status of cortisol findings in post-traumatic stress disorder. *Psychiatric Clinics of North America, 25*(2), 341–368, vii.

Yehuda, R., Siever, L. J., Teicher, M. H., Levengood, R. A., Gerber, D. K., Schmeidler, J., et al. (1998). Plasma norepinephrine and 3-methoxy-4-hydroxyphenylglycol concentrations and severity of depression in combat posttraumatic stress disorder and major depressive disorder. *Biological Psychiatry, 44*(1), 56–63.

Young, S. N., Smith, S. E., Phil, P. O., & Ervin, F. R. (1985). Tryptophan depletion causes a rapid lowering of mood in normal males. *Psychopharmacology, 87,* 173–177.

Zahrt, J., Taylor, J. R., Mathew, R. G., & Arnsten, A. F. T. (1997). Supranormal stimulation of dopamine D1 receptors in the rodent prefrontal cortex impairs spatial working memory performance. *Journal of Neuroscience, 17,* 8528–8535.

Zigmond, M. J., Finlay, J. M., & Sved, A. F. (1995). Neurochemical studies of central noradrenergic responses to acute and chronic stress. In M. J. Friedman, D. Charney, & A. Y. Deutch (Eds.), *Neurobiological and clinical consequences of stress: From normal adaptation to PTSD* (pp. 45–60). Philadelphia: Lippincott-Raven.

CHAPTER 3

Structural and Functional Anatomy of PTSD

Findings from Neuroimaging Research

LISA M. SHIN, SCOTT L. RAUCH,
and ROGER K. PITMAN

Over the past decade, neuroimaging research has helped to illuminate structural and functional abnormalities associated with posttraumatic stress disorder (PTSD) and to advance neurobiological models of this disorder. In this chapter, we highlight three brain regions of interest and describe a functional neuroanatomical model of PTSD. Next, we summarize the techniques and paradigms used in neuroimaging studies of PTSD. Finally, we review relevant findings from neuroimaging studies and offer suggestions for future research. Our review is selective, highlighting findings related to the amygdala, medial prefrontal cortex, and hippocampus. Earlier relevant reviews can be found elsewhere (e.g., Bremner, 2002; Elzinga & Bremner, 2002; Grossman, Buchsbaum, & Yehuda, 2002; Hull, 2002; Pitman, Shin, & Rauch, 2001; Tanev, 2003).

BRAIN REGIONS OF INTEREST IN PTSD

Findings from basic science research have highlighted at least three brain regions that may play an important role in the pathophysiology of PTSD: the amygdala, medial prefrontal cortex, and hippocampus. The amygdala is a medial temporal lobe structure that appears to be involved in the assessment of threat-related stimuli (Davis & Whalen, 2001; Morris, Ohman, & Dolan, 1998; Paradiso et al., 1999; Whalen, Rauch, et al., 1998) and plays a crucial role in the process of fear conditioning (Davis & Whalen, 2001; LeDoux, 2000). Interestingly, individuals with PTSD have shown heightened acquisition of conditioned fear in Pavlovian fear-conditioning paradigms (Orr et al., 2000; Peri, Ben-Shakhar, Orr, & Shalev, 2000). In the text below, we review evidence suggesting that the amygdala may be hyperresponsive in individuals with this disorder.

A second region of interest is the medial prefrontal cortex (including the anterior cingulate gyrus, medial frontal gyrus, and subcallosal cortex). Portions of this brain region send projections to the amygdala in primates (Aggleton, Burton, & Passingham, 1980; Chiba, Kayahara, & Nakano, 2001; Ghashghaei & Barbas, 2002; Stefanacci & Amaral, 2002) and may be critically involved in the process of extinction of fear conditioning and the retention of extinction (Milad & Quirk, 2002; Morgan, Romanski, & LeDoux, 1993; Quirk, Russo, Barron, & Lebron, 2000). Patients with PTSD exhibit abnormal extinction of conditioned fear responses in the laboratory (Orr et al., 2000; Rothbaum, Kozak, Foa, & Whitaker, 2001). Clinically, many PTSD patients experience only minimal declines in fear responses over repeated presentations of traumatic reminders. In addition, recent neuroimaging studies have reported reduced neuronal integrity and cortical volumes in medial prefrontal structures in this disorder (De Bellis, Keshavan, Spencer, & Hall, 2000; Rauch et al., 2003). As we discuss later in the chapter, existing neuroimaging data are consistent with the hypothesis that the medial prefrontal cortex is hyporesponsive in PTSD.

A third region of interest is the hippocampus, a medial temporal lobe structure that is involved in memory processes (Eichenbaum, 2000; Schacter, 1997). Classic research on animals has indicated that severe stressors and high levels of stress-related hormones can be associated with memory impairment and hippocampal cell damage (Sapolsky, 2000; Sapolsky, Uno, Rebert, & Finch, 1990; Uno, Tarara, Else, Suleman, & Sapolsky, 1989; Watanabe, Gould, & McEwen, 1992; Woolley, Gould, & McEwen, 1990). We review recent findings of reduced hippocampal volumes and abnormal hippocampal function in PTSD.

We have previously presented a neurocircuitry model of PTSD (Rauch, Shin, Whalen, & Pitman, 1998) that emphasizes the role of the amygdala, as well as its interactions with medial prefrontal cortex and the hippocampus. Briefly, this model hypothesizes hyperresponsivity within the amygdala to threat-related stimuli, with inadequate top–down governance over the amygdala by the medial prefrontal cortex and the hippocampus. According to this model, amygdala hyperresponsivity mediates symptoms of hyperarousal and explains the indelible quality of the emotional memory for the traumatic event; inadequate influence by medial prefrontal cortex underlies deficits of extinction; and decreased hippocampal function underlies deficits in identifying safe contexts, as well as explicit memory difficulties (see also Elzinga & Bremner, 2002; Hamner, Lorberbaum, & George, 1999; Layton & Krikorian, 2002).

OVERVIEW OF NEUROIMAGING TECHNIQUES AND PARADIGMS

Neuroimaging Techniques

Neuroimaging studies of PTSD have examined brain structure, neurochemistry, and function. Structural neuroimaging studies of PTSD have used morphometric magnetic resonance imaging (mMRI), which involves automated or semiautomated segmentation of brain structures of interest, enabling investigators to calculate volume or features of shape. Imaging studies of neurochemistry have employed positron emission tomography (PET) and single photon emission computed tomography (SPECT) methods in conjunction with radiolabeled high-affinity ligands to characterize region receptor number or affinity. Other approaches include the use of magnetic resonance spectroscopy (MRS) to measure the regional relative concentration of select compounds such as N-acetyl aspartate (NAA), a purported marker of healthy neuronal tissue. Functional neuroimaging studies of PTSD have utilized PET with tracers that measure regional cerebral blood flow (rCBF) (e.g., oxygen-15-labeled carbon dioxide), SPECT with tracers that measure correlates of blood flow (e.g., technetium-99-labeled hexamethyl propylene amine oxime [TcHMPAO]), and functional magnetic resonance imaging (fMRI) to measure blood oxygenation level dependent (BOLD) signal changes. Each of these techniques yields maps that reflect regional brain activity.

Neuroimaging Paradigms

Functional neuroimaging paradigms can be categorized based upon the type of conditions in which participants are studied and the main statistical analyses employed. In neutral state paradigms, participants are studied during a nominal "resting" state, or while performing a nonspecific continuous task, and between-group comparisons of regional brain activity are conducted. In symptom provocation paradigms, participants are scanned during a symptomatic state as well as during control conditions. Behavioral and/or pharmacological challenges can be used to induce symptoms. Within-group comparisons can be made to test hypotheses regarding the mediating anatomy of the symptomatic state; group-by-condition interactions distinguish responses in patient versus control groups. In cognitive activation paradigms, participants are studied while performing cognitive tasks that specifically activate brain systems of interest. Group-by-condition interactions are sought to test the functional responsivity or integrity of specific brain systems in patients versus control participants. In the following text, we review recent findings from imaging studies of brain structure, chemistry, and function in PTSD. In this review, we highlight findings relevant to the amygdala, medial prefrontal cortex, and hippocampus in PTSD.

AMYGDALA

Structural Neuroimaging Studies

To our knowledge, no studies in the literature to date have revealed abnormal amygdala volumes in PTSD. Although none of the participants met diagnostic criteria for PTSD, Matsuoka, Yamawaki, Inagaki, Akechi, and Uchitomi (2003) found that left amygdala volumes were 5.7% smaller in 35 breast cancer survivors with intrusive recollections compared to 41 breast cancer survivors without intrusive recollections.

Functional Neuroimaging Studies

Neutral State

In a PET study, Semple et al. (2000) studied regional cerebral blood flow during an auditory continuous performance task in seven PTSD patients with histories of cocaine and alcohol abuse and six healthy comparison participants. The PTSD group had higher rCBF in the right amygdala compared to the healthy comparison group.

Symptom Provocation

Rauch et al. (1996) used PET and script-driven imagery to examine rCBF patterns in eight individuals with PTSD. In separate conditions, participants were prompted by audiotaped narratives (i.e., scripts) to recall and imagine neutral and traumatic autobiographical events. Heart rate and subjective ratings of negative emotions were higher in the traumatic condition than in the neutral condition. In the traumatic versus control conditions, significant rCBF increases occurred in the right amygdala, among other paralimbic regions. However, this study was limited by the absence of a comparison group. Using a similar paradigm, Shin, Orr, et al. (2004) found that, compared to nine healthy male combat veterans, seven male combat veterans with PTSD had greater left amygdala responses to traumatic versus neutral script-driven imagery. In addition, PTSD symptom severity was positively correlated with rCBF within the right amygdala in the traumatic condition.

Using SPECT and TcHMPAO, Liberzon et al. (1999) studied rCBF in 14 Vietnam veterans with PTSD, 11 combat veteran control participants, and 14 healthy nonveteran participants. In separate scanning sessions, participants listened to combat sounds and white noise. In the combat sounds versus white noise comparison, only the PTSD group exhibited activation in the left amygdaloid region. Using PET, Pissiota et al. (2002) also measured rCBF during the presentation of combat sounds versus neutral sounds in seven veterans with PTSD. Heart rate and anxiety increased during the combat versus neutral-sound condition. Regional CBF in the right amygdala region of interest was greater during combat versus neutral-sound condition. Furthermore, rCBF in the right amygdala was positively correlated with self-reported anxiety (see also Fredrikson & Furmark, 2003).

In an fMRI study, Driessen et al. (2004) presented six patients with PTSD and borderline personality disorder (BPD) with personalized trauma-related and generally negative words that cued the participant to recall corresponding autobiographical events. In the traumatic versus generally negative recall comparison, participants with both PTSD and BPD showed activation of the amygdala, among other regions.

In contrast, a number of functional neuroimaging studies have failed to find amygdala activation during symptom provocation (Bremner, Narayan, et al., 1999; Bremner, Staib, et al., 1999; Lanius et al., 2001; Shin et al., 1999). Although the precise reasons for this failure to replicate are not clear, in general, amygdala activation may be more difficult to detect (1) in small groups of participants, especially with high variability, (2) when temporal and spatial resolution are relatively poor, (3) if an optimal symptomatic state is not achieved, and/or (4) if blood flow in the amygdala is moderately elevated in control conditions as well as in experimental conditions in PTSD. Fortunately, some of these issues can be addressed in future functional neuroimaging studies of PTSD.

Cognitive Activation

Shin et al. (1997) studied visual perception and visual mental imagery in seven combat veterans with PTSD and seven combat veterans without PTSD. In the perception conditions, participants viewed and evaluated pictures; in the imagery conditions, participants imagined and evaluated pictures. Within the perception and imagery conditions, participants saw neutral, negative, and combat-related pictures. In the combat-imagery versus combat-perception conditions, only the PTSD group exhibited rCBF increases in the right amygdala. Hendler et al. (2003) found greater amygdala responses to combat and neutral pictures in combat veterans with PTSD compared to combat veterans without PTSD.

Rauch et al. (2000) sought to determine whether exaggerated amygdala activation could be demonstrated using affective stimuli, unrelated to trauma. During fMRI scanning, eight combat veterans with PTSD and eight combat veterans without PTSD were shown fearful and happy facial expressions that were backwardly masked with neutral facial expressions so as to prevent explicit processing of the emotional facial expressions (Whalen, Rauch, et al., 1998). In the masked-fear versus masked-happy comparison, amygdala activation was greater in the PTSD group compared to the control group. In addition, amygdala activation was positively correlated with PTSD symptom severity. Exaggerated amygdala responses in PTSD also can be demonstrated using overtly presented fearful versus happy facial expressions (Shin et al., in press).

In summary, functional neuroimaging studies have provided evidence in support of heightened amygdala responsivity in PTSD. Across studies, exaggerated amygdala activation has been found in response to both traumatic reminders and more general predictors of threat (i.e., fearful facial expressions). In addition, three separate studies have reported a positive relationship between symptom severity and amygdala activation (Pissiota et al., 2002; Rauch et al., 2000; Shin, Orr, et al., 2004).

MEDIAL PREFRONTAL CORTEX

Structural Neuroimaging Studies

Several MRI studies have reported decreased volumes of frontal cortex in PTSD (Carrion et al., 2001; De Bellis et al., 2002; Fennema-Notestine, Stein, Kennedy, Archibald, & Jernigan, 2002). However, only a few studies have examined the structural aspects of medial prefrontal cortex specifically. Rauch et al. (2003) used MRI and cortical parcellation techniques to examine volumes of medial prefrontal cortical regions in nine women with PTSD and nine trauma-exposed women without PTSD. The PTSD group exhibited decreased volumes in pregenual anterior cingulate cortex and subcallosal cortex. Yamasue et al. (2003) used MRI and voxel-based morphometry to study 25 survivors of a Tokyo subway sarin attack: 9 with PTSD and 16 without PTSD. Relative to the control group, the PTSD group had significantly smaller gray matter volumes in dorsal anterior cingulate cortex. In the PTSD group, severity of PTSD was inversely correlated with gray-matter volumes in anterior cingulate cortex.

Neurochemistry Studies

In an MRS study, DeBellis et al. (2000) examined NAA/creatine ratios in pregenual anterior cingulate cortex in 11 maltreated children and adolescents with PTSD and 11 matched healthy control participants. The PTSD group had lower NAA/creatine ratios in pregenual anterior cingulate than the control group, consistent with decreased neuronal integrity in that region in PTSD. According to one case report, NAA/creatine ratios in a maltreated boy with PTSD increased following successful treatment with clonidine (De Bellis, Keshavan, & Harenski, 2001).

In a SPECT study, Bremner et al. (2000) used [^{123}I]iomazenil to investigate benzodiazepine receptor binding in 13 combat veterans with PTSD and 13 healthy comparison participants. Compared to the control group, the PTSD group had lower binding in anterior medial prefrontal cortex. The investigators noted that this finding is consistent with preclinical studies showing decreased benzodiazepine binding in the frontal cortex of chronically stressed animals and may be related to the decreased activity of medial prefrontal structures in PTSD (discussed later in the chapter).

Functional Neuroimaging Studies

Neutral State

In a study described above, Semple et al. (2000) found that seven PTSD patients with histories of cocaine and alcohol abuse had lower rCBF in the anterior cingulate gyrus/medial frontal gyrus during rest and an auditory continuous performance task, compared to six healthy comparison participants. In contrast, Sachinvala, Kling, Suffin, Lake, and Cohen (2000) used TcHMPAO and SPECT to study resting regional cerebral perfusion in 17 patients with PTSD and 8 healthy comparison subjects. Relative to the comparison group, the PTSD group had relatively greater perfusion in bilateral anterior cingulate cortex.

Symptom Provocation

Several symptom provocation studies have reported either diminished activation or deactivation in medial prefrontal cortex in PTSD. Bremner, Staib, et al. (1999) used PET to study rCBF in 10 combat veterans with PTSD and 10 without PTSD. During exposure to combat-related versus neutral pictures and sounds, the PTSD group exhibited rCBF decreases in subcallosal cortex and a failure to activate anterior cingulate gyrus. In a script-driven imagery PET study conducted by Bremner, Narayan, et al. (1999), 10 women with PTSD and 12 women without PTSD underwent PET scanning while they listened to scripts describing abuse-related and neutral events. In the PTSD group, abuse imagery was associated with decreased rCBF in subcallosal cortex (Brodmann's area 25) and a failure to activate anterior cingulate gyrus. Using a similar design, Shin et al. (1999) examined rCBF in 16 female survivors of childhood sexual abuse: 8 with PTSD and 8 without PTSD. In the traumatic versus neutral-imagery comparison, the PTSD group failed to activate anterior cingulate gyrus. Using script-driven imagery and PET in a study of Vietnam veterans, Liberzon, Britton, and Phan (2003) reported deactivation in anterior cingulate gyrus in the traumatic versus neutral-imagery condition. Finally, Shin, Orr, et al. (2004) found that 17 veterans with PTSD exhibited rCBF decreases in medial frontal gyrus in the traumatic versus neutral-imagery comparison. Such decreases were not seen in 19 veterans without PTSD. Furthermore, symptom severity was inversely related to rCBF in medial frontal gyrus in the traumatic-imagery condition. That is, as symptom severity increased, rCBF in medial frontal gyrus in the traumatic condition decreased.

In an fMRI symptom provocation study of PTSD, Lanius et al. (2001) studied nine patients with PTSD and nine trauma-exposed participants without PTSD. In the traumatic script-driven imagery versus implicit baseline contrast, the PTSD group showed less activation than the comparison group in medial frontal gyrus, anterior cingulate gyrus, thalamus, and right occipital lobe. The findings of relatively smaller fMRI signal responses in anterior cingulate gyrus and thalamus in PTSD were also observed in other negative emotional states (sadness and anxiety) in PTSD (Lanius et al., 2003). Interestingly, PTSD patients who dissociated during script-driven imagery had *greater* activation than control participants in medial frontal gyrus and anterior cingulate gyrus (Lanius et al., 2002). This suggests that reexperiencing and dissociation may be associated with opposite responses in medial prefrontal regions, and that participants' dissociative state during script-driven imagery should be monitored.

In contrast, using PET, Rauch et al. (1996) found increased activation in anterior cingulate cortex during traumatic imagery in PTSD, although whether this rCBF increase was normal or blunted is unknown due to the absence of a comparison group. In a SPECT study, Zubieta et al. (1999) found greater blood flow increases in medial prefrontal cortex in 12 PTSD patients compared to 12 healthy control participants during the presentation of combat sounds versus white noise. Liberzon et al. (1999) reported no group differences in anterior cingulate activation in PTSD. Possible reasons for these discrepant results might include the different imaging technique used in these latter two reports (i.e., SPECT) and/or the dissociative state of the participants studied.

Cognitive Activation

To test the functional integrity of medial prefrontal regions in PTSD using a cognitive activation paradigm, Shin et al. (2001) administered the emotional counting Stroop task (Whalen, Bush, et al., 1998) during fMRI to eight combat veterans with PTSD and eight combat veterans without PTSD. In this task, participants viewed words of different valence (neutral, generally negative, and combat-related) on a computer screen, counted the number of words presented at each trial, and then pressed the corresponding response button. In contrast to the control group, the PTSD group failed to activate anterior cingulate gyrus in the combat versus general-negative condition.

Preliminary analyses of an fMRI study in our laboratory have revealed diminished medial prefrontal cortex responses to overtly presented fearful versus happy facial expressions in 13 individuals with PTSD compared to 13 trauma-exposed control participants without PTSD. In this study, symptom severity was negatively correlated with medial prefrontal cortex responses (Shin et al., in press).

In a PET study of the neural correlates mediating the retrieval of negatively valenced and neutral word pairs, Bremner, Vythilingam, Vermetten, Southwick, McGlashan, Staib, et al. (2003) studied 10 abused women with PTSD and 11 healthy comparison participants. PET data were gathered as participants completed a paired associates retrieval task with shallowly encoded neutral word pairs, deeply encoded neutral word pairs, and deeply encoded negatively valenced word pairs. During the retrieval of deeply encoded emotional words versus deeply encoded neutral words, the PTSD group showed greater rCBF decreases in medial prefrontal regions (including subcallosal gyrus and anterior cingulate/medial frontal gyrus), relative to the comparison group.

In summary, both symptom provocation and cognitive activation studies have reported either diminished activation or deactivation in medial prefrontal structures in PTSD, including anterior cingulate, subcallosal, and medial frontal cortices. Two studies have reported an inverse correlation between PTSD symptom severity and medial prefrontal cortex responses. Additional research is needed to determine the relationship between the volumetric and functional findings in medial prefrontal cortex in this disorder.

AMYGDALA/MEDIAL PREFRONTAL CORTEX INTERACTIONS

Using correlational and more complex multivariate analyses, researchers have begun to determine the brain regions that covary together in functional networks (e.g., Lanius et al., 2004). Critical tests of neuroanatomical models of PTSD will come from studies examining the relationship between the amygdala and medial prefrontal cortex in this disorder. The studies below have suggested a relationship between these two regions in PTSD.

In a script-driven imagery PET study mentioned above, Shin, Orr, et al. (2004) found that in the PTSD group, rCBF changes in medial frontal gyrus were significantly inversely related to rCBF changes in bilateral amygdala. That is, as rCBF changes in medial frontal gyrus decreased, rCBF changes in amygdala increased. This suggests a reciprocal relationship between medial prefrontal cortex and amygdala function in PTSD, although the direction of causality remains undetermined. The finding of an inverse relationship between these two regions in PTSD has been replicated in an independent sample using a paradigm involving the presentation of fearful versus happy facial expressions (Shin et al., in press). In both studies, the inverse correlation remained even when participants with comorbid depression were removed from the analyses. Furthermore, a recent symptom provocation PET study reported a very different pattern of relationships between these two brain regions in patients with major depressive disorder (without PTSD) (Dougherty et al., 2004). Thus, the inverse relationship between the amygdala and medial prefrontal cortex in PTSD does not appear to be attributable to comorbid major depression.

Gilboa et al. (2004) studied functional networks associated with traumatic mental imagery in 10 patients with PTSD and 10 trauma-exposed individuals who never had PTSD. PET data were analyzed with partial least squares, which identifies groups of brain regions that covary with a particular region of interest, and structural equation modeling, which is used to test models of the direction of influence between regions. Two groups of brain regions were associated with amygdala activity. The first group of brain regions included positive associations with the hippocampus, medial frontal cortex, and anterior cingulate gyrus in both the PTSD and control groups. The second group of brain regions associated with amygdala activity differed between the PTSD and control groups. Unlike the control group, the PTSD group exhibited a positive relationship between the amygdala, anterior cingulate gyrus, and posterior subcallosal cortex, among other regions. The authors noted that their findings are consistent with the notion that amygdala directly influences medial prefrontal regions.

In summary, there is preliminary evidence for a functional relationship between the amygdala and the medial prefrontal cortex in PTSD. Additional research will be required to determine the direction of this relationship and to identify other important relationships among brain systems in this disorder.

HIPPOCAMPUS

Structural Neuroimaging Studies

In the first volumetric MRI study of PTSD, Bremner et al. (1995) measured hippocampal volume in 26 Vietnam combat veterans with PTSD and 22 noncombat veteran control participants. The results indicated an 8% decrease in right hippocampal volume in the PTSD group relative to the control group, with no significant group differences for left hippocampus, caudate nucleus, or temporal lobe. Deficits in short-term verbal memory as measured by the Logical Memory subtest of the Wechsler Memory Scale—Revised (Wechsler, 1987) were associated with decreased right hippocampal volume in the PTSD patients. Likewise, Gurvits et al. (1996) found a 26% decrease in left hippocampal volume and a 22% decrease in right hippocampal volume in seven Vietnam veterans with PTSD, compared to seven combat veterans without PTSD. Hippocampal volumes were inversely correlated with self-reported combat exposure severity.

Similar results have been reported in studies of abuse-related PTSD. Stein, Koverola, Hanna, Torchia, and McClarty (1997) found a 5% reduction in left hippocampal volume in 21 women with PTSD who had suffered repeated childhood sexual abuse (15 of whom had PTSD) compared to nonabused women. Left-sided hippocampal volume correlated (inversely) with dissociative symptom severity but not with explicit memory functioning. Similarly, Bremner, Randall, et al. (1997) found a 12% decrease in left hippocampal volume in 17 adult survivors of child physical and sexual abuse, compared to 17 nonabused, healthy participants. Finally, Bremner, Vythilingam, Vermetten, Southwick, McGlashan, Nazeer, et al. (2003) reported smaller hippocampal volumes bilaterally in a group of women with childhood sexual abuse histories and PTSD (n = 10), compared to both abused women without PTSD (n = 12) and nonabused, psychiatrically healthy women (n = 11). Hippocampal volumes were 16% smaller in the women with abuse and PTSD, compared to women with abuse but without PTSD. Left hippocampal volumes were significantly inversely related to dissociative symptom severity, whereas right hippocampal volumes were significantly inversely related to PTSD symptom severity.

In a mixed trauma cohort, Villarreal, Hamilton, et al. (2002) found smaller left (13%) and right (10%) hippocampal volumes in 12 participants with PTSD compared to 10 healthy participants. Group differences persisted even after hippocampal volumes were normalized to total brain tissue volumes and after lifetime number of weeks of alcohol intoxication was statistically controlled. PTSD and depression scores were inversely correlated with left hippocampal volume.

To determine whether smaller hippocampal volume might be a preexisting risk factor for the development of PTSD, Gilbertson et al. (2002) studied hippocampal volumes in monozygotic twins, discordant for trauma exposure. They found that 17 unexposed co-twins of veterans with PTSD had smaller hippocampal volumes compared to the 23 unexposed co-twins of veterans without PTSD. In addition, PTSD symptom severity in the exposed twin was inversely correlated with hippocampal volume in both the exposed and unexposed identical co-twin. The authors interpreted these findings as being consistent with the hypothesis that smaller hippocampal volume is a preexisting risk factor for the development of pathological stress responses.

One recent study has investigated the change in hippocampal volume associated with treatment. Vermetten, Vythilingam, Southwick, Charney, and Bremner (2003) studied memory and hippocampal volumes before and after 9 to 12 months of treatment with paroxetine in 20 men and women with PTSD. Treatment was associated with significant improvements in symptom severity and verbal memory, and a 4.6% mean increase in hippocampal volume. The authors speculated that selective serotonin reuptake inhibitors might reverse hippocampal atrophy by promoting neurogenesis.

In contrast to the results reviewed above, several cross-sectional studies have failed to reveal PTSD-related differences in hippocampal volume. De Bellis et al. (1999) found no significant hippocampal volume differences in 44 maltreated children and adolescents with PTSD compared to 61 matched, healthy, nonabused controls, although the PTSD group had lower overall cerebral volume, lower corpus callosum volume, and greater ventricular and CSF volumes. Likewise, no group difference in hippocampal volume emerged in an independent sample of 28 psychotropic naïve maltreated children and adolescents with PTSD (De Bellis et al., 2002). Carrion et al. (2001) found no significant hippocampal volume differences between a group of 24 children with PTSD symptoms (12 of whom had PTSD) and 24 healthy comparison participants, although the symptomatic group had smaller total brain volumes and total brain gray matter volumes and attenuated frontal gray matter volume asymmetry compared to the control group. Finally, Fennema-Notestine et al. (2002) failed to find differences in hippocampal volumes between 22 victims of intimate partner violence (11 with and 11 without PTSD), and 17 nonvictimized comparison participants, although intimate partner violence participants had smaller supratentorial cranial vaults and frontal and occipital gray matter volumes compared to nontraumatized control participants.

The findings of two prospective longitudinal studies have not supported the hypothesis of diminished hippocampal volumes over time in PTSD. De Bellis, Hall, Boring, Frustaci, and Moritz (2001) studied hippocampal volumes before and after a 2-year follow-up period in nine prepubertal maltreated participants with PTSD and nine healthy participants without histories of maltreatment. Although there was a trend for hippocampal volume to decline over time in both groups, there were no significant group differences in hippocampal volumes at baseline, follow-up, or across time. Bonne et al. (2001) examined hippocampal volumes in 37 survivors of traumatic events, 10 who had PTSD at 6 months posttrauma and 27 who did not. Hippocampal volume did not differ between groups at

1 week or 6 months posttrauma and did not decrease over 6 months in either group.

Neurochemistry Studies

Several studies have utilized MRS to measure NAA in the medial temporal lobes of individuals with PTSD. Freeman, Cardwell, Karson, and Komoroski (1998) reported significantly lower NAA/creatine ratios in right medial temporal lobe in 21 PTSD veterans compared to 8 non-PTSD veterans. Menon, Nasrallah, Lyons, Scott, and Liberto (2003) reported decreased NAA/creatine ratios in the left hippocampal region in 14 veterans with PTSD and 7 comparison participants without PTSD. In a study combining MRS and mMRI techniques, Schuff et al. (2001) found a 23% reduction in NAA bilaterally in the hippocampal region and a 26% decrease in choline in the right hippocampus in 18 male combat veterans with PTSD compared to 19 male control participants. However, the groups had similar volumes of the hippocampus and entorhinal cortex, suggesting that NAA may be a more sensitive measure of hippocampal pathology than volumetric measures. The authors interpreted their finding of reduced hippocampal NAA in the absence of volumetric loss in PTSD as reflecting either neuron loss in the presence of glial proliferation and/or neuronal metabolic impairments.

Other MRS studies failed to reveal significant group differences but have indicated trends suggesting altered hippocampal neurochemistry in PTSD. In a preliminary report, Villarreal, Petropoulos, et al. (2002) found a trend for reduced left hippocampal NAA and creatine in eight civilian patients with PTSD compared to five participants without PTSD, although groups did not differ with regard to occipital lobe NAA levels. Likewise, Brown, Freeman, Kimbrell, Cardwell, and Komoroski (2003) found a trend for smaller left medial temporal lobe NAA/creatine ratios in former prisoners of war with PTSD compared to those without PTSD.

In summary, over half of the volumetric MRI studies reviewed above reported smaller hippocampal volumes in PTSD. Hippocampal volume reductions have been associated with greater PTSD symptom severity (Bremner, Vythilingam, Vermetten, Southwick, McGlashan, Nazeer, et al., 2003; Gilbertson et al., 2002; Villarreal, Hamilton, et al., 2002), dissociative symptom severity (Bremner, Vythilingam, Vermetten, Southwick, McGlashan, Nazeer, et al., 2003; Stein et al., 1997), and poorer memory performance (Bremner et al., 1995). The results of the MRS studies indicated that medial temporal lobe NAA/creatine ratios are also lower in PTSD, suggesting decreased neuronal integrity in hippocampus, although two of the MRS studies reported only trends in this direction.

Whether hippocampal volumetric changes precede or follow the onset of PTSD remains to be determined. (For further discussion on this topic, see

Bremner, 2001; Pitman, 2001; Sapolsky, 2001; Yehuda, 2001). The results of a twin study suggested that smaller hippocampal volumes may be a pre-existing risk factor for the development of PTSD (Gilbertson et al., 2002). Further twin and longitudinal studies are needed to effectively address this question.

It is important to note, however, that several of the MRI studies did not replicate the finding of decreased hippocampal volumes in PTSD. These mixed results suggest that hippocampal volumetric changes may be restricted to only some subgroups (e.g., adults with chronic PTSD), that they may be secondary to comorbid conditions (e.g., depression, alcohol dependence), or that hippocampal pathology may be relatively subtle and not always detectable by standard mMRI procedures. The latter possibility is consistent with the finding of decreased hippocampal region NAA in the absence of volumetric changes in a sample of veterans with PTSD (Schuff et al., 2001).

Functional Neuroimaging Studies

Neutral State

Semple et al. (1993) reported a trend for decreased left/right ratios of hippocampal blood flow during a word-generation task in six veterans with PTSD and substance abuse histories compared with seven healthy participants. This research group later found that PTSD patients with histories of cocaine and alcohol abuse had higher rCBF in left parahippocampal gyrus during an auditory continuous performance task compared to a healthy comparison group (Semple et al., 2000). Sachinvala et al. (2000) used TcHMPAO and SPECT to study regional cerebral perfusion in 17 patients with PTSD and 8 healthy comparison subjects. Relative to the comparison group, the PTSD group had relatively greater perfusion in the left hippocampal region.

Symptom Provocation

Several early functional neuroimaging studies reported abnormal blood flow in the hippocampus or parahippocampal gyrus in PTSD. In a PET study described above, Bremner, Narayan, et al. (1999) found that abuse-related traumatic imagery was associated with rCBF decreases in the right hippocampus of abused women with PTSD relative to abused women without PTSD. Shin et al. (1999) reported a similar finding of greater rCBF decreases in the parahippocampal gyrus in PTSD. Bremner, Innis, et al. (1997) found decreased glucose metabolism in the hippocampus bilaterally following administration of yohimbine versus placebo in PTSD. In a script-driven imagery study of PTSD, Osuch et al. (2001) reported a positive correlation between flashback intensity and rCBF in a left perihippocampal region in patients with chronic PTSD.

Cognitive Activation

Recently, functional neuroimaging studies using cognitive activation paradigms have contributed to our understanding of hippocampal function in PTSD. Bremner, Vythilingam, Vermetten, Southwick, McGlashan, Nazeer, et al. (2003) used MRI and PET to study the structure and function of the hippocampus in 22 women with histories of childhood sexual abuse: 10 with PTSD and 12 without PTSD. As noted previously, analysis of structural MRI scans revealed smaller hippocampal volumes bilaterally in the PTSD group. During PET scanning, participants heard narratives and were asked to either count the number of times they heard the letter *d* (control condition) or to form a mental image of the described events and to remember as much of the narrative as possible (verbal memory encoding condition). Recall measures did not differ significantly between the PTSD and comparison groups. In the verbal memory encoding versus control condition comparison, women without PTSD showed rCBF increases in the left hippocampus, but women with PTSD failed to show such increases. Regional CBF in the control condition did not differ between groups. There were no significant correlations between symptom severity and left hippocampal blood flow or between left hippocampal volume and left hippocampal blood flow. Using PET and a verbal paired-associates task (described earlier), Bremner, Vythilingam, Vermetten, Southwick, McGlashan, Staib, et al. (2003) found that during the retrieval of deeply encoded emotional versus neutral words, the group of abused women with PTSD had greater rCBF decreases in the left hippocampus, relative to the healthy group.

Shin, Shin, et al. (2004) used a word-stem completion task to study rCBF in the hippocampus in eight firefighters with PTSD and eight without PTSD. During PET scanning, participants viewed three-letter word stems on a computer screen and completed each stem with a word they had previously encoded either deeply (high-recall condition) or shallowly (low-recall condition) (Schacter, Alpert, Savage, Rauch, & Albert, 1996). Relative to the control group, the PTSD group exhibited significantly smaller rCBF increases in the left hippocampus in the high- versus low-recall comparison. However, this finding reflected relatively elevated rCBF in the low-recall condition in the PTSD group. Collapsing across conditions, the PTSD group had higher rCBF bilaterally in the hippocampus and in the left amygdala than the control group. In addition, within the PTSD group, symptom severity was positively associated with rCBF in the hippocampus and the parahippocampal gyrus, consistent with the findings of Osuch et al. (2001). The groups did not significantly differ with regard to accuracy scores on the word-stem completion task. Although the PTSD group had significantly smaller right (and a trend for smaller left) hippocampal volumes than the control group, hippocampal volumes were not significantly related to hippocampal rCBF.

In summary, several neuroimaging studies of hippocampal function revealed relatively diminished hippocampal activation during script-driven imagery and memory encoding and retrieval tasks. However, two PET studies reported a positive correlation between symptom severity measures and rCBF in hippocampal regions in PTSD (Osuch et al., 2001; Shin, Shin, et al., 2004), one PET study reported greater rCBF in the parahippocampal gyrus in PTSD (Semple et al., 2000), one PET study reported greater hippocampal rCBF across conditions in PTSD (Shin, Shin, et al., 2004), and one resting SPECT study reported increased perfusion in the hippocampal region in PTSD (Sachinvala et al., 2000). These findings raise the question of whether a "failure to activate" the hippocampus in PTSD may be attributable to increased baseline activity in the hippocampus (but see also Bremner, Vythilingam, Vermetten, Southwick, McGlashan, Nazeer, et al., 2003; Bonne et al., 2003). Further studies examining resting perfusion or glucose metabolism in the hippocampus would be needed to address this question. Two studies have reported no significant correlations between hippocampal volumes and rCBF changes (Bremner, Vythilingam, Vermetten, Southwick, McGlashan, Nazeer, et al., 2003; Shin, Shin, et al., 2004). Additional studies with larger sample sizes will be needed to adequately explore the relationship between hippocampal structure and function in PTSD.

GENERAL SUMMARY AND CONCLUSIONS

Neuroimaging research concerning brain structure, chemistry, and function in PTSD has provided evidence consistent with exaggerated responsivity in the amygdala, diminished responsivity in medial prefrontal cortex, and an inverse relationship between these two regions. Neuroimaging data have also suggested diminished volumes, neuronal integrity, and functional integrity of the hippocampus in PTSD.

The interpretation of neuroimaging findings should be tempered by a consideration of several methodological issues, similar to those discussed by Duke and Vasterling (Chapter 1, this volume). Most neuroimaging studies have included relatively small samples of individuals with chronic PTSD; whether the findings summarized above generalize to acute PTSD remains to be determined. In the neuroimaging literature, comorbidity has been addressed either via analysis of covariance or by temporary exclusion of participants with a specific comorbid disorder (e.g., depression). Future studies might seek to include either psychiatric comparison groups (e.g., depression without PTSD) or larger numbers of PTSD patients with and without comorbidity to permit adequate statistical comparison of these subgroups. Lastly, methodology varies greatly across studies in the functional neuroimaging literature. Variability in technique (e.g., PET, fMRI), tasks implemented during scanning (e.g., resting, symptom provocation, Stroop task), design (e.g., blocked, event-related), and data analytic method (e.g., voxelwise, region of interest) may complicate a comparison of results across studies.

Although knowledge concerning the neurobiology of PTSD has increased over the past decade, many questions remain unanswered. What is the precise relationship between abnormalities in the amygdala, medial prefrontal cortex, and hippocampus? Are these abnormalities preexisting risk factors for, or consequences of, the development of PTSD? Does treatment correct the abnormal structure or function of these three brain regions? Future studies utilizing twin, longitudinal, and/or treatment designs are needed to address these remaining questions.

REFERENCES

Aggleton, J. P., Burton, M. J., & Passingham, R. E. (1980). Cortical and subcortical afferents to the amygdala of the rhesus monkey (Macaca mulatta). *Brain Research, 190*, 347–368.

Bonne, O., Brandes, D., Gilboa, A., Gomori, J. M., Shenton, M. E., Pitman, R. K., & Shalev, A. Y. (2001). Longitudinal MRI study of hippocampal volume in trauma survivors with PTSD. *American Journal of Psychiatry, 158*, 1248–1251.

Bonne, O., Gilboa, A., Louzoun, Y., Brandes, D., Yona, I., Lester, H., Barkai, G., Freedman, N., Chisin, R., & Shalev, A. Y. (2003). Resting regional cerebral perfusion in recent posttraumatic stress disorder. *Biological Psychiatry, 54*, 1077–1086.

Bremner, J. D. (2001). Hypotheses and controversies related to effects of stress on the hippocampus: An argument for stress-induced damage to the hippocampus in patients with posttraumatic stress disorder. *Hippocampus, 11*, 75–81; discussion 82–74.

Bremner, J. D. (2002). Neuroimaging studies in post-traumatic stress disorder. *Current Psychiatry Reports, 4*, 254–263.

Bremner, J. D., Innis, R. B., Ng, C. K., Staib, L. H., Salomon, R. M., Bronen, R. A., Duncan, J., Southwick, S. M., Krystal, J. H., Rich, D., Zubal, G., Dey, H., Soufer, R., & Charney, D. S. (1997). Positron emission tomography measurement of cerebral metabolic correlates of yohimbine administration in combat-related posttraumatic stress disorder. *Archives of General Psychiatry, 54*, 246–254.

Bremner, J. D., Innis, R. B., Southwick, S. M., Staib, L., Zoghbi, S., & Charney, D. S. (2000). Decreased benzodiazepine receptor binding in prefrontal cortex in combat-related posttraumatic stress disorder. *American Journal of Psychiatry, 157*, 1120–1126.

Bremner, J. D., Narayan, M., Staib, L. H., Southwick, S. M., McGlashan, T., & Charney, D. S. (1999). Neural correlates of memories of childhood sexual abuse in women with and without posttraumatic stress disorder. *American Journal of Psychiatry, 156*, 1787–1795.

Bremner, J. D., Randall, P., Scott, T. M., Bronen, R. A., Seibyl, J. P., Southwick, S. M., Delaney, R. C., McCarthy, G., Charney, D. S., & Innis, R. B. (1995). MRI-based measurement of hippocampal volume in patients with combat-related posttraumatic stress disorder. *American Journal of Psychiatry, 152*, 973–981.

Bremner, J. D., Randall, P., Vermetten, E., Staib, L., Bronen, R. A., Mazure, C., Capelli, S., McCarthy, G., Innis, R. B., & Charney, D. S. (1997). Magnetic resonance imaging-based measurement of hippocampal volume in posttraumatic stress disorder related to childhood physical and sexual abuse—A preliminary report. *Biological Psychiatry, 41*, 23–32.

Bremner, J. D., Staib, L. H., Kaloupek, D., Southwick, S. M., Soufer, R., & Charney, D. S. (1999). Neural correlates of exposure to traumatic pictures and sound in Vietnam combat veterans with and without posttraumatic stress disorder: a positron emission tomography study. *Biological Psychiatry, 45*, 806–816.

Bremner, J. D., Vythilingam, M., Vermetten, E., Southwick, S. M., McGlashan, T., Nazeer, A., Khan, S., Vaccarino, L. V., Soufer, R., Garg, P. K., Ng, C. K., Staib, L. H., Duncan, J. S., & Charney, D. S. (2003). MRI and PET study of deficits in hippocampal structure and function in women with childhood sexual abuse and posttraumatic stress disorder. *American Journal of Psychiatry, 160*, 924–932.

Bremner, J. D., Vythilingam, M., Vermetten, E., Southwick, S. M., McGlashan, T., Staib, L. H., Soufer, R., & Charney, D. S. (2003). Neural correlates of declarative memory for emotionally valenced words in women with posttraumatic stress disorder related to early childhood sexual abuse. *Biological Psychiatry, 53*, 879–889.

Brown, S., Freeman, T., Kimbrell, T., Cardwell, D., & Komoroski, R. (2003). In vivo proton magnetic resonance spectroscopy of the medial temporal lobes of former prisoners of war with and without posttraumatic stress disorder. *Journal of Neuropsychiatry and Clinical Neuroscience, 15*, 367–370.

Carrion, V. G., Weems, C. F., Eliez, S., Patwardhan, A., Brown, W., Ray, R. D., & Reiss, A. L. (2001). Attenuation of frontal asymmetry in pediatric posttraumatic stress disorder. *Biological Psychiatry, 50*, 943–951.

Chiba, T., Kayahara, T., & Nakano, K. (2001). Efferent projections of infralimbic and prelimbic areas of the medial prefrontal cortex in the Japanese monkey, Macaca fuscata. *Brain Research, 888*, 83–101.

Davis, M., & Whalen, P. J. (2001). The amygdala: Vigilance and emotion. *Molecular Psychiatry, 6*, 13–34.

De Bellis, M. D., Hall, J., Boring, A. M., Frustaci, K., & Moritz, G. (2001). A pilot longitudinal study of hippocampal volumes in pediatric maltreatment-related posttraumatic stress disorder. *Biological Psychiatry, 50*, 305–309.

De Bellis, M. D., Keshavan, M. S., Clark, D. B., Casey, B. J., Giedd, J. N., Boring, A.

M., Frustaci, K., & Ryan, N. D. (1999). A.E. Bennett Research Award. Developmental traumatology. Part II: Brain development. *Biological Psychiatry, 45,* 1271–1284.

De Bellis, M. D., Keshavan, M. S., & Harenski, K. A. (2001). Anterior cingulate N-acetylaspartate/creatine ratios during clonidine treatment in a maltreated child with posttraumatic stress disorder. *Journal of Child and Adolescent Psychopharmacology, 11,* 311–316.

De Bellis, M. D., Keshavan, M. S., Shifflett, H., Iyengar, S., Beers, S. R., Hall, J., & Moritz, G. (2002). Brain structures in pediatric maltreatment-related posttraumatic stress disorder: A sociodemographically matched study. *Biological Psychiatry, 52,* 1066–1078.

De Bellis, M. D., Keshavan, M. S., Spencer, S., & Hall, J. (2000). N-Acetylaspartate concentration in the anterior cingulate of maltreated children and adolescents with PTSD. *American Journal of Psychiatry, 157,* 1175–1177.

Dougherty, D. D., Rauch, S. L., Deckersbach, T., Marci, C., Loh, R., Shin, L. M., Alpert, N. M., Fischman, A. J., & Fava, M. (2004). Ventromedial prefrontal cortex and amygdala dysfunction during an anger induction PET study in patients with major depression with anger attacks. *Archives of General Psychiatry, 61,* 795–804.

Driessen, M., Beblo, T., Mertens, M., Piefke, M., Rullkoetter, N., Silva-Saavedra, A., Reddemann, L., Rau, H., Markowitsch, H. J., Wulff, H., Lange, W., & Woermann, F. G. (2004). Posttraumatic stress disorder and fMRI activation patterns of traumatic memory in patients with borderline personality disorder. *Biological Psychiatry, 55,* 603–611.

Eichenbaum, H. (2000). A cortical–hippocampal system for declarative memory. *Nature Reviews Neuroscience, 1,* 41–50.

Elzinga, B. M., & Bremner, J. D. (2002). Are the neural substrates of memory the final common pathway in posttraumatic stress disorder (PTSD)? *Journal of Affective Disorders, 70,* 1–17.

Fennema-Notestine, C., Stein, M. B., Kennedy, C. M., Archibald, S. L., & Jernigan, T. L. (2002). Brain morphometry in female victims of intimate partner violence with and without posttraumatic stress disorder. *Biological Psychiatry, 52,* 1089–1101.

Fredrikson, M., & Furmark, T. (2003). Amygdaloid regional cerebral blood flow and subjective fear during symptom provocation in anxiety disorders. *Annals of the New York Academy of Sciences, 985,* 341–347.

Freeman, T. W., Cardwell, D., Karson, C. N., & Komoroski, R. A. (1998). In vivo proton magnetic resonance spectroscopy of the medial temporal lobes of subjects with combat-related posttraumatic stress disorder. *Magnetic Resonance Medicine, 40,* 66–71.

Ghashghaei, H. T., & Barbas, H. (2002). Pathways for emotion: Interactions of prefrontal and anterior temporal pathways in the amygdala of the rhesus monkey. *Neuroscience, 115,* 1261–1279.

Gilbertson, M. W., Shenton, M. E., Ciszewski, A., Kasai, K., Lasko, N. B., Orr, S. P., & Pitman, R. K. (2002). Smaller hippocampal volume predicts pathologic vulnerability to psychological trauma. *Nature Neuroscience, 5,* 1242–1247.

Gilboa, A., Shalev, A. Y., Laor, L., Lester, H., Louzoun, Y., Chisin, R., & Bonne, O.

(2004). Functional connectivity of the prefrontal cortex and the amygdala in posttraumatic stress disorder. *Biological Psychiatry, 55*, 263–272.

Grossman, R., Buchsbaum, M. S., & Yehuda, R. (2002). Neuroimaging studies in post-traumatic stress disorder. *Psychiatric Clinics of North America, 25*, 317–340, vi.

Gurvits, T. V., Shenton, M. E., Hokama, H., Ohta, H., Lasko, N. B., Gilbertson, M. W., Orr, S. P., Kikinis, R., Jolesz, F. A., McCarley, R. W., & Pitman, R. K. (1996). Magnetic resonance imaging study of hippocampal volume in chronic, combat-related posttraumatic stress disorder. *Biological Psychiatry, 40*, 1091–1099.

Hamner, M. B., Lorberbaum, J. P., & George, M. S. (1999). Potential role of the anterior cingulate cortex in PTSD: Review and hypothesis. *Depression and Anxiety, 9*, 1–14.

Hendler, T., Rotshtein, P., Yeshurun, Y., Weizmann, T., Kahn, I., Ben-Bashat, D., Malach, R., & Bleich, A. (2003). Sensing the invisible: Differential sensitivity of visual cortex and amygdala to traumatic context. *Neuroimage, 19*, 587–600.

Hull, A. M. (2002). Neuroimaging findings in post-traumatic stress disorder. Systematic review. *British Journal of Psychiatry, 181*, 102–110.

Lanius, R., Williamson, P., Boksman, K., Densmore, M., Gupta, M., Neufeld, R., Gati, J., & Menon, R. (2002). Brain activation during script-driven imagery induced dissociative responses in PTSD: A functional magnetic resonance imaging investigation. *Biological Psychiatry, 52*, 305.

Lanius, R. A., Williamson, P. C., Densmore, M., Boksman, K., Gupta, M. A., Neufeld, R. W., Gati, J. S., & Menon, R. S. (2001). Neural correlates of traumatic memories in posttraumatic stress disorder: A functional MRI investigation. *American Journal of Psychiatry, 158*, 1920–1922.

Lanius, R. A., Williamson, P. C., Densmore, M., Boksman, K., Neufeld, R., Gati, J. S., & Menon, R. S. (2004). The nature of traumatic memories: A 4-T fMRI functional connectivity analysis. *American Journal of Psychiatry, 160*, 1–9.

Lanius, R. A., Williamson, P. C., Hopper, J., Densmore, M., Boksman, K., Gupta, M. A., Neufeld, R. W., Gati, J. S., & Menon, R. S. (2003). Recall of emotional states in posttraumatic stress disorder: An fMRI investigation. *Biological Psychiatry, 53*, 204–210.

Layton, B., & Krikorian, R. (2002). Memory mechanisms in posttraumatic stress disorder. *Journal of Neuropsychiatry and Clinical Neuroscience, 14*, 254–261.

LeDoux, J. E. (2000). Emotion circuits in the brain. *Annual Review of Neuroscience, 23*, 155–184.

Liberzon, I., Britton, J. C., & Phan, K. L. (2003). Neural correlates of traumatic recall in posttraumatic stress disorder. *Stress, 6*, 151–156.

Liberzon, I., Taylor, S. F., Amdur, R., Jung, T. D., Chamberlain, K. R., Minoshima, S., Koeppe, R. A., & Fig, L. M. (1999). Brain activation in PTSD in response to trauma-related stimuli. *Biological Psychiatry, 45*, 817–826.

Matsuoka, Y., Yamawaki, S., Inagaki, M., Akechi, T., & Uchitomi, Y. (2003). A volumetric study of amygdala in cancer survivors with intrusive recollections. *Biological Psychiatry, 54*, 736–743.

Milad, M. R., & Quirk, G. J. (2002). Neurons in medial prefrontal cortex signal memory for fear extinction. *Nature, 420*, 70–74.

Menon, P. M., Nasrallah, H. A., Lyons, J. A., Scott, M. F., & Liberto, V. (2003). Single-voxel proton MR spectroscopy of right versus left hippocampi in PTSD. *Psychiatry Research: Neuroimaging, 123*, 101–108.

Morgan, M. A., Romanski, L. M., & LeDoux, J. E. (1993). Extinction of emotional learning: Contribution of medial prefrontal cortex. *Neuroscience Letters, 163*, 109–113.

Morris, J. S., Ohman, A., & Dolan, R. J. (1998). Conscious and unconscious emotional learning in the human amygdala. *Nature, 393*, 467–470.

Orr, S. P., Metzger, L. J., Lasko, N. B., Macklin, M. L., Peri, T., & Pitman, R. K. (2000). De novo conditioning in trauma-exposed individuals with and without posttraumatic stress disorder. *Journal of Abnormal Psychology, 109*, 290–298.

Osuch, E. A., Benson, B., Geraci, M., Podell, D., Herscovitch, P., McCann, U. D., & Post, R. M. (2001). Regional cerebral blood flow correlated with flashback intensity in patients with posttraumatic stress disorder. *Biological Psychiatry, 50*, 246–253.

Paradiso, S., Johnson, D. L., Andreasen, N. C., O'Leary, D. S., Watkins, G. L., Ponto, L. L., & Hichwa, R. D. (1999). Cerebral blood flow changes associated with attribution of emotional valence to pleasant, unpleasant, and neutral visual stimuli in a PET study of normal subjects. *American Journal of Psychiatry, 156*, 1618–1629.

Peri, T., Ben-Shakhar, G., Orr, S. P., & Shalev, A. Y. (2000). Psychophysiologic assessment of aversive conditioning in posttraumatic stress disorder. *Biological Psychiatry, 47*, 512–519.

Pissiota, A., Frans, O., Fernandez, M., von Knorring, L., Fischer, H., & Fredrikson, M. (2002). Neurofunctional correlates of posttraumatic stress disorder: A PET symptom provocation study. *European Archives of Psychiatry and Clinical Neuroscience, 252*, 68–75.

Pitman, R. K. (2001). Hippocampal diminution in PTSD: More (or less?) than meets the eye. *Hippocampus, 11*, 73–74.

Pitman, R. K., Shin, L. M., & Rauch, S. L. (2001). Investigating the pathogenesis of posttraumatic stress disorder with neuroimaging. *Journal of Clinical Psychiatry, 62*(Suppl. 17), 47–54.

Quirk, G. J., Russo, G. K., Barron, J. L., & Lebron, K. (2000). The role of ventromedial prefrontal cortex in the recovery of extinguished fear. *Journal of Neuroscience, 20*, 6225–6231.

Rauch, S. L., Shin, L. M., Segal, E., Pitman, R. K., Carson, M. A., McMullin, K., Whalen, P. J., & Makris, N. (2003). Selectively reduced regional cortical volumes in post-traumatic stress disorder. *Neuroreport, 14*, 913–916.

Rauch, S. L., Shin, L. M., Whalen, P. J., & Pitman, R. K. (1998). Neuroimaging and the neuroanatomy of PTSD. *CNS Spectrums, 3*(Suppl. 2), 30–41.

Rauch, S. L., van der Kolk, B. A., Fisler, R. E., Alpert, N. M., Orr, S. P., Savage, C. R., Fischman, A. J., Jenike, M. A., & Pitman, R. K. (1996). A symptom provocation study of posttraumatic stress disorder using positron emission tomography and script-driven imagery. *Archives of General Psychiatry, 53*, 380–387.

Rauch, S. L., Whalen, P. J., Shin, L. M., McInerney, S. C., Macklin, M. L., Lasko, N. B., Orr, S. P., & Pitman, R. K. (2000). Exaggerated amygdala response to masked facial stimuli in posttraumatic stress disorder: A functional MRI study. *Biological Psychiatry, 47*, 769–776.

Rothbaum, B. O., Kozak, M. J., Foa, E. B., & Whitaker, D. J. (2001). Posttraumatic stress disorder in rape victims: Autonomic habituation to auditory stimuli. *Journal of Traumatic Stress, 14*, 283–293.

Sachinvala, N., Kling, A., Suffin, S., Lake, R., & Cohen, M. (2000). Increased regional cerebral perfusion by 99mTc hexamethyl propylene amine oxime single photon emission computed tomography in post-traumatic stress disorder. *Military Medicine, 165*, 473–479.

Sapolsky, R. M. (2000). Glucocorticoids and hippocampal atrophy in neuropsychiatric disorders. *Archives of General Psychiatry, 57*, 925–935.

Sapolsky, R. M. (2001). Atrophy of the hippocampus in posttraumatic stress disorder: How and when? *Hippocampus, 11*, 90–91.

Sapolsky, R. M., Uno, H., Rebert, C. S., & Finch, C. E. (1990). Hippocampal damage associated with prolonged glucocorticoid exposure in primates. *Journal of Neuroscience, 10*, 2897–2902.

Schacter, D. L. (1997). The cognitive neuroscience of memory: Perspectives from neuroimaging research. *Philosophical Transactions of the Royal Society of London. Series B, Biological Sciences, 352*, 1689–1695.

Schacter, D. L., Alpert, N. M., Savage, C. R., Rauch, S. L., & Albert, M. S. (1996). Conscious recollection and the human hippocampal formation: Evidence from positron emission tomography. *Proceedings of the National Academy of Sciences of the United States of America, 93*, 321–325.

Schuff, N., Neylan, T. C., Lenoci, M. A., Du, A. T., Weiss, D. S., Marmar, C. R., & Weiner, M. W. (2001). Decreased hippocampal N-acetylaspartate in the absence of atrophy in posttraumatic stress disorder. *Biological Psychiatry, 50*, 952–959.

Semple, W. E., Goyer, P., McCormick, R., Morris, E., Compton, B., Muswick, G., Nelson, D., Donovan, B., Leisure, G., Berridge, M., Miraldi, F., & Schulz, S.C. (1993). Preliminary report: Brain blood flow using PET in patients with posttraumatic stress disorder and substance-abuse histories. *Biological Psychiatry, 34*, 115–118.

Semple, W. E., Goyer, P. F., McCormick, R., Donovan, B., Muzic, R. F., Jr., Rugle, L., McCutcheon, K., Lewis, C., Liebling, D., Kowaliw, S., Vapenik, K., Semple, M. A., Flener, C. R., & Schulz, S. C. (2000). Higher brain blood flow at amygdala and lower frontal cortex blood flow in PTSD patients with comorbid cocaine and alcohol abuse compared with normals. *Psychiatry, 63*, 65–74.

Shin, L. M., Kosslyn, S. M., McNally, R. J., Alpert, N. M., Thompson, W. L., Rauch, S. L., Macklin, M. L., & Pitman, R. K. (1997). Visual imagery and perception in posttraumatic stress disorder. A positron emission tomographic investigation. *Archives of General Psychiatry, 54*, 233–241.

Shin, L. M., McNally, R. J., Kosslyn, S. M., Thompson, W. L., Rauch, S. L., Alpert, N. M., Metzger, L. J., Lasko, N. B., Orr, S. P., & Pitman, R. K. (1999). Regional cerebral blood flow during script-driven imagery in childhood sexual abuse-related PTSD: A PET investigation. *American Journal of Psychiatry, 156*, 575–584.

Shin, L. M., Orr, S. P., Carson, M. A., Rauch, S. L., Macklin, M. L., Lasko, N. B., Marzol Peters, P., Metzger, L., Dougherty, D. D., Cannistraro, P. A., Alpert, N. M., Fischman, A. J., & Pitman, R. K. (2004). Regional cerebral blood flow in amygdala and medial prefrontal cortex during traumatic imagery in male and female Vietnam veterans with PTSD. *Archives of General Psychiatry, 61,* 168–176.

Shin, L. M., Shin, P. S., Heckers, S., Krangel, T. S., Macklin, M. L., Orr, S. P., Lasko, N. B., Segal, E., Makris, N., Richert, K., Levering, J., Schacter, D. L., Alpert, N. M., Fischman, A. J., Pitman, R. K., & Rauch, S. L. (2004). Hippocampal function in posttraumatic stress disorder. *Hippocampus, 14,* 292–300.

Shin, L. M., Whalen, P. J., Pitman, R. K., Bush, G., Macklin, M. L., Lasko, N. B., Orr, S. P., McInerney, S. C., & Rauch, S. L. (2001). A fMRI study of anterior cingulate function in posttraumatic stress disorder. *Biological Psychiatry, 50,* 932–942.

Shin, L. M., Wright, C. I., Cannistraro, P., Wedig, M., McMullin, K., Martis, B., Macklin, M. L., Lasko, N. B., Cavanagh, S., Krangel, T. S., Orr, S. P., Pitman, R. K., Whalen, P. J., & Rauch, S. L. (in press). A functional magnetic resonance imaging study of amygdala and medial prefrontal cortex responses to overtly presented fearful faces in posttraumatic stress disorder. *Archives of General Psychiatry.*

Stefanacci, L., & Amaral, D. G. (2002). Some observations on cortical inputs to the macaque monkey amygdala: An anterograde tracing study. *Journal of Comparative Neurology, 451,* 301–323.

Stein, M. B., Koverola, C., Hanna, C., Torchia, M. G., & McClarty, B. (1997). Hippocampal volume in women victimized by childhood sexual abuse. *Psychological Medicine, 27,* 951–959.

Tanev, K. (2003). Neuroimaging and neurocircuitry in post-traumatic stress disorder: What is currently known? *Current Psychiatry Reports, 5,* 369–383.

Uno, H., Tarara, R., Else, J. G., Suleman, M. A., & Sapolsky, R. M. (1989). Hippocampal damage associated with prolonged and fatal stress in primates. *Journal of Neuroscience, 9,* 1705–1711.

Vermetten, E., Vythilingam, M., Southwick, S. M., Charney, D. S., & Bremner, J. D. (2003). Long-term treatment with paroxetine increases verbal declarative memory and hippocampal volume in posttraumatic stress disorder. *Biological Psychiatry, 54,* 693–702.

Villarreal, G., Hamilton, D. A., Petropoulos, H., Driscoll, I., Rowland, L. M., Griego, J. A., Kodituwakku, P. W., Hart, B. L., Escalona, R., & Brooks, W. M. (2002). Reduced hippocampal volume and total white matter volume in posttraumatic stress disorder. *Biological Psychiatry, 52,* 119–125.

Villarreal, G., Petropoulos, H., Hamilton, D. A., Rowland, L. M., Horan, W. P., Griego, J. A., Moreshead, M., Hart, B. L., & Brooks, W. M. (2002). Proton magnetic resonance spectroscopy of the hippocampus and occipital white matter in PTSD: Preliminary results. *Canadian Journal of Psychiatry, 47,* 666–670.

Watanabe, Y., Gould, E., & McEwen, B. S. (1992). Stress induces atrophy of apical dendrites of hippocampal CA3 pyramidal neurons. *Brain Research, 588,* 341–345.

Wechsler, D. (1987). *WMS-R: Wechsler Memory Scale–Revised Manual*. San Antonio, TX: Psychological Corporation.

Whalen, P. J., Bush, G., McNally, R. J., Wilhelm, S., McInerney, S. C., Jenike, M. A., & Rauch, S. L. (1998). The emotional counting Stroop paradigm: A functional magnetic resonance imaging probe of the anterior cingulate affective division. *Biological Psychiatry, 44,* 1219–1228.

Whalen, P. J., Rauch, S. L., Etcoff, N. L., McInerney, S. C., Lee, M. B., & Jenike, M. A. (1998). Masked presentations of emotional facial expressions modulate amygdala activity without explicit knowledge. *Journal of Neuroscience, 18*, 411–418.

Woolley, C. S., Gould, E., & McEwen, B. S. (1990). Exposure to excess glucocorticoids alters dendritic morphology of adult hippocampal pyramidal neurons. *Brain Research, 531*, 225–231.

Yamasue, H., Kasai, K., Iwanami, A., Ohtani, T., Yamada, H., Abe, O., Kuroki, N., Fukuda, R., Tochigi, M., Furukawa, S., Sadamatsu, M., Sasaki, T., Aoki, S., Ohtomo, K., Asukai, N., & Kato, N. (2003). Voxel-based analysis of MRI reveals anterior cingulate gray-matter volume reduction in posttraumatic stress disorder due to terrorism. *Proceedings of the National Academy of Sciences of the United States of America, 100*, 9039–9043.

Yehuda, R. (2001). Are glucocortoids responsible for putative hippocampal damage in PTSD? How and when to decide. *Hippocampus, 11*, 85–89; discussion 82–84.

Zubieta, J. K., Chinitz, J. A., Lombardi, U., Fig, L. M., Cameron, O. G., & Liberzon, I. (1999). Medial frontal cortex involvement in PTSD symptoms: A SPECT study. *Journal of Psychiatric Research, 33*, 259–264.

CHAPTER 4

Electrophysiology of PTSD

LINDA J. METZGER, MARK W. GILBERTSON,
and SCOTT P. ORR

Nearly 15 years ago, Paige and colleagues (Paige, Reid, Allen, & Newton, 1990) published the first study of posttraumatic stress disorder (PTSD) that used event-related brain potential (ERP) methodology to investigate central nervous system function. This study examined cortical responses measured from the scalp surface to tones presented at four different intensity levels in male Vietnam veterans with and without PTSD. Paige and colleagues found that as tones increased in intensity, veterans with PTSD showed a pattern of brain response that leveled off or decreased, whereas their non-PTSD counterparts showed an increasing pattern of brain response. The researchers interpreted their findings as supporting heightened nervous system sensitivity in PTSD, and suggested that individuals with this disorder experienced cortical "dampening" or inhibition of cortical activity when faced with an aversive stimulus. Since this original study, there have been at least 20 additional published reports of studies employing ERP methodology to examine both sensory and cognitive processing in PTSD. This work has revealed evidence consistent with impaired sensory gating, increased sensitivity to stimulus change, heightened orienting responses, impaired attention to neutral stimuli, and heightened attention to trauma related, stimuli in PTSD. We review this work in detail following a brief introduction to ERPs and a discussion of their usefulness in the study of cognitive dysfunction. We also discuss the link between ERP and neuropsychology findings in PTSD and present examples of how these measures might be used together in future research efforts (for a general review of the use of ERPs in neuropsychological assessment, see Reinvang, 1999).

THE CLINICAL UTILITY OF EVENT-RELATED POTENTIALS

In contrast to neuropsychological methods, which approach the study of brain function by measuring process and outcome via behavioral performance or output, ERPs provide a temporally linked process approach by mapping the temporal flow of sensory and cognitive stages involved in the processing of discrete stimulus events. ERPs are measured within the context of an electroencephalogram (EEG) by placing electrodes on the surface of the scalp and recording and amplifying microvolt signals. Unlike a standard EEG, the recorded signals are time-locked to the presentation of a stimulus, thereby capturing "event-related" cortical activity. Because most ERPs are relatively small (1–30 millionths of a volt, i.e., μV) compared to background cortical activity, the time-locked EEG segments are averaged over repeated trials involving the same or similar stimulus events. The process of averaging eliminates random background activity and preserves the underlying response. The resulting averaged ERP "waveform" consists of a sequence of positive and negative voltage deflections. These deflections are referred to as components and are typically labeled according to their polarity (P = positive; N = negative) and to their ordinal position within the waveform or the latency of their peak (in milliseconds). For example, the P3 (also known as P300) component is the third going positive deflection in the ERP waveform and reaches its maximum deflection at approximately 300 milliseconds poststimulus onset. There are a few idiosyncratic exceptions to this traditional nomenclature. Mismatch negativity (MMN), for example, is named for a negative going component that begins at approximately 120 milliseconds in response to a stimulus that is different (i.e., "mismatch") from a series of identical stimuli.

Although their meaning or psychological interpretation largely depends on the experimental context in which they are elicited, each component of the ERP waveform is presumed to reflect a discrete stage of information processing, with earlier components representing sensory and later components representing cognitive operations. A component's peak amplitude, which is most often defined as the voltage difference between the prestimulus baseline and largest point of the component, is believed to reflect the amount of neural resources recruited during that particular stage. The latency of the peak, as measured from stimulus onset, provides a measure of the processing speed. For example, the most widely studied ERP component, the parietally dominant P3 component (hereafter referred to as P3b to distinguish it from the earlier and more frontally distributed P3a component) is evoked in tasks involving the discrimination of stimulus events (e.g., the "oddball" task), and is generated in response to low probability and task-relevant (e.g., "target") or subjectively meaningful stimulus events. P3b amplitude is popularly held to index the amount of attentional resources devoted to stimulus evaluation (Polich, 1996) and its latency indexing the timing of this process (Coles, Smid, Scheffers, & Otten, 1995).

Clinical researchers have long recognized the potential utility of ERPs for elucidating the nature and source of cognitive impairment associated with psychopathological disorders (see Pfefferbaum, Roth, & Ford, 1995). Although there was early hope that ERP component abnormalities might provide a diagnostic tool, similar ERP abnormalities have been found across neurological and psychiatric disorders, and even in normal aging (Polich, 1996). For example, diminished P3b amplitudes have been reported in Alzheimer's disease (Holt et al., 1995); alcoholism (Polich, Pollock, & Bloom, 1994); depression (e.g., Bruder et al., 1995); schizophrenia (see Ford, 1999); and obsessive–compulsive (e.g., Beech, Ciesielski, & Gordon, 1983), attention-deficit/hyperactivity (e.g., Young, Perros, Price, & Sadler, 1995), and reading (Holcomb, Ackerman, & Dykman, 1985) disorders; as well as in PTSD (Charles et al., 1995; Felmingham, Bryant, Kendall, & Gordon, 2002; Galletly, Clark, McFarlane, & Weber, 2001; McFarlane, Weber, & Clark, 1993; Metzger, Orr, Lasko, Berry, & Pitman, 1997; Metzger, Orr, Lasko, & Pitman, 1997). Nonetheless, the clinical utility of ERPs remains strong. Regardless of its lack of clinical specificity, P3b is viewed as a general index of cognitive function or "efficiency" that provides a useful measure for tracking the decline in cognitive function associated with age, dementing illness, and clinical disorders (Polich & Herbst, 2000).

P3b amplitude and other ERP component measures have also been found to be useful in predicting and tracking improvements following pharmacological and clinical intervention. For example, ERP component measures have been shown to successfully predict treatment response in schizophrenia (Schall, Catts, Karayanidis, & Ward, 1999), depression (see Hegerl & Juckel, 1993; Paige, Fitzpatrick, Kline, Balogh, & Hendricks, 1994; Paige, Hendricks, Fitzpatrick, Balogh, & Burke, 1995) and attention-deficit disorder (e.g., Young et al., 1995). ERP abnormalities have also been found to "normalize" in individuals with depression (see Hegerl & Juckel, 1993), dysthymia (Murthy, Gangadhar, Janakiramaiah, & Subbakrishna, 1997), attention-deficit/hyperactivity disorder (ADHD; e.g., Young et al., 1995) and obsessive–compulsive disorder (OCD; Sanz, Molina, Martin-Loeches, Calcedo, & Rubia, 2001) following drug treatment, and during remission from schizophrenia (see Ford, 1999). One study of PTSD reviewed below (Metzger, Orr, Lasko, & Pitman, 1997) suggests that medications might normalize P3b amplitudes in individuals with this disorder as well.

Finally, and perhaps most pertinent here, several studies of normal individuals have found that measures of "fluid" intelligence (i.e., active reasoning and problem solving for which familiar solutions are not available) as opposed to "crystal" intelligence (i.e., overlearned, well-practiced and familiar skills or knowledge) are related to P3b amplitude and latency in expected directions (Egan et al., 1994; Fjell & Walhovd, 2001, 2003; Jausovec & Jausovec, 2000; O'Donnell, Friedman, Swearer, & Drachman, 1992; Reinvang, 1999; Walhovd & Fjell, 2001), supporting the view that these ERP measures reflect the speed and efficiency of allocating attentional resources (Polich & Martin, 1992). However, only a few clinical studies have attempted to link specific ERP deficits to performance on neurocognitive tests involving attention. Two studies of Parkinson's (Hansch et al., 1982; O'Donnell, Squires, Martz, Chen, & Phay, 1987) and one of alcoholic (Parsons, Sinha, & Williams, 1990) patients found that poorer performance on perceptual–motor tests that are highly dependent on attentional functioning (e.g., Digit Symbol Test) was associated with longer P3b component latencies. Parsons et al. additionally found that poorer performance was also associated with reduced P3b amplitude. These studies provide encouraging support for the use of ERP measures as a supplement to standard neuropsychological assessment.

EVENT-RELATED POTENTIAL ABNORMALITIES IN PTSD

The formal diagnosis of PTSD (*Diagnostic and Statistical Manual of Mental Disorders* [DSM IV]; American Psychiatric Association, 1994) includes two symptoms that are clearly suggestive of information processing abnormalities, viz, hypervigilance and concentration difficulties (PTSD arousal criteria D4 and D3, respectively). Hypervigilance involves staying watchful and alert to danger whereas difficulties in concentration pertain to one's ability to stay focused on and complete a particular mental task. Below are ERP studies of PTSD that offer additional insight into these information processing abnormalities.

Impaired Sensory Gating: Increased P50 Ratios

Sensory gating mechanisms in the brain function to attenuate cortical responses to repetitive, and therefore noninformative, environmental events. ERP studies of the integrity of sensory gating processes generally examine the early P50, also known as the P1, component in the context of a procedure that presents a series of paired-clicks (e.g., one pair every 5 seconds) with the intraclick interval between 250 and 500 milliseconds. In normal individuals, the amplitude of the P50 component produced to the second click of the pair is appreciably smaller than the amplitude produced to the first click. The reduction in amplitude is presumed to be the result of a central inhibitory function or sensory gating response at the neuronal level and is typically expressed as a ratio score of the average P50 amplitude to the second click divided by the average P50 amplitude to the first click.

Abnormalities of the P50 response have been reported for several clinical disorders. For example, individuals with schizophrenia (e.g., Clementz, Blumenfeld, & Cobb, 1997; Clementz, Geyer, & Braff, 1997; Freedman, Adler, Waldo, Pachtman, & Franks, 1983), acute bipolar and depressive disorder (Baker et al., 1987; Franks, Adler, Waldo, Alpert, & Freedman, 1983), cocaine abuse (Fein, Biggins, & MacKay, 1996), as well as traumatic brain injury (Arciniegas et al., 2000) have been found to show abnormally increased P50 ratio responses. At least three studies have found that individuals with PTSD also fail to show a normal P50 ratio response, including studies of male Vietnam combat veterans (Gillette et al., 1997; Neylan et al., 1999) and female rape victims (Skinner et al., 1999).

Only one study of P50 ratio in PTSD (Metzger et al., 2002) did not find support for abnormal gating responses in this disorder. Female Vietnam nurse veterans with PTSD did not differ in their P50 ratio from nurses without PTSD. However, P50 ratios were related to self-report measures of general psychopathology when examined for the entire sample. This finding is consistent with the observation that P50 ratios are increased in several other clinical disorders, particularly schizophrenia.

According to Arciniegas et al. (2000), hypervigilance and attentional impairments are most likely the clinical manifestations of reduced sensory gating. Individuals producing abnormally large P50 ratios, including those with PTSD, may have difficulty selectively attending to any stimulus because of an inability to filter out irrelevant environmental stimuli. Instead, they continue to interpret or respond to repetitive stimuli as though they might maintain some significance. One interesting question is whether this ERP abnormality observed in PTSD reflects a trait-like or stable impairment in brain function or a transitory impairment related to fluctuations in stress or anxiety. For example, transient increases in noradrenergic activity (Waldo et al., 1992), sympathetic arousal (Johnson & Adler, 1993), and brief psychological stress (White & Yee, 1997) have each been found to be associated with abnormal P50 responses. Kisley et al. (2003) have recently addressed this issue in schizophrenia by examining P50 responses both during a waking recording and during rapid eye movement (REM) sleep. Compared with controls, they found that patients with schizophrenia failed to show normal levels of P50 suppression across both wake- and sleep-recording periods. Kisley and colleagues concluded that the P50 gating deficit observed in schizophrenia is a state-independent abnormality.

Increased Sensitivity to Stimulus Intensity: P2 Slope Abnormalities

Typically, individuals show increasingly larger brain response as the intensity of a stimulus increases. This is referred to as an "augmenting" response pattern. However, with a very intense (e.g., loud) stimulus, individuals will begin to show a smaller brain response. This "reducing" response is believed to reflect the operation of a central mechanism that protects the cortex from over stimulation (Buchsbaum, 1971). Two studies of male Vietnam combat veterans suggest that individuals with PTSD begin to show the reducing pattern of brain response at lower sound intensity levels compared to individuals without this disorder. Using a four-tone stimulus-intensity modulation (i.e., augmenting–reducing) procedure, Paige et al. (1990) measured the slope of the function relating P2 (also know as the P200) amplitude to increasing sound intensity levels (i.e., 74-, 84-, 94-, and 104-decibel 500-millisecond tones) in male Vietnam combat veterans with and without PTSD. The amplitude of this component is believed to index the tuning properties of a gating mechanism that regulates sensory input to the cerebral cortex. Based on the notion that PTSD is associated with heightened nervous system sensitivity, Paige and colleagues predicted that veterans with PTSD would more readily enter a state of protective inhibition as evidenced by a reducing pattern of P2 responses. Consistent with their predictions, male veterans with combat-related PTSD had significantly lower P2 slopes compared to veterans without PTSD. They found that 75% of combat veterans with PTSD produced a P2-reducing pattern whereas 83% of veterans without PTSD produced a P2-augmenting pattern.

Lewine et al. (2002) have recently replicated Paige et al.'s (1990) findings in a sample of male combat veterans with PTSD. They found that 58% of veterans with PTSD showed a reducing pattern of P2 responses, whereas 95% of the mentally healthy nonveteran control group showed a P2-augmenting response pattern. Lewine and colleagues also examined P2 response patterns in a group of male combat veterans who had a history of major depression and a group of veterans with a history of chronic alcohol use. Unlike Veterans with PTSD, 100% of participants in both groups showed an augmenting pattern of P2 responses. In fact, the veterans with major depression (and without comorbid PTSD) showed greater augmentation of P2 responses than the mentally healthy control group, a finding that has been previously documented in the literature (Paige et al., 1994). As is typically the case, many of the veterans with PTSD also had comorbid major depression. However, in subsidiary analyses, Lewine and colleagues found that PTSD participants showing both N1 and P2 reducing patterns were the most depressed, leading the authors to speculate that "depression in PTSD has different neurobiological correlates than depression in the absence of PTSD" (p. 1694).

Two studies have not found the reducing pattern of P2 response in PTSD samples. In one of the studies which used a paradigm nearly identical to that employed by Paige et al. (1990), Metzger et al. (2002) found that female Vietnam nurse veterans with PTSD showed an augmenting pattern of P2 responses (i.e., increased P2 slope) to tones of increasing intensities, compared to nurse veterans without PTSD. The authors speculated that this finding of an opposite P2 response abnormality might reflect sex differences in PTSD. However, depression comorbidity also might have played a role. In contrast to findings reported by Lewine et al. (2002), subsidiary analyses in the Metzger et al. study found that nurses with PTSD and comorbid major depression showed somewhat greater P2 augmentation than nurses who had PTSD without comorbid major depression. However, Metzger and colleagues also found that the nurses with PTSD and comorbid major depression had significantly more severe PTSD symptoms than nurses with PTSD alone. This raises the unanswerable question of whether the augmenting responses were due to depressive comorbidity, more severe PTSD, or a combination of these factors. Additionally, following removal of nurses with comorbid PTSD and major depression, the group comparison in P2 slope between nurses with and without PTSD was marginally significant. The contrasting pattern of findings in the Lewine et al. and Metzger et al. studies suggests the importance of considering gender and comorbid depression in future studies of P2 response abnormalities in PTSD.

The final study that has examined P2 response abnormalities found that children with PTSD related to physical and/or sexual abuse showed an augmenting pattern of P2 response (i.e., increased P2 slopes) compared to those without PTSD (McPherson, Newton, Ackerman, Oglesby, & Dykman, 1997). However, when groups were formed based on the number of PTSD arousal symptoms, McPherson and colleagues found that children with the highest, compared to those with the lowest, number of arousal symptoms showed a significant reducing pattern of P2 slope (i.e., decreased P2 slope). The general procedure employed by McPherson and colleagues deviates substantially from the passive listening procedure used in the studies described above, thereby making it difficult to compare findings across studies. Specifically, the children were required to make a button-press response to all tones and were provided with feedback and a monetary reward for responding quickly and without blinking.

Heightened Sensitivity to Stimulus Change and Novelty: Mismatch Negativity and P3a

The ability to rapidly detect and respond to a changing environment has fundamental survival value. Two ERP components have been identified as markers of the detection of stimulus change or deviance: mismatch negativity (MMN) and the novelty P3 response (also designated as the P3a). MMN is a negative going deflection that is elicited in response to a deviant stimulus when it is embedded in a series of identical stimuli. This ERP component is believed to reflect the operation of a "change detector" (Näätänen, 1992) or comparator mechanism. It is not elicited by stimuli that are positioned at the beginning of a sequence or by an infrequent stimulus without a series of intervening standard stimuli. Occurring between 100 and 250 milliseconds following a deviant stimulus, MMN appears to reflect an automatic and preconscious process. This view is supported by the fact that MMN occurs in response to consciously undetected deviant stimuli (Näätänen, 1992).

The typical procedure for eliciting and measuring MMN involves a passive listening task in which frequently occurring "standard" (probability = 90%) and infrequent "deviant" (probability = 10%) tones are presented. The standard and deviant tones differ only in their pitch. Subjects are instructed either to ignore the stimuli or to perform some unrelated task such as reading a book or magazine. In contrast to the baseline-to-peak method typically employed for scoring ERP component amplitudes and latencies, MMN is scored from a difference waveform that is produced by subtracting the averaged ERP waveform to the deviant stimulus from the averaged ERP waveform to the standard stimulus.

Given that MMN is sensitive to increased cortical activation and vigilance (Näätänen, 1992), it is not surprising that evidence exists for larger MMN in individuals with PTSD. Using a typical MMN procedure, Morgan and Grillon (1999) found that females with sexual-assault-related PTSD produced larger MMN amplitude responses compared to a female mentally healthy control group. Furthermore, for PTSD participants, amplitudes of the component responses positively correlated with Mississippi scores. As pointed out by these researchers, the augmented MMN responses produced by participants with PTSD are consistent with symptoms of hypervigilance and feelings of being "on alert" and "on guard."

MMN does not appear to reflect an orienting or "what-is-it?" response, although it may be a precursor (Friedman, Cycowicz, & Gaeta, 2001). Instead, a later positive component has been linked to the brain's evaluation of novelty. Specifically, if a stimulus event is sufficiently deviant, a frontally distributed positive potential is generated as early as 280 milliseconds following stimulus presentation. This component, termed the "novelty P3" or P3a, is believed to index the orienting response and is presumed to indicate that the event has involuntarily captured attentional focus (Friedman, Kazmerski, & Cycowicz, 1998). The P3a component is distinguished from the more parietally distributed P3b component, which is viewed as an index of the ability to sustain voluntary attention. This latter component is discussed below in the next section.

The P3a component has been studied using a procedure that is a slight modification of the popular three-tone auditory "oddball" task (Pfefferbaum, Wenegrat, Ford, Roth, & Kopell, 1984). In this procedure, which is similar in principle to a continuous performance task, individuals are instructed to selectively attend and respond to a low-frequency "target" (i.e., oddball) tone (probability = 14%) that is embedded in a series of high-frequency "common" tones (probability = 72%) and low-frequency "distractor" (probability = 14%) tones. Target, distractor, and common tones differ only in their pitch, and participants are taught to correctly discriminate amongst the different tones prior to starting the procedure. During the task, participants are instructed to respond to target tones by making a button-press response or keeping a mental count, and to ignore the other tones. To study the novelty P3 response, researchers have replaced the distractor tone trials with unique computer-generated sounds so that no two distractor trials are the same. ERP responses are averaged across the novelty trials, as they are for target and common trials, providing a measure of the brain's average response to novel environmental events.

Using this novelty oddball procedure, as well as the traditional three-tone auditory oddball task, Kimble, Kaloupek, Kaufman, and Deldin (2000) compared P3a responses to repeated presentations of a distractor tone with P3a responses to unique computer-generated distractor sounds in male Vietnam veterans with and without PTSD. In contrast to somewhat diminished responses to the repeated, non-novel distractors, veterans with PTSD produced relatively larger P3a responses to the novel distractors, whereas veterans without PTSD showed more comparable P3a responses to the novel and non-novel distractors. Kimble et al. interpreted their findings of relatively enhanced cortical responses to novel stimuli as consistent with the position that PTSD is characterized by heightened orienting responses, which might reflect symptoms of hypervigilance. However, the limitation of Kimble et al.'s findings is that the effect was only evident in a group by task (i.e., novel vs. repeated distractor) interaction. A direct comparison of the group differences in P3a response to novel distractors was not significant. In another study involving both a novel auditory and a novel visual oddball task, Neylan et al. (2003) compared P3a amplitudes to the novel distractors in male Vietnam veterans with and without PTSD. Similar to Kimble et al., there were no significant group differences in P3a amplitude to novel auditory or visual distractors. Because Neylan and colleagues did not include a repeated distractor stimulus, there is no way to determine whether veterans with PTSD would have shown the interaction effect reported by Kimble et al., that is, relatively larger P3a responses to the novel compared to repeated distractors.

Disturbances in Attention-Related Processes: P3b Response Abnormalities

The most studied and replicated ERP finding in PTSD to date is that of diminished P3b response amplitudes to target stimuli in the context of the auditory oddball (described previously) or oddball-like paradigms. The P3b component generated within this task usually occurs 250 to 400 millisec-

onds following presentation of the target stimulus and has its maximum
amplitude at the midline parietal site. Mixed-trauma (Felmingham et al.,
2002; Galletly et al., 2001; McFarlane et al., 1993) and recent assault
(Charles et al., 1995) victims, male Vietnam combat veterans (Metzger, Orr,
Lasko, & Pitman, 1997), and adult females sexually abused during childhood (Metzger, Orr, Lasko, Berry, et al., 1997) with PTSD have been found
to produce smaller P3b response amplitudes to target stimuli relative to
their comparison groups. Given that the amplitude of the P3b component is
generally accepted to reflect the amount of capacity-limited attentional resources devoted to stimulus evaluation (Polich, 1996), most have interpreted this finding as providing electrophysiological evidence for the DSM-
IV (American Psychiatric Association, 1994) PTSD symptom of disturbed
concentration.

Some of these studies have found behavioral evidence of increased difficulty with the target detection task. Both McFarlane et al. (1993) and
Felmingham et al. (2002) found that PTSD participants took significantly
longer to make a button-press response to targets. Galletly et al. (2001)
found comparable response times to targets, but PTSD participants in this
study missed more targets than controls. Although one study (Charles et
al., 1995) did not record behavioral responses because participants silently
counted targets, the remaining two studies (Metzger, Orr, Lasko, Berry, et
al., 1997; Metzger, Orr, Lasko, & Pitman, 1997) found smaller P3b amplitudes to target tones in PTSD participants with no evidence of diminished
behavioral performance in speed or in accuracy. The observation of ERP
abnormalities in the absence of behavioral-response deficits is consistent
with the position that ERPs provide a more sensitive measure of cognitive
functioning than traditional behavioral indices.

Not all studies have found diminished P3b amplitudes in individuals
with PTSD. Rather, several factors appear to influence P3b amplitude findings, including the presence of comorbid anxiety disorders and psychoac-
tive medication use. Metzger, Orr, Lasko, and Pitman (1997) found that a
small sample of unmedicated Vietnam combat veterans with PTSD and
comorbid panic disorder tended to have larger, rather than smaller, P3b
amplitudes to targets. Two studies that included PTSD participants on
psychotropic medications failed to replicate smaller P3b amplitudes to auditory (Kimble et al., 2000) and visual (Neylan et al., 2003) target stimuli.
Furthermore, after subdividing their PTSD sample into medicated and unmedicated subgroups, Metzger, Orr, Lasko, and Pitman (1997) found that
the medication-free subsample showed diminished P3b amplitudes, whereas
the medicated subsample had "normal" P3b amplitudes. Most of the veterans in the medicated subsample were receiving treatment with selective
serotonin reuptake inhibitors (SSRIs). The absence of diminished P3 amplitudes in the medicated subsample of veterans with PTSD is consistent with

the general clinical literature showing that medications tend to normalize P3b and other ERP component abnormalities. In particular, a recent study demonstrated that SSRI treatment had a normalizing effect on P3b amplitudes in individuals with OCD (Sanz et al., 2001).

Finally, a recent study of unmedicated female Vietnam nurse veterans found significantly larger, rather than smaller, target P3b amplitudes in nurse veterans with PTSD, compared to nurses who never had PTSD (Metzger et al., 2002). The difference remained significant even after removing individuals with comorbid panic disorder. This finding is particularly difficult to explain given that P3b amplitude abnormalities in clinical populations are typically associated with reduced, rather than augmented, responses. One possible explanation is that the larger P3b amplitudes in the nurse veterans with PTSD represent an effortful "overcompensation" or increase in cognitive effort to compensate for limitations associated with having PTSD.

Recent findings from an auditory oddball study (Bruder et al., 2002) suggest that depression, anxiety, the comorbidity of depression and anxiety, and possibly even gender, might differently modulate frontal and parietal P3 amplitude findings. Specifically, Bruder and colleagues compared responses in individuals having depressive disorder alone, an anxiety disorder alone, or comorbidity of these disorders, with mentally healthy controls. They found that individuals with an anxiety disorder alone produced larger frontocentral P3 (i.e., P3a) response amplitudes compared with the other groups, a finding also reported in individuals with panic disorder (Clark, McFarlane, Weber, & Battersby, 1996). Bruder et al. interpreted this finding as suggesting that the somatic arousal found in anxiety disorders may be associated with an increased orienting response to the oddball stimuli. Conversely, for the parietal P3b component amplitude, Bruder et al. found that individuals having comorbid depressive and anxiety disorders produced the largest amplitude compared to the remaining groups. It is noteworthy, however, that this comorbid patient group was comprised of 67% females, whereas the anxiety disorder alone and depressive disorder alone groups were comprised of 41% and 48% females, respectively. Similar to studies of P2 slope, the somewhat mixed pattern of findings both within and across studies highlights the importance of examining the role of medication status, gender, and comorbid anxiety and depression in future studies of P3b amplitude in PTSD.

Finally, because the standard interpretation of reduced P3b amplitude in clinical disorders has been as a marker of an attention-related cognitive deficit, the most salient PTSD symptom tied to diminished P3b amplitudes is concentration difficulties. From this perspective, the findings of larger P3b amplitudes in female nurses with PTSD would suggest the unlikely scenario of greater concentration abilities. Another factor implicated in diminished P3b amplitude in clinical disorders is reduced motivation (Ford, 1999; Friedman, 1990). This view is largely based on research by Begleiter and colleagues (Begleiter, Porjesz, Chou, & Aunon, 1983; Brecher & Begleiter, 1983) demonstrating that manipulating the incentive value of a target stimulus leads to corresponding changes in P3b amplitude in normal individuals. They found that individuals produced significantly larger P3b amplitudes under incentive conditions (i.e., in response to stimuli associated with the potential to earn money) than under baseline, nonincentive conditions. Consistent with a motivation-based explanation, Felmingham et al. (2002) found that within their sample of nonsexual assault and accident victims with PTSD, smaller P3b amplitudes were associated with increased numbing symptom scores. This finding raises the possibility that reduced P3b amplitude in PTSD reflects disinterest or lack of emotional engagement with the task, rather than a primary disturbance in attention. Charles et al. (1995) suggested that reductions in P3b amplitude in individuals with PTSD might be attributable to emotional numbing symptoms and their potential for adversely impacting the meaningfulness of target stimuli. This explanation is also consistent with the position that depression or depressive symptoms are responsible for the findings of smaller P3b amplitudes in individuals with PTSD.

Attentional Bias to Trauma-Relevant Information: Augmented P3a and P3b Amplitude Responses

Although task relevance and subjective probability of a stimulus are considered to be key modulating variables of P3b or P3b-like component amplitudes (Johnson, 1993), the intrinsic motivational significance or emotional value of a stimulus has been found to influence their amplitude as well. For example, in studies of normal individuals (see Schupp et al., 2000) both pleasant and unpleasant emotional pictures produce a more widely distributed (i.e., found at frontal, central, and parietal recording sites) and larger "P3" response than neutral pictures. The P3 component generated in response to emotional stimuli is often referred to as a late positive potential and is interpreted as reflecting motivational engagement and the subsequent allocation of attentional resources to the eliciting stimulus.

Several studies have now examined such P3 component responses to combat-related words (Stanford, Vasterling, Mathias, Constans, & Houston, 2001) and pictures (Attias, Bleich, Furman, & Zinger, 1996; Attias, Bleich, & Gilat, 1996; Bleich, Attias, & Furman, 1996) in veterans with PTSD. Using an "emotional" oddball procedure, combat-related pictures or words were presented as infrequent, to-be-ignored distractors and were interspersed among common (e.g., home furnishings) and target (e.g., domestic animals) stimuli. In each study, combat veterans with PTSD produced larger P3 amplitudes to the trauma-related stimuli, compared to veterans without PTSD. This effect appeared across frontal, central, and parietal recording sites for studies involving combat pictures but was found only at frontal recording sites in the study of combat words. Because participants were asked to ignore all nontarget stimuli in each of these studies, the larger P3 amplitudes appeared to reflect an automatic, involuntary attentional response. Stanford and colleagues have raised the possibility that the augmented P3 responses to trauma-related stimuli represent a P3a-orienting response rather than a P3b-voluntary-attentional response because group differences in their study were limited to frontal recording sites. However, Attias, Bleich, Furman, and Zinger (1996) separately examined P3a and P3b components and found that PTSD participants produced both significantly larger P3a and P3b amplitude responses to combat pictures across recording sites. Overall, these findings suggest that PTSD is characterized by "selective cognitive sensitivity" to stimuli reminiscent of the traumatic event (Stanford et al., 2001) involving both early (i.e., orienting) and later (i.e., voluntary) attentional processes (see Attias, Bleich, Furman, & Zinger, 1996).

In the study by Stanford et al. (2001), social-threat words replaced combat-related words as distractors in a second emotional oddball task. Combat veterans with PTSD did not show larger P3a amplitudes to these negatively-valenced distractors. Larger P3a amplitudes to combat-related, but not social-threat words suggest that the heightened attentional bias in PTSD is specific to trauma-related cues, and does not generalize across all negative emotional cues.

To date, only one published study (Metzger, Orr, Lasko, McNally, & Pitman, 1997) has not found evidence of larger P3a or P3b amplitude responses to trauma-related words in PTSD. In this study, individuals with and without PTSD related to various traumatic events completed an emotional Stroop color-naming task. This procedure involved indicating the color of computer-presented neutral, positive, and trauma-related words (via button press), while ignoring a word's meaning. Compared to the group without PTSD, those with PTSD produced smaller P3 amplitudes (and longer P3 latencies) across frontal, central, and parietal sites to all three word types. The generally smaller and later P3 responses are suggestive of attentional difficulties with the overall task, and might reflect poorer performance due to the more difficult format of the emotional Stroop task for the individuals with PTSD. Importantly, while PTSD participants did not show selective differences in P3 amplitudes to trauma-related words, behaviorally they did take longer to indicate the color of trauma-related words. These reaction-time findings are consistent with the presence of a cognitive bias for trauma-related information.

Finally, there is some evidence that ERP responses to trauma-specific

96   BIOLOGICAL PERSPECTIVES

stimuli might provide a useful diagnostic tool. Attias, Bleich, and Gilat
(1996) found that parietal P3b responses to trauma-related stimuli correctly classified 90% of Israeli combat veterans with PTSD and 85% of the
veterans without PTSD. These sensitivity and specificity values are in line
with those obtained for autonomic measures (Orr, Metzger, Miller, &
Kaloupek, 2004) supporting the potential diagnostic utility of this ERP
procedural measure.

FUTURE DIRECTIONS:
MERGING NEUROPSYCHOLOGY AND ELECTROPHYSIOLOGY

Like ERP studies, findings from clinical neuropsychological and behavioral
information processing studies also support disturbances in attention-related process in individuals with PTSD (for reviews see Golier & Yehuda,
2002; Horner & Hamner, 2002; Constans, Chapter 5, this volume;
Vasterling & Brailey, Chapter 8, this volume). For example, Vasterling,
Brailey, Constans, and Sutker (1998) found that male Gulf War veterans
with PTSD showed deficits in sustained attention, mental manipulation,
and initial acquisition of information, and a heightened sensitivity to retroactive interference. According to these researchers, the errors of commission and false alarms produced by the veterans with PTSD could reflect a
general pattern of disinhibition. More specifically, and in line with P50 ratio findings in PTSD, they contend that the increased error rate might result
from the inability to inhibit inaccurate responses and filter out irrelevant
information (cf., Vasterling et al., 2002). There is also some evidence that
findings of generalized cognitive impairment in PTSD might be secondary
to disturbances in attention (see Horner & Hamner, 2002). Gilbertson,
Gurvits, Lasko, Orr, and Pitman (2001) found that male Vietnam veterans
with PTSD showed deficits not only in attention, but memory, perceptual–
motor, visuospatial skill, and executive "frontal lobe" functioning as well.
However, statistically adjusting for levels of attentional impairment eliminated group differences for many of these neuropsychological measures.
Finally, neuropsychological findings suggest that attention deficits in PTSD
might be related to arousal symptomatology. Specifically, Vasterling et al.
(1998) found that the cognitive impairments identified in male Gulf War
veterans were most consistent with a pattern of disrupted arousal and dysfunction of frontal subcortical systems. The notion that dysregulated
arousal might be at the root of cognitive dysfunction in PTSD is intriguing,
in light of the fact that most of the ERP component abnormalities identified
in individuals with this disorder have also been experimentally and/or theoretically tied to levels of cortical arousal or stress during testing.
    The converging findings from neuropsychological and electrophysiol-

ogical investigations of PTSD, as well as the unique and shared questions generated by these fields of inquiry, strongly support the integration of these methodologies. Our understanding of cognitive dysfunction in PTSD should be notably advanced by combining neuropsychological and electrophysiological measurements into a single, unified investigation. This could be accomplished by examining the correlations among these measures, as well as by the direct concurrent measurement of ERP and behavioral responses within amendable neuropsychological test procedures (e.g., continuous performance and card sorting tasks; see Reinvang, 1999). For example, studies documenting executive dysfunction in PTSD using the Wisconsin Card Sorting Task (WCST; Heaton, 1981), have found differing patterns of perseverative and nonperseverative errors (Gilbertson et al., 2001; Gurvits et al., 1993). One study measuring ERPs during WCST performance in mentally healthy individuals found that perseverative and nonperseverative errors evoked distinctly different abnormal ERP response patterns, including significantly larger P3b responses to perseverative than nonperseverative errors (Barcelo, 1999). Given these findings and the potential for ERPs to provide a more sensitive measure of cognitive functioning, an informative starting place may be the measurement of ERPs during WCST performance. Finally, according to Horner and Hamner (2002) an important next step for neuropsychological research in PTSD is the examination of subtypes of attention, including focused, sustained and divided attention. This is also an important direction for ERP research in PTSD and might be addressed by studies employing both neuropsychological and electrophysiological measures.

REFERENCES

American Psychiatric Association. (1994). *Diagnostic and statistical manual of mental disorders* (4th ed.). Washington, DC: Author.

Arciniegas, D., Olincy, A., Topkoff, J., McRae, K., Cawthra, E., Filley, C. M., Reite, M., & Adler, L. E. (2000). Impaired auditory gating and P50 nonsuppression following traumatic brain injury. *Journal of Neuropsychiatry and Clinical Neurosciences, 12*, 77–85.

Attias, J., Bleich, A., Furman, V., & Zinger, Y. (1996). Event-related potentials in posttraumatic stress disorder of combat origin. *Biological Psychiatry, 40*, 373–381.

Attias, J., Bleich, A., & Gilat, S. (1996). Classification of veterans with post-traumatic stress disorder using visual brain evoked P3s to traumatic stimuli. *British Journal of Psychiatry, 168*, 110–115.

Baker, N., Adler, L. E., Franks, R. D., Waldo, M., Berry, S., Nagamoto, H., Muckle, A., & Freedman, R. (1987). Neurophysiological assessment of sensory gating in psychiatric inpatients: Comparison between schizophrenia and other diagnosis. *Biological Psychiatry, 22*, 603–617.

Barcelo, F. (1999). Electrophysiological evidence of two different types of error in the Wisconsin Card Sorting Test. *NeuroReport, 10,* 1299–1303.

Beech, H., Ciesielski, K., & Gordon, P. (1983). Further observations of evoked potentials in obsessional patients. *British Journal of Psychiatry, 142,* 605–609.

Begleiter, H., Porjesz, B., Chou, C. L., & Aunon, J. I. (1983). P3 and stimulus incentive value. *Psychophysiology, 20,* 95–101.

Bleich, A., Attias, J., & Furman, V. (1996). Effect of repeated visual traumatic stimuli on the event related P3 brain potential in post-traumatic stress disorder. *International Journal of Neuroscience, 85,* 45–55.

Brecher, M., & Begleiter, H. (1983). Event-related brain potentials to high-incentive stimuli in unmedicated schizophrenic patients. *Biological Psychiatry, 18,* 661–674.

Bruder, G. E., Kayser, J., Tanke, C. E., Leite, P., Schneier, F. R., Stewart, J. W., & Quitkin, F. M. (2002). Cognitive ERPs in depressive and anxiety disorders during tonal and phonetic oddball tasks. *Clinical Electroencephalography, 33,* 119–124.

Bruder, G. E., Tenke, C. E., Stewart, J. W., Towey, J. P., Leite, P., Voglmaier, M., & Quitkin, F. M. (1995). Brain event-related potentials to complex tones in depressed patients: Relations to perceptual asymmetry and clinical features. *Psychophysiology, 32,* 373–381.

Buchsbaum, M. (1971). Neural events and psychophysical law. *Science, 172,* 502.

Charles, G., Hansenne, M., Ansseau, M., Pitchot, W., Machowski, R., Schittecatte, M., & Wilmotte, J. (1995). P300 in posttraumatic stress disorder. *Neuropsychobiology, 32,* 72–74.

Clark, C. R., McFarlane, A. C., Weber, D. L., & Battersby, M. (1996). Enlarged frontal P300 to stimulus change in panic disorder. *Biological Psychiatry, 39,* 845–856.

Clementz, B. A., Blumenfeld, L. D., & Cobb, S. (1997). The gamma band response may account for poor P50 suppression in schizophrenia. *Neuroreport, 8,* 3889–3893.

Clementz, B. A., Geyer, M. A., & Braff, D. L. (1997). P50 suppression among schizophrenia and normal comparison subjects: A methodological analysis. *Biological Psychiatry, 41,* 1035–1044.

Coles, M.G. H., Smid, H.G.O.M., Scheffers, M. K., & Otten, L. J. (1995). Mental chronometry and the study of human information processing. In M. D. Rugg & M.G. H. Coles (Eds.), *Electrophysiology of mind* (pp. 86–131). New York: Oxford University Press.

Egan, V., Chiswick, A., Santosh, C., Naidu, K., Rimmington, J. E., & Best, J. J. (1994). Size isn't everything: A study of brain volume, intelligence, and auditory evoked potentials. *Personality and Individual Differences, 17,* 357–367.

Fein, G., Biggins, C., & MacKay, S. (1996). Cocaine abusers have reduced auditory P50 amplitude and suppression compared to both normal controls and alcoholics. *Biological Psychiatry, 39,* 955–965.

Felmingham, K. L., Bryant, R. A., Kendall, C., & Gordon, E. (2002). Event-related potential dysfunction in posttraumatic stress disorder: The role of numbing. *Psychiatry Research, 109,* 171–179.

Fjell, A. M., & Walhovd, K. B. (2001). P300 and neuropsychological tests as measures of aging: Scalp topography and cognitive changes. *Brain Topography, 14,* 25–40.

Fjell, A. M., & Walhovd, K. B. (2003). Effects of auditory stimulus intensity and hearing threshold on the relationship among P300, age, and cognitive function. *Clinical Neurophysiology, 114,* 799–807.

Ford, J. M. (1999). Schizophrenia: The broken P300 and beyond. *Psychophysiology, 36,* 667–682.

Franks, R. B., Adler, L. E., Waldo, M. C., Alpert, J., & Freedman, R. (1983). Neurophysiological studies of sensory gating in mania: Comparison with schizophrenia. *Biological Psychiatry, 18,* 989–1005.

Freedman, R., Adler, L. E., Waldo, M. C., Pachtman, E., & Franks, R. D. (1983). Neurophysiological evidence for a defect in inhibitory pathways in schizophrenia: Comparison of medicated and drug-free patients. *Biological Psychiatry, 18,* 537–551.

Friedman, D. (1990). Event-related potentials in populations at genetic risk: A methodological review. In J. W. Rohrbaugh, R. Parasuraman, & R. Johnson (Eds.), *Event-related brain potentials: Basic issues and applications* (pp. 310–332). New York: Oxford University Press.

Friedman, D., Cycowicz, Y. M., & Gaeta, H. (2001). The novelty P3: An event-related brain potential (ERP) sign of the brain's evaluation of novelty. *Neuroscience and Biobehavioral Reviews, 25,* 355–373.

Friedman, D., Kazmerski, V. A., & Cycowicz, Y. M. (1998). Effects of aging on the novelty P3 during attend and ignore oddball tasks. *Psychophysiology, 35,* 508–520.

Galletly, C., Clark, C. R., McFarlane, A. C., & Weber, D. L. (2001). Working memory in posttraumatic stress disorder: An event-related potential study. *Journal of Traumatic Stress, 14,* 295–309.

Gilbertson, M. W., Gurvits, T. V., Lasko, N. B., Orr, S. P., & Pitman, R. K. (2001). Multivariate assessment of explicit memory function in combat veterans with postraumatic stress disorder. *Journal of Traumatic Stress, 14,* 413–432.

Gillette, G., Skinner, R., Rasco, L., Fielstein, E., Davis, D., Pawelak, J., Freeman, T., Karson, C., Boop, F., & Garcia-Rill, E. (1997). Combat veterans with posttraumatic stress disorder exhibit decreased habituation of the p1 midlatency auditory evoked potential. *Life Sciences, 61,* 1421–1434.

Golier, J., & Yehuda, R. (2002). Neuropsychological processes in post-traumatic stress disorder. *Psychiatric Clinics of North America, 25,* 295–315.

Gurvits, T. V., Lasko, N. B., Schachter, S. C., Kuhne, A. A., Orr, S. P., & Pitman, R. K. (1993). Neurological status of Vietnam veterans with chronic posttraumatic stress disorder. *The Journal of Neuropsychiatry and Clinical Neurosciences, 5,* 183–188.

Hansch, E. C., Syndulko, K., Cohen, S. N., Goldberg, Z. I., Potvin, A. R., & Tourtellotte, W. W. (1982). Cognition in Parkinson disease: An event-related potential perspective. *Annals of Neurology, 11,* 599–607.

Heaton, R. K. (1981). *The Wisconsin Card Sorting Test Manual.* New York: Psychological Assessment Resources.

Hegerl, U., & Juckel, G. (1993). Intensity dependence of auditory evoked potentials as an indicator of central serotonergic neurotransmission: A new hypothesis. *Biological Psychiatry, 33,* 173–187.

Holcomb, P., Ackerman, P. T., & Dykman, R. (1985). Cognitive event-related brain potentials in children with attention and reading deficits. *Psychophysiology, 22,* 656–667.

Holt, L. E., Raine, A., Pa, G., Schneider, L. S., Henderson, V. W., & Pollock, V. (1995). P300 topography in Alzheimer's disease. *Psychophysiology, 32,* 257–265.

Horner, M. D., & Hamner, M. B. (2002). Neurocognitive functioning in posttraumatic stress disorder. *Neuropsychology Review, 12,* 15–30.

Jausovec, N., & Jausovec, K. (2000). Correlations between ERP parameters and intelligence: A reconsideration. *Biological Psychology, 55,* 137–154.

Johnson, M. R., & Adler, L. E. (1993). Transient impairment of P50 auditory sensory gating induced by a cold-pressor test. *Biological Psychiatry, 33,* 380–387.

Johnson, R., Jr. (1993). On the neural generators of the P300 component of the event-related potential. *Psychophysiology, 30,* 90–77.

Kimble, M., Kaloupek, D., Kaufman, M., & Deldin, P. (2000). Stimulus novelty differentially affects attentional allocation in PTSD. *Biological Psychiatry, 47,* 880–890.

Kisley, M. A., Olincy, A., Robbins, E., Polk, S., Adler, L. E., Waldo, M. C., & Freedman R. (2003). Sensory gating impairment associated with schizophrenia persists into REM sleep. *Psychophysiology, 40,* 29–38.

Lewine, J. D., Thoma, R. J., Provencal, S. L., Edgar, C., Miller, G. A., & Canive, J. M. (2002). Abnormal stimulus–response intensity functions in posttraumatic stress disorder: An electrophysiologic investigation. *American Journal of Psychiatry, 159,* 1689–1695.

McFarlane, A. C., Weber, D. L., & Clark, C. R. (1993). Abnormal stimulus processing in posttraumatic stress disorder. *Biological Psychiatry, 34,* 311–320.

McPherson, W. B., Newton, J. E., Ackerman, P., Oglesby, D. M., & Dykman, R. A. (1997). An event-related brain potential investigation of PTSD and PTSD symptoms in abused children. *Integrative Physiological and Behavioral Science, 32,* 31–42.

Metzger, L. J., Carson, M. A., Paulus, L. A., Lasko, N. B., Paige, S. R., Pitman, R. K., & Orr, S. P. (2002). Event-related potentials to auditory stimuli in female Vietnam nurse veterans with post-traumatic stress disorder. *Psychophysiology, 39,* 49–63.

Metzger, L. J., Orr, S. P., Lasko, N. B., Berry, N. J., & Pitman, R. K. (1997). Evidence for diminished P3 amplitudes in PTSD. In *Psychobiology of Posttraumatic Stress Disorder, 821,* 499–503. New York: Annals of the New York Academy of Sciences.

Metzger, L. J., Orr, S. P., Lasko, N. B., McNally, R. J., & Pitman, R. K. (1997). Seeking the source of emotional Stroop interference effects in PTSD: A study of P3s to traumatic words. *Integrative Physiological and Behavioral Science, 32,* 43–51.

Metzger, L. J., Orr, S. P., Lasko, N. B., & Pitman, R. K. (1997). Auditory event-related potentials to tone stimuli in combat-related posttraumatic stress disorder. *Biological Psychiatry, 42,* 1006–1015.

Morgan, C. A., III, & Grillon, C. (1999). Abnormal mismatch negativity in women with sexual assault-related posttraumatic stress disorder. *Biological Psychiatry, 45,* 827–832.

Murthy, P. J., Gangadhar, B. N., Janakiramaiah, N., & Subbakrishna, D. K. (1997). Normalization of P300 amplitude following treatment in dysthymia. *Biological Psychiatry, 42,* 740–743.

Näätänen, R. (1992). *Attention and brain function.* Hillsdale, NJ: Erlbaum.

Neylan, T. C., Fletcher, D. J., Lenoci, M., McCallin, K., Weiss, D. S., Schoenfeld, F. B.,

Marmar, C. R., & Fein, G. (1999). Sensory gating in chronic posttraumatic stress disorder: Reduced auditory P50 suppression in combat veterans. *Biological Psychiatry, 46,* 1656–1664.

Neylan, T. C., Jasiukaitis, P. A., Lenoci, M., Scott, J. C., Metzler, T. J., Weiss, D. S., Schoenfeld, F. B., & Marmar, C. R. (2003). Temporal instability of auditory and visual event-related potentials in posttraumatic stress disorder. *Biological Psychiatry, 53,* 216–225.

O'Donnell, B. F., Friedman, S., Swearer, J. M., & Drachman, D. A. (1992). Active and passive P3 latency and psychometric performance: Influence of age and individual differences. *International Journal of Psychophysiology, 12,* 187–195.

O'Donnell, B. F., Squires, N. K., Martz, M. J., Chen, J., & Phay, A. J. (1987). Evoked potential changes and neuropsychological performance in Parkinson's disease. *Biological Psychiatry, 24,* 23–37.

Orr, S. P., Metzger, L. J., Miller, M. W., & Kaloupek, D. G. (2004). Psychophysiological assessment of PTSD. In J. P. Wilson & T. M. Keane (Eds.), *Assessing psychological trauma and PTSD, 2nd edition* (pp. 289–343). New York: Guilford Press.

Paige, S. R., Fitzpatrick, D. F., Kline, J. P., Balogh, S. E., & Hendricks, S. E. (1994). Event-related potential amplitude/intensity slopes predict response to antidepressants. *Neuropsychobiology, 30,* 197–201.

Paige, S. R., Hendricks, S. E., Fitzpatrick, D. F., Balogh, S., & Burke, W. J. (1995). Amplitude/intensity functions of auditory event-related potentials predict responsiveness to bupropion in major depressive disorder. *Psychopharmacology Bulletin, 31,* 243–248.

Paige, S. R., Reid, G. M., Allen, M. G., & Newton, J. E. (1990). Psychophysiological correlates of posttraumatic stress disorder in Vietnam veterans. *Biological Psychiatry, 27,* 419–430.

Parsons, O. A., Sinha, R., & Williams, H. L. (1990). Relationships between neuropsychological test performance and event-related potentials in alcoholic and nonalcoholic samples. *Alcoholism: Clinical and Experimental Research, 14,* 746–755.

Pfefferbaum, A., Roth, W. T., & Ford, J. M. (1995). Event-related potentials in the study of psychiatric disorders. *Archives of General Psychiatry, 52,* 559–563.

Pfefferbaum, A., Wenegrat, B. G., Ford, J. M., Roth, W. T., & Kopell, B. S. (1984). Clinical application of the P3 component of event-related potentials: II. Dementia, depression and schizophrenia. *Electroencephalography and Clinical Neurophysiology, 59,* 104–124.

Polich, J. (1996). Meta-analysis of P300 normative aging studies. *Psychophysiology, 33,* 334–353.

Polich, J., & Herbst, K. L. (2000). P300 as a clinical assay: Rationale, evaluation, and findings. *International Journal of Pyschophysiology, 38,* 3–19.

Polich, J. M., & Martin, S. (1992). P300, cognitive capability, and personality: A correlational study of university undergraduates. *Personality and Individual Differences, 13,* 533–543.

Polich, J. M., Pollock, V. E., & Bloom, F. E. (1994). Meta-analysis of P300 amplitude from males at risk for alcoholism. *Psychological Bulletin, 115,* 55–73.

Reinvang, I. (1999). Cognitive event-related potentials in neuropsychological assessment. *Neuropsychology Review, 9,* 231–248.

Sanz, M., Molina, V., Martin-Loeches, M., Calcedo, A., & Rubia, F. J. (2001). Auditory P300 event related potential and serotonin reuptake inhibitor treatment in obsessive–compulsive disorder patients. *Psychiatry Research, 101,* 75–81.

Schall, U., Catts, S. V., Karayanidis, F., & Ward, P. B. (1999). Auditory event-related potential indices of fronto-temporal information processing in schizophrenia syndromes: Valid outcome prediction of clozapine therapy in a three-year follow-up. *International Journal of Neuropsychopharmacology, 2,* 83–93.

Schupp, H. T., Cuthbert, B. N., Bradley, M. M., Cacioppo, J. T., Ito, T., & Lang, P. J. (2000). Affective picture processing: The late positive potential is modulated by motivational relevance. *Psychophysiology, 37,* 257–261.

Skinner, R. D., Rasco, L. M., Fitzgerald, J., Karson, C. N., Matthew, M., Williams, D. K., & Garcia-Rill, E. (1999). Reduced sensory gating of the P1 potential in rape victims and combat veterans with posttraumatic stress disorder. *Depression and Anxiety, 9,* 122–130.

Stanford, M. S., Vasterling, J. J., Mathias, C. W., Constans, J. I., & Houston, R. J. (2001). Impact of threat relevance on P3 event-related potentials in combat-related post-traumatic stress disorder. *Psychiatry Research, 102,* 125–137.

Vasterling, J. J., Brailey, K., Constans, J. I., & Sutker, P. B. (1998). Attention and memory dysfunction in posttraumatic stress disorder. *Neuropsychology, 12,* 125–133.

Vasterling, J. J., Duke, L. M., Brailey, K., Constans, J. I., Allain, Jr., A. N., & Sutker, P. B. (2002). Attention, learning, and memory performances and intellectual resources in Vietnam veterans: PTSD and no disorder comparisons. *Neuropsychology, 16,* 5–14.

Waldo, M., Gerhardt, G., Baker, N., Drebing, C., Adler, L., & Freedman, R. (1992). Auditory sensory gating and catecholamine metabolism in schizophrenic and normal subjects. *Psychiatry Research, 44,* 21–31.

Walhovd, K. B., & Fjell, A. M. (2001). Two- and three-stimuli auditory oddball ERP tasks and neuropsychological measures in aging. *NeuroReport, 12,* 3149–3153.

White, P. M., & Yee, C. M. (1997). Effects of attentional and stressor manipulations on the P50 gating response. *Psychophysiology, 34,* 703–711.

Young, E. S., Perros, P., Price, G. W., & Sadler, T. (1995). Acute challenge ERP as a prognostic of stimulant therapy outcome in attention-deficit hyperactivity disorder. *Biological Psychiatry, 37,* 25–33.

PART III

Cognitive and Information-Processing Perspectives

CHAPTER 5

Information-Processing
Biases in PTSD

JOSEPH I. CONSTANS

A contemporary understanding of posttraumatic stress disorder (PTSD) from a neuropsychological perspective requires knowledge of how information-processing paradigms have been used to study PTSD. The information-processing approach is based in the cognitive–experimental tradition, but unlike traditional cognitive psychology, the experimental methods are modified to allow assessment of disorder-based differences. Modifications typically include the use of affective stimuli to assess for disorder-based differences in processing emotional information. For example, while cognitive and neuropsychologists have used the Stroop (1935) color-naming task to study attention, psychopathology researchers have modified the task to include emotional words as the target stimuli, as opposed to the neutral color-congruent and color-incongruent stimuli associated with the standard Stroop. Similar to the neuropsychological assessment approach described in Vasterling and Brailey (Chapter 8, this volume), information-processing investigations are concerned with cognitive processes such as attention, memory, and executive control. To assess these mental processes and products, both information-processing and neuropsychological approaches avoid introspective strategies and instead rely on performance-based methods. Information-processing paradigms also have significant relevance for PTSD research when using technologies such as fMRI (see Shin, Rauch, & Pitman, Chapter 3, this volume) or electrophysiology (see Metzger, Gilbertson, & Orr, Chapter 4, this volume) that assess neural activation. These approaches have frequently included cognitive–experimental designs, and thus, information-processing paradigms have increasingly come to be viewed within the broader neuroscience context.

Finally, an information-processing approach to the study of PTSD has a number of clinical implications. The paradigms allow for the testing of reported PTSD-related phenomena such as hypervigilance for threat or unwanted processing of trauma cues. As described in this chapter, information-processing approaches have led to the identification of a number of cognitive biases that are associated with PTSD, supporting some clinical observations but failing to validate others. Potential treatment implications are predicated in the assumption that information-processing biases are not merely byproducts of a negative mood state, but rather are important factors in the causation and maintenance of PTSD (Brewin, 2001; Ehlers & Clark, 2000). Although data demonstrating these biases as causative factors in PTSD are currently lacking, research with nonpathological anxiety has recently established that changes in how emotional stimuli are processed can in fact lead to changes in emotional state (MacLeod, Rutherford, Campbell, Ebsworthy, & Holker, 2002; Mathews & Mackintosh, 2000). This suggests that future clinical interventions may involve attempts to change information-processing biases and thus remediate the pathological emotional response in PTSD.

Because there are a number of reviews of information-processing studies in PTSD (Buckley, Blanchard, & Neill, 2000; McNally, 1998; Thrasher & Dalgleish, 1999), the current chapter highlights recent investigations and discusses how the extant literature addresses issues important to a neurocognitive understanding of PTSD. Following a traditional information-processing approach to the study of emotional disorders (Williams, Watts, MacLeod, & Mathews 1997), this review is grouped into sections on attentional, judgment, and memory biases.

ATTENTIONAL BIAS

There is a long history of investigating attentional processes in individuals with emotional disorders (Mathews & MacLeod, 1994). In general, this research has found that certain forms of psychopathology, particularly anxiety-related disorders, are associated with an attentional bias to threatening information. Attentional bias refers to a phenomenon whereby a mild threat stimulus leads to a disruption of ongoing cognitive activities due to an involuntary redirection of attentional resources to that stimulus. Whereas strong threats likely lead to attentional capture for all individuals regardless of their emotional state (Mogg & Bradley, 1998), mild threat stimuli appear to lead to a reallocation of attentional resources only for individuals with either elevated levels of trait anxiety or with certain emotional disorders (Mathews & MacLeod, 1994).

Attentional bias is believed to be important to the development and maintenance of emotional disorders, such as PTSD, as the constant attention directed to mild threat increases salience of innocuous stimuli that in turn may lead to chronic overarousal and increased stress vulnerability (MacLeod et al., 2002; Mathews & MacLeod, 2002). To study attentional bias in PTSD, the vast majority of investigations have typically used trauma-relevant words to represent mild threat stimuli. When the performance of PTSD subjects is specifically influenced by the presence of trauma-related words in an attentional task, this group difference is assumed to be a function of an attentional bias to trauma-relevant stimuli. To date, two information-processing paradigms, the dot probe paradigm and the emotional Stroop task, have been used to investigate issues of attentional bias in PTSD,[1] and studies that have included these paradigms are reviewed in this chapter.

Dot Probe Paradigm

The dot probe task requires the subject to identify one of two probes (e.g., * or **) and respond with a key press that is consistent with the presented probe. Prior to the presentation of the probe, a threat and nonthreat word are simultaneously displayed on the computer monitor (MacLeod, Mathews, & Tata, 1986), and immediately after offset of the two words, the probe is presented in place of one of the words. A relatively faster response when the probe is preceded by the threat word is taken as evidence of attentional bias. This faster response presumably occurs because the participant's visual attention is directed toward the threat word, and thus an attentional shift is not required when the probe is presented. With respect to PTSD, there is only one published study with adults that has incorporated the dot probe paradigm. In a study of motor vehicle accident (MVA) victims, Bryant and Harvey (1997) found that, compared to MVA survivors without PTSD, those with PTSD showed faster responses when the probe was preceded by a word related to driving threats. Dalgleish, Taghavi, et al. (2003) compared the performance of children and adolescents with depression, PTSD, or generalized anxiety disorder (GAD) on a dot probe task that included general threat words on the critical trials. In this study, adolescents with GAD, but not those with PTSD or depression, showed relative response speeding when the probe was preceded by a threat word.

---

[1]Trandel and McNally (1987) used the dichotic listening task to assess for attentional bias. Because there are many threats to the internal validity of this paradigm, it is unclear if the dichotic listening paradigm serves as an accurate measure of attentional bias, and therefore, this study will not be reviewed.

Emotional Stroop Task

In contrast to the limited evidence of attentional bias in PTSD using the dot probe paradigm, there is strong and abundant evidence of attentional bias in PTSD when using the emotional Stroop task. The emotional Stroop task refers to a variant of the traditional Stroop color-naming task (Stroop, 1935). In the classic Stroop task, subjects are presented with color-congruent and color-incongruent words, and relative decrements in response time are found during color-incongruent trials. When the Stroop task is modified to study biases associated with processing of emotional stimuli, the critical trials involve color naming emotional, rather than color-incongruent, words. In the study of PTSD, evidence of attentional bias is found when PTSD subjects, but not controls, are slower to color name trauma-related words as compared to emotionally neutral words or emotional words unrelated to the trauma.

There is now ample evidence showing that, regardless of the type of trauma experienced by the individual, PTSD is associated with an attentional bias when using the emotional Stroop task. Individuals with PTSD due to combat trauma have been shown to be significantly slower when color naming combat-relevant words (Constans, McCloskey, Vasterling, Brailey, & Mathews, 2004; Kaspi, McNally, & Amir, 1995; McNally, Amir, & Lipke, 1996; McNally, English, & Lipke, 1993; McNally, Kaspi, Riemann, & Zeitlin, 1990; Vrana, Roodman, & Beckman, 1995). Litz et al. (1996) also found that Vietnam veterans with PTSD were slower in color naming threat words but, unlike the other studies, they failed to find that interference was specifically related to trauma words. Research with crime victims has found that individuals with PTSD are slower in color naming crime-relevant words than crime victims without PTSD. This effect appears to be strongest for rape victims who show significant slowing when color naming rape-related words (Cassiday, McNally, & Zeitlin, 1992; Foa, Feske, Murdock, Kozak, & McCarthy, 1991). Paunovic, Lundh, and Ost (2002) also found that crime victims with varied traumatic experiences were slower when color naming general crime words as opposed to neutral words. However, the PTSD group in Cassiday et al. (1992) and Paunovic et al. (2002) were also slower when color naming positive words.

Accident victims with PTSD have also been found to show color-naming interference for trauma-relevant words including ferry accident victims (Thrasher, Dalgleish, & Yule, 1994) and motor vehicle accident victims (Bryant & Harvey, 1995; Buckley, Blanchard, & Hickling, 2002). Whereas the emotional Stroop effect in Bryant and Harvey (1995) and Thrasher et al. (1994) was specific to trauma words, Buckley et al. (2002) found that PTSD was associated with response slowing for both panic and trauma words. Finally, Metzger, Orr, Lasko, McNally, and Pitman (1997) found evidence of a trauma-specific bias when participants with varied trauma experiences (combat, childhood sexual abuse, MVA) were tested on an emotional Stroop task that included trauma and positive words that were individually chosen for each participant based on their history of traumatic and positive events.

Emotional Stroop and PTSD: Theoretical Issues

In sum, there is strong evidence of attentional bias using the emotional Stroop task, and the majority of these studies indicate that PTSD is associated with particularly slow responses when color naming trauma-relevant, as opposed to general-threat, words. This effect is not solely associated with any particular type of trauma. Furthermore, the emotional Stroop effect in PTSD does not appear to be dependent on the methodological strategy used in the color-naming procedure. Whereas a somewhat larger effect is found when emotional words are presented in a block (McNally et al., 1996; Williams, Mathews, & MacLeod, 1996), attentional bias effects persist when the word type is randomly varied on a trial-to-trial basis.

Although attentional bias in PTSD appears to be a robust phenomenon, the explanation for this effect remains debatable. The most influential account of the emotional Stroop effect (Williams et al., 1996) is based on a model of the classic Stroop interference effect proposed by Cohen, Dunbar, and McClelland (1990). Cohen et al. (1990) suggested that exposure to a colored word in a standard Stroop task activates two response options— naming the color and reading the word. Although the participant is instructed to attend to the color, the word-reading response is automatically activated. If the automatic response (word reading) is incongruent with the task demand (name color), then conflict between the two response options must be resolved, leading to the behavioral interference effect. When imaging techniques have been used to study the Stroop effect, investigators have found that incongruent conditions, as compared with congruent or neutral conditions, are associated with greater anterior cingulate cortex (ACC) activation (e.g., Bush et al., 1998). As the dorsal ACC is believed to be associated with resolution of conflict on cognitive tasks (Drevets & Raichle, 1998), imaging data offer some support for this model.

To account for emotional Stroop effects, Williams et al. (1996) modified the Cohen et al. (1990) model with the additional stipulation that certain fear-related stimuli are awarded processing priority in subsequent cognitive tasks. With respect to PTSD, this would mean that trauma-related stimuli, such as mild trauma words, would receive processing priority because of the evolutionary advantages associated with attending to fear-producing stimuli. In the context of an emotional Stroop task involving PTSD participants, exposure to mild trauma-related words would activate a word-reading response, which would then interfere with the individual's attempt to name the color of the word. Consistent with this model, Shin et al. (2001) conducted an fMRI study involving a counting Stroop task and found that PTSD participants, but not non-PTSD controls, showed increased dorsal ACC activation when exposed to combat-related words.[2] Increased activation of dorsal ACC could represent increased efforts to comply with the demands of the task (i.e., counting) to overcome interference due to activation of a competing response (i.e., word reading).

A feature of the Williams et al. (1996) model that has been tested with PTSD samples is the hypothesis that the emotional Stroop effect represents an automatic process. The concept of an automatic behavior is one that (1) cannot be strategically controlled, (2) is impervious to other cognitive demands, and (3) can occur without conscious awareness (Shiffrin & Schneider, 1977). In an attempt to address one component of the automaticity hypothesis, namely that emotional Stroop effects cannot be strategically controlled, Constans et al. (2004) required male combat veterans with PTSD to complete the emotional Stroop task under a variety of testing conditions. In a "reward" condition, each PTSD participant was told that he would receive additional compensation if his performance on the color-naming task was exceptionally fast and accurate. Despite this financial incentive, the response time was similar for the "reward" and control conditions across all word-type conditions. In other words, PTSD participants were unable to override the emotional Stroop when motivated to do so with a financial reward.

Approaching the issue of volitional control from a different perspective, Buckley, Galovski, Blanchard, and Hickling (2003) had psychologists familiar with PTSD and a method-acting coach train six actors to feign a PTSD presentation. These actors, along with six participants with MVA-related PTSD and six control participants, completed a thorough assessment of PTSD involving completion of an interview, self-report, and emotional Stroop task. The response of the actors was similar to the response of the PTSD participants on self-report and interview assessments. On the emotional Stroop task, actors and PTSD participants showed similar response times to neutral words. However, only PTSD participants showed specific slowing to trauma-related words (i.e., attentional bias).

The studies by Buckley et al. (2003) and Constans et al. (2004) suggest

---

[2]Shin et al. (2001) also found *decreased* activation of rostral ACC when PTSD participants were exposed to trauma-related stimuli, and this decreased activation in the rostral region could be related to an inability to down-regulate amygdala response. This finding is discussed in greater detail in Shin, Rauch, and Pitman (Chapter 3, this volume).

emotional Stroop effects in PTSD are automatic in the sense that the response is not under volitional control. However, other studies have found that PTSD-related attentional bias may not be automatic in that emotional Stroop effects are eliminated by certain cognitive or emotional demands and may not occur unless the individual is consciously aware of the threat stimuli. In Constans et al. (2004), some combat veterans also completed an emotional Stroop under threat conditions that were designed to increase anticipatory anxiety. In the two threat conditions, participants were told either that a combat video would be shown after the Stroop task or that they would be videotaped while giving a speech after the Stroop task. The basic finding from this study was that both threat conditions led to a suppression of attentional bias to combat threat stimuli, although inhibition was slightly larger in the combat video condition. To account for the counterintuitive finding that an upcoming threat suppresses attentional bias, Constans et al. (2004) suggested that anticipatory anxiety leads to a restriction of attentional resources such that only the central component of the stimulus (i.e., font color) receives attention. Alternate explanations could include that, when multiple stressors are encountered, attention is awarded only to the most significant fear-related event (i.e., upcoming combat video) or that multiple threats lead to increased effort and concentration devoted to color naming (MacLeod & Rutherford, 1992). Regardless of the etiology of the suppression effect, Constans et al. (2004) showed that emotional Stroop effects for unmasked stimuli are not inevitable and can be moderated by contextual features of the task.

Other studies have addressed automaticity by investigating whether threat-related biases emerge when using masked stimuli. Masking a word stimulus following its brief presentation (typically less than 33 milliseconds) allows the investigator to assess the degree to which conscious awareness of the stimulus is necessary to produce attentional bias effects. Current models of attentional bias suggest that the bias occurs at a preattentive level, and evidence in support of this hypothesis has been found for other anxiety disorders and for nondisorder individuals with high levels of "trait" anxiety (Williams et al., 1996). With regard to PTSD, only one study found support for the preattentive bias hypothesis. Harvey, Bryant, and Rapee (1996) found that MVA victims with PTSD showed an attentional bias to threat-related words that were masked and presented at speeds preventing conscious awareness. However, three other studies failed to find evidence of attentional bias using masked stimuli despite providing evidence of attentional bias in the unmasked condition (Buckley et al., 2002; McNally et al., 1996; Paunovic et al., 2002). Although emotional Stroop effects are generally less robust when using masked stimuli (Fox, 1996), investigators appear to have particular difficulty identifying masked

Stroop effects in PTSD. For example, Lundh, Wikstrom, Westerlund, and Ost (1999) found evidence of attentional bias in participants with panic disorder when using both masked and unmasked stimuli. However, when the same research group replicated the procedures to study information-processing biases associated with acute MVA-related PTSD (Paunovic et al., 2002), attentional bias for trauma-related words was evident in the unmasked, but not masked, condition.

Summary

PTSD-related biases emerge when the Stroop paradigm is modified to include trauma-related and emotionally neutral words. Despite motivated attempts to comply with instructions to name a color and ignore word meaning, individuals with PTSD are unable to avoid processing trauma-related words, and this inability to control either the emotional or attentional response to trauma-relevant stimuli leads to a disruption of ongoing cognitive processes. The clinical relevance associated with this effect is clear. Attentional bias to threat is consistent with reported hypervigilance, and this body of research suggests that this attentional response may not be under direct volitional control. Furthermore, the attention awarded to trauma-related cues can lead to difficulties concentrating on other tasks, a problem that is frequently described by individuals with PTSD. As described in Vasterling and Brailey (Chapter 8, this volume), PTSD-related deficits emerge only in a subset of the neuropsychological assessment tasks. The information-processing research suggests that, when emotionally neutral stimuli are used in an attentional task, performance interference would be observed only on tasks that allow sufficient time for intrusive trauma-related cognitions to interfere with performance. This hypothesis could potentially account for the failure to find PTSD-related performance deficits in the classic Stroop task.

Although the emotional Stroop provides a demonstration of how trauma-related stimuli can disrupt performance, the reasons for this effect are not entirely clear. Current models suggest the emotional Stroop effect is due to relative increased activation of the word-reading response when a trauma-related word is presented. However, other investigators have suggested emotional Stroop effects may be due to cognitive or behavioral inhibition occurring secondary to exposure to negatively valenced stimuli (McKenna & Sharma, 2004). Furthermore, although response slowing to disorder-related words is present for many emotional disorders, the degree of interference is significantly larger for PTSD. This robustness of the emotional Stroop effect in PTSD has led some to speculate that the mechanism for response slowing in PTSD may be different from other anxiety disorders (Williams et al., 1996).

JUDGMENT BIAS

Some conceptualizations of PTSD theories suggest that judgmental biases may contribute to elevated anxiety and arousal in PTSD and are therefore important in the maintenance of the disorder (e.g., Ehlers & Clark, 2000). Increased anxiety could arise if individuals with PTSD routinely process emotionally ambiguous events as threatening, thus increasing feelings of vulnerability and vigilance for possible threats. For example, if an individual with PTSD routinely judges ambiguous noises outside of his or her home to be threatening (e.g., possible criminal) rather than innocuous (e.g., cat), this process may maintain beliefs of vulnerability, levels of heightened arousal, and hypervigilance. To assess potential judgment bias in a laboratory setting, emotion researchers have used information-processing paradigms that assess perceived risk associated with possible negative events (subjective risk bias) or the interpretation of ambiguous events or stimuli (interpretive bias). In the study of PTSD, however, there are currently only four published studies that have used subjective risk or interpretive bias paradigms.

Subjective Risk Bias

There is significant evidence suggesting that high levels of negative affect, particularly anxiety, are associated with increased perception of risk in the environment (Butler & Mathews, 1983; Constans, 2001). To assess bias in risk estimation, investigators typically administer questionnaires that ask the participant to estimate the likelihood that certain negative and positive events will occur in the future. The questionnaires may also assess whether risk is biased for self or others and whether there are biases associated with the perceived cost associated with certain negative events. In general, biased risk estimates have been found across multiple anxiety disorders (Williams et al., 1997).

Two studies have investigated subjective risk biases associated with trauma-related psychopathology. Warda and Bryant (1998) found that compared to MVA survivors without acute stress disorder (ASD), individuals with ASD overestimated both the probability and cost associated with future negative events that could potentially have adverse consequences (e.g., getting a flat tire). Similarly, Dalgleish (as cited in Thrasher & Dalgleish, 1999) found that ferry disaster survivors with high levels of PTSD symptoms overestimated the likelihood of experiencing negative events when their responses were compared with ferry disaster survivors who had low levels of PTSD or control participants. PTSD symptom elevation was associated with biased risk for uncertain events both related and unrelated to the traumatic event.

Interpretive Bias

Unlike subjective risk paradigms that require participants to make judgments about future events, interpretive bias paradigms require participants to interpret experimental stimuli that are ambiguous with regard to their meaning. As compared to subjective risk paradigms, interpretive bias paradigms are believed to reflect more precisely the process of how individuals judge ongoing events. Different methodological strategies have been used to assess interpretive bias, including requiring participants to spell an auditorily presented word that could be construed as either threatening or nonthreatening (e.g., die/dye; Eysenck, MacLeod, & Mathews, 1987) and requiring participants to make interpretations of ambiguous sentences or paragraphs (Constans, Penn, Ihen, & Hope, 1999). However, these paradigms allow susceptibility to demand effects, thus limiting inferences that the data reflect true judgmental biases. For example, in the aforementioned homophone paradigm, a participant could access both word meanings but chose to report only the threatening word due to a self-imposed belief that anxious individuals should report the threat word. To reduce possible demand effects, other paradigms have been developed in which reading response time serves as the dependent variable. In these paradigms, the participant reads an ambiguous sentence that is followed by a word or sentence that disambiguates the preceding sentence in either a threatening or nonthreatening manner (e.g., Calvo, Eysenck, & Estevez, 1994). Relatively faster reading times for the threatening word or sentence suggests that a negative interpretation had been made of the ambiguous sentence. The results of this body of research show that individuals with anxiety-related psychopathology make more negative interpretations of ambiguous stimuli.

There are two studies involving PTSD patients that have included paradigms assessing potential biases in interpretive style. Kimble et al. (2002) recruited combat veterans with and without PTSD to participate in a sentence completion task. The sentence fragments were created such that either a military-related or nonmilitary word could meaningfully complete the sentence. The investigators found that PTSD participants completed the sentences with significantly more military words than combat veterans without PTSD. Although Kimble et al. (2002) argued that the results of this study indicate PTSD is characterized by active trauma schema, the nature of the task does not preclude a demand explanation.

In an attempt to eliminate demand explanations, Amir, Coles, and Foa (2002) required traumatized participants with and without PTSD to read a sentence and then decide whether a subsequent target word was related to the sentence. The word was presented either 100 milliseconds or 850 milliseconds following offset of the sentence. Of particular interest to the investigators was latency of decision when the threat word was preceded by a sentence ending in a homograph that had both a threat and nonthreat meaning. On these critical trials, the sentence meaning always reflected the safe interpretation of the homograph while the target word always related to the threat meaning of the homograph. On comparison trials, the same critical threat word was preceded by a nonthreatening sentence that did not end in a homograph. The investigators hypothesized that individuals with PTSD would be slower because the threat meaning of the homograph could not be inhibited, even when preceded by a nonthreatening sentence. The predicted effect of slower decision latency for PTSD patients emerged only in the 850-millisecond condition. In fact, in the 100-millisecond condition, the opposite pattern emerged with non-PTSD patients showing significantly slower response latencies in the critical condition involving the homograph. The investigators concluded that interpretive bias in PTSD patients occurs only during later, more strategic stages of information processing.

Summary

Only a handful of studies have assessed possible PTSD-related bias in judgment and decision processes. In general, this research is consistent with the clinical view that individuals with PTSD are more likely to judge emotionally ambiguous events as threatening. In particular, PTSD is associated with a heightened risk perception such that potential negative events, even those unrelated to the trauma, are viewed as more likely to occur. This pattern of responding could be due to general negative affect associated with trauma-related psychopathology (Constans & Mathews, 1993) rather than specifically to PTSD. Individuals with PTSD also appear to be characterized by a negative interpretive bias when exposed to homographs. However, because this bias only emerges in delay conditions, it is unlikely that the judgment bias is automatic but instead follows elaboration on the potential meaning of the ambiguous stimuli.

The finding that judgment bias occurs only after the stimulus has been processed in an elaborative manner is inconsistent with both specific models of PTSD (Ehlers & Clark, 2000) and models of fear processing (Ohman & Mineka, 2001). In an fMRI study that required PTSD and control participants to passively view masked faces, Rauch et al. (2000) found that PTSD participants showed increased amygdala response to the masked angry faces suggesting that PTSD-related bias in emotional processing can occur outside of conscious awareness. In contrast to the passive viewing of masked faces included in the fMRI study, the behavioral studies reviewed in this chapter all included complex word or sentence stimuli that required subjects to make conscious inferences or predictions. Therefore, either the stimuli or processes used in these behavioral studies may have prevented detection of automatic judgmental biases.

MEMORY BIAS

Although PTSD is characterized by unwanted recall of the traumatic event, individuals with PTSD also experience mild impairments in recall of newly acquired information. A number of information-processing paradigms have been used to study hypothesized PTSD-related biases in memory functioning. The majority of this experimental research has involved variations on one of two paradigms: (1) tests involving memory for trauma-relevant and trauma-irrelevant words and (2) tests of autobiographical memory.

Memory Studies Involving Word Stimuli

Explicit Memory Biases

There is a long history of using word stimuli to investigate recall biases associated with different emotional disorders. In general, investigators using explicit memory tasks have found that depression is associated by a mood-congruent memory bias. In other words, when required to remember word lists involving emotional and nonemotional stimuli, individuals with depression recall relatively more negative words than individuals without depression (e.g., Bradley, Mogg, & Williams, 1995). In contrast, there is no clear consensus that anxiety disorders are associated with mood-congruent memory biases (Coles & Heimberg, 2002).

Five published studies to date have assessed whether PTSD is associated with a mood-congruent (or trauma-congruent) memory bias. In four of the five studies, memory was assessed for words that had been displayed within the context of an earlier color-naming task, thus allowing for incidental learning of the stimuli. In three of the studies using the incidental learning approach (Kaspi et al., 1995; Paunovic et al., 2002; Vrana et al., 1995), the investigators administered a free-recall test, whereas Litz et al. (1996) assessed recognition memory. In all three studies using the free-recall task, PTSD participants recalled more trauma-related words than control participants. However, because false positives (i.e., reporting trauma-related words that were not presented) were not reported, it is unclear whether the recall bias reflected increased sensitivity to the trauma words or a response bias to report more trauma-related stimuli, regardless of whether the word had been presented.

Litz et al. (1996) attempted to address this issue by using signal detection theory to analyze responses on a recognition task. Their analysis suggested that PTSD participants were characterized by an increased response bias to acknowledge having seen any military-related word, regardless of whether the word was in fact presented. However, this increased response bias was present only when the PTSD sample was compared with an emotionally healthy sample but not when the PTSD group was compared to other psychiatric patients. No group differences emerged on measures of sensitivity, suggesting that explicit memory bias may be due to a tendency to report exposure to any trauma-related word.

Golier, Yehuda, Lupien, and Harvey (2003) assessed putative PTSD-related bias in recall of trauma-related words with a sample of Holocaust survivors. However, their encoding task differed from previous studies in that the word stimuli were presented in pairs, and all participants were aware that memory would be assessed. Participants were exposed to a block of neutral word pairs that were either highly associated or unassociated with one another. An additional block of word pairs that consisted of a personalized Holocaust word and a neutral word pair were also presented. In the test of explicit memory, the investigators presented one word in the word pair and asked the subject to recall the word with which it was paired during the earlier encoding phase. Whereas Holocaust survivors with PTSD showed general deficits in paired associated recall, the PTSD group recalled more words from the Holocaust word-pair set than neutral word-pair sets. Holocaust survivors without PTSD and age-matched controls failed to show the same enhancement effects for Holocaust word pairs, thus suggesting that PTSD facilitates associative learning of trauma-related information.

Implicit Memory Bias

Because fear-related disorders may be associated with perceptual biases, emotion researchers have investigated whether anxiety disorders are characterized by a bias in implicit memory. In a typical test of implicit memory, critical words are presented without expectation of a later memory task and the participant later completes a seemingly unrelated task (i.e., word-stem completion; tachistoscopic identification). As performance on the identification or word-completion tasks are strongly influenced by the physical features of previously exposed word stimuli, group differences in performance are assumed to reflect enhanced perceptual priming of the word stimuli. However, because word stimuli are used, it is difficult to rule out the possible contribution of semantic-related priming in implicit memory performance.

Although there is limited support that some anxiety disorders are associated with enhanced implicit memory for threat words (Coles & Heimberg, 2002), the evidence supporting a PTSD-related bias is weak. There are two published studies that assessed for PTSD-related biases in perceptual priming using a tachistoscopic identification task. McNally and Amir (1996) exposed Vietnam combat veterans with and without PTSD to word stimuli for a period of 3 seconds and later asked them to complete a tachistoscopic identification task that included a subset of the presented words as well as "new" words. In the tachistoscopic task, the word stimulus appeared on the screen for 100 milliseconds, and the participant was instructed to read aloud the target word. Although "old" words were read more easily than "new" words, no disorder or word type effects or interactions emerged. Paunovic et al. (2002) also used a tachistoscopic identification task but tailored the stimulus duration to reflect the briefest exposure in which the participant identified a target word during an earlier pretest. This study also differed from McNally and Amir (1996) in that the exposure phase was embedded within the context of an emotional Stroop task. Nevertheless, the findings of Paunovic et al. (2002) were similar in that they also failed to find evidence of an implicit memory bias.

Using a word-stem completion task, Golier et al. (2003) assessed implicit memory for Holocaust words in the previously described sample of Holocaust survivors. The word stem completion task was administered after the test of explicit memory and a distraction task. Similar to the previous studies, these investigators found no evidence of a PTSD-related implicit memory bias for Holocaust words.

A different paradigm was used in the one study that did find evidence for a PTSD-related bias in implicit memory. Amir, McNally, and Wiegartz (1996) employed a "white noise paradigm" that required Vietnam veterans to rate the perceived loudness of a background noise that was presented simultaneously with a prerecorded sentence characterized as either trauma-relevant or trauma-irrelevant. Half of the sentences had been previously presented to the participants without the white noise background. Results revealed that at the highest levels of background noise, PTSD participants rated the noise as lower than individuals without PTSD when trauma-related sentences were presented. Amir et al. (1996) argued that the lower noise ratings for trauma-relevant sentences reflected enhanced *conceptual*, as opposed to perceptual, priming of this material.

The DRM and Directed Forgetting Paradigms

A number of clinical theories suggest that the narrative memory of the traumatic event is likely to be disorganized (e.g., Foa, Molnar, & Cashman, 1995) and omit sensory details (Brewin, 2001) in individuals who develop PTSD. This has led to the suggestion (e.g., McNally, Metzger, Lasko, Clancy, & Pitman, 1998) that patients with PTSD might be particularly good at forgetting or be open to suggestion. To address this issue using a cognitive–experimental approach, two specific versions of a word learning task, the DRM and directed forgetting paradigms, have been applied to the study of biased recall of trauma-related stimuli.

In the DRM paradigm, so named because of its development by Deese (1959) and modification by Roediger and McDermott (1995), participants are asked to learn, and later recall, lists of words that are semantically related. In each list, certain words that are highly associated with the theme of the list are intentionally not included (critical lures). Research with normal participants shows that critical lures are often recalled or recognized with fairly high confidence despite their noninclusion during the learning phase. Two studies have now used this paradigm to assess for PTSD-related biases in producing "false memories" of the critical lure (Bremner, Shobe, & Kihlstrom, 2000; Zoellner, Foa, Brididi, & Przeworski, 2000). These studies had a number of similarities including the use of nontraumatized and traumatized control participants, the use of word lists that had been modified by Roediger and McDermott (1995), and assessments of recall and recognition of critical lures. The studies differed slightly in the nature of the traumatized participants as Bremner et al. (2000) included women with childhood sexual abuse histories and Zoellner et al. (2000) included women who had been victims of crime involving either sexual or physical assault. Bremner et al. (2000) found that PTSD participants recognized critical lures more often than either abused women without PTSD or control participants but failed to find differences in recall of critical lures. Zoellner et al. (2000) found that trauma history, rather than the presence or absence of PTSD, was associated with increased recall of critical lures.

In sum, these experiments offer very limited support for the hypothesis that PTSD or a trauma history is associated with an increased generation of false memories. However, as the word lists involved emotionally neutral topics, it is unclear if this predisposition to false memory generation would differ for emotional or trauma-relevant stimuli. Furthermore, because this paradigm has not been incorporated into the study of other anxiety or depressive disorders, it is unclear if the false memory effects are due to increased levels of distress or depression rather than PTSD or trauma history.

Another laboratory-based strategy that has been used to assess possible PTSD-related biases in recall of trauma-related material is the directed forgetting task. In this paradigm, individual words or word lists are first presented. Following presentation of a word or word list, the participant is instructed to either remember or forget the previously presented information. However, in subsequent recall and recognition tests, the participant is asked to recall *all* words that were presented and disregard any previous instructions to forget certain stimuli. In the study of PTSD, the word lists are typically modified to include emotionally neutral, trauma-related, and positive words.

Three studies have been published that have used the directed forgetting paradigm with a PTSD sample (Cloitre, 1998; McNally et al., 1998; Zoellner, Sacks, & Foa, 2003), all including women with chronic PTSD as participants. Two studies found that either presence of trauma (Cloitre, 1998) or presence of PTSD (McNally et al., 1998) was associated with a relative enhancement in recalling trauma-related words. The third study (Zoellner et al., 2003) failed to find that any group differences in recall were related to either PTSD or trauma history. In sum, there is no current support for the hypothesis that individuals with *chronic* PTSD show enhanced forgetting of trauma-related words presented in a memory task.

However, in a study of acutely traumatized individuals, Moulds and Bryant (2002) found that ASD participants recalled fewer trauma-related words in the to-be-forgotten condition than did traumatized individuals without ASD. The investigators speculated that this effect might be related to a tendency for individuals who develop ASD to use avoidant cognitive strategies such as dissociation when confronted with threatening information. Consistent with this hypothesis, Myers, Brewin, and Power (1998) found that undergraduate participants classified as "repressors" showed enhanced forgetting of negative words in the to-be-forgotten condition. DePrince and Freyd (2004) found that undergraduates who were classified as high dissociators (and who report more past trauma) showed relative deficits in recalling trauma-related words in the to-be-remembered condition, but this effect was only present when experimental conditions required attention be divided between two tasks during encoding. Thus, individuals with more acute trauma-related psychopathology or with a predisposition to dissociate may show enhanced forgetting of trauma stimuli.

Autobiographical Memory Studies

It has been suggested that studies involving word lists might not allow an accurate assessment of bias associated with highly personal events. Therefore, to increase the ecological validity of a laboratory-based memory assessment, a number of investigators have used a version of the Autobiographical Memory Test (AMT; Williams & Broadbent, 1986) to assess PTSD-related biases in memory for personal events. In this paradigm, participants are asked to recall a specific memory in response to a cue word. Despite instructions to report a specific event, certain groups of patients, particularly depressives, tend to produce an "overgeneral" memory (see Williams, 1996, for review). Overgeneral memory refers to a description of a category of events rather than one specific episode from the past. For example, when presented with the cue word "candle," an individual with depression may report the memory "birthday parties" rather than relating the memory of one particular birthday party.

In the earliest of four studies investigating autobiographical memory bias in PTSD, McNally, Litz, Prassas, Shin, and Weathers (1994) found that Vietnam veterans with PTSD produced overgeneral memories to positive, neutral, and negative cue words. The frequency of overgeneral memory production was further enhanced following a negative mood induction involving viewing a combat video. McNally, Lasko, Macklin, and Pitman (1995) replicated the overgeneral memory effect for combat-related PTSD with a modified AMT that included words reflecting positive or negative personal characteristics but, in a post hoc analysis, found overgeneral memory only occurred for those PTSD veterans wearing war regalia. Harvey, Bryant, and Dang (1998) found an overgeneral memory bias for MVA victims with ASD when their responses were compared to MVA victims without ASD, and the degree of overgeneral memory bias served as a positive predictor of later PTSD development. However, an overgeneral memory effect was observed only for positive cue words in this study. Finally, Wessel, Merckelbach, and Dekkers (2002) found that psychiatric patients (40% with PTSD) who had experienced war atrocities in childhood produced less specific memories than nonpatients with childhood exposure to war atrocities.

It remains unclear why individuals with PTSD experience autobiographical memory bias. As autobiographical memory bias is frequently associated with presence of depression, it is possible that overgeneral memory in PTSD is a function of comorbid depressive symptoms. In fact, for non-PTSD anxiety disorders, overgeneral memory biases are not typically found unless depression is comorbid to the anxiety disorder (Burke & Mathews, 1992; Wilhelm, McNally, Baer, & Florin, 1997).

Although autobiographical memory biases in PTSD could be due to comorbid depression, other research implicates trauma history as an important etiological factor. Dalgleish, Tchanturia, et al. (2003), Kuyken and Brewin (1995), and Hermans et al. (2004) each found that self-reported history of abuse, rather than mood disturbance per se, was associated with overgeneral memory in samples of eating disordered or depressed patients. In one of the earlier models of overgeneral memory bias, Williams (1996) proposed that individuals who have negative life events, particularly in childhood, learn to manage their mood state by avoiding specific memories, thus decreasing the chance of experiencing the associated negative emotion. Repeated practice of this strategy leads to a retrieval process for personal memories that is characterized by a lack of specificity. In support of this hypothesis, Brewin and colleagues (Brewin, Watson, McCarthy, Hyman, & Dayson, 1998; Brewin, Reynolds, & Tata, 1999) found in naturalistic studies that the severity of overgeneral memory bias was related to the extent of intrusion and avoidance of stressful memories in samples of depressed patients. This finding suggests unwanted reexperiencing and subsequent cognitive avoidance of upsetting memories may lead to an overgeneral memory bias, regardless of whether the patient's diagnostic status is PTSD or depression. To date, however, the experimental investigation of this hypothesis has involved only nonclinical participants, and the findings have been mixed (Philippot, Schaefer, & Herbette, 2003; Raes, Hermans, Decker, Williams, & Eelen, 2003).

One potential criticism associated with the use of the AMT is that it does not directly assess recall of traumatic memories because specific trauma-related cue words are not typically included in the protocol and the participant can choose any memory to report. In fact, Harvey et al. (1998) found group differences for positive cue words but not for negative cue words, possibly suggesting that trauma-related psychopathology is characterized by lack of specificity for positive rather than negative events. In none of the completed investigations did the PTSD or trauma participants produce more overgeneral memories to the negative, as opposed to positive, cue words.

Summary

PTSD appears to be characterized by an explicit memory bias as evidenced by enhanced recall of trauma-related words. In fact, even when directed to do so, participants with PTSD have difficulty forgetting trauma-related words. This bias is consistent with the suggestion that PTSD is characterized by a trauma-congruent bias in explicit memory possibly due to an involuntary process of elaborating on trauma-related stimuli. In contrast, tachistoscopic identification tasks have failed to find evidence of implicit memory biases. Only implicit memory tasks that purport to measure conceptual, rather than perceptual, processing have found PTSD-related differences. Finally, when asked to recall specific memories that occur in response to cue words, PTSD participants tend to report an overgeneral memory, but it is unclear if this bias extends to memories of trauma.

In general, memory paradigms using emotional stimuli are consistent with clinical reports that individuals with PTSD have difficulty controlling trauma-related thoughts, particularly following exposure to trauma cues. This research, however, fails to support the suggestion that PTSD is characterized by increased susceptibility to intentionally forgetting or suppressing trauma-related material. It is notable that, whereas information-processing studies show that PTSD is associated with relative enhancements in recall for trauma stimuli, neuropsychological studies often find impaired performance for PTSD participants in tests involving emotionally neutral stimuli. Correlational data suggest that unwanted processing of emotional memories may reflect a more general cognitive gating deficit (Vasterling, Brailey, Constans, & Sutker, 1998). It may be that deficits in prefrontal cortical regulatory control of limbic structures such as the amygdala lead to increased elaboration of trauma-related stimuli. Increased activation of trauma-related cognitions may in turn result in impairments in learning emotionally neutral stimuli because the prioritization of trauma-related material may limit the availability of cognitive resources for processing emotionally neutral stimuli. An alternative, but not mutually exclusive, explanation is that frontal system or hippocampal dysfunction leads more directly to general memory deficits. However, these memory impairments are overcome when processing trauma-related stimuli because the emotional associations with this trauma material promote increased elaboration and thus improved recall.

CONCLUSIONS AND FUTURE DIRECTIONS

A review of the information-processing literature shows that a number of PTSD-related biases emerge in the processing of emotional stimuli. Whereas the most powerful effect has been found with the emotional Stroop task, PTSD-related biases have also been found for explicit memory tests involving trauma-related words and recall of autobiographical memories. Although very few studies have investigated possible subjective risk or interpretive biases, the available evidence suggests that individuals with PTSD are characterized by threat-related judgmental bias when the duration of the stimulus presentation allows for conscious elaboration.

In contrast to the effects found for consciously accessible stimuli, there is very little evidence of PTSD-related bias on the masked Stroop task or on measures of implicit memory that assess for enhanced perceptual priming of lexical stimuli. This failure to find attentional and memory bias for barely perceptible stimuli is somewhat surprising given that perceptual–emotional associations are believed to be important in both general models of fear-related psychopathology (e.g., Ohman & Soares, 1994) as well as specific models of PTSD (Brewin, 2001; Ehlers & Clark, 2000). Models of fear-related psychopathology assume that anxiety disordered individuals will show emotional, cognitive, and physiological responses to perceptual features of fear-related stimuli. This response is presumably based on biases associated with "an evolved module for fear elicitation and fear learning" that confers an evolutionary advantage to developing emotional responses to the perceptual, rather than conceptual, features of threatening stimuli (Ohman & Mineka, 2001). Similarly, contemporary models of PTSD suggest that this disorder is characterized by enhanced perceptual processing of the traumatic event (Brewin, Dalgleish, & Joseph, 1996; Brewin, 2001; Ehlers & Clark, 2000).

It is possible that the failure to find biases in perceptual processing could be due to the almost exclusive use of lexical stimuli. McNally, et al. (1996) speculated that, because there is no evolutionary advantage associated with early word identification, perceptual biases may only emerge when using stimuli that are directly, rather than conceptually, related to the traumatic event. However, evidence of enhanced perceptual processing has been found for other anxiety disorders when lexical stimuli have been used in both subliminal Stroop (e.g., Bradley et al., 1995) and implicit memory paradigms (Coles & Heimberg, 2002). It is, therefore, unclear why perceptually based biases would emerge for some anxiety disorders but not for PTSD, unless this is related to the relatively greater importance of intrusive images versus verbal thoughts in PTSD. Additionally, PTSD may differ from other anxiety disorders in that aberrant conceptual, as opposed to perceptual, processing of the traumatic event is associated with development of the disorder (Ehlers & Clark, 2000).

An alternative explanation for the failure to find enhanced perceptual processing is that depression, which frequently co-occurs with PTSD, interferes either with response time data (Lawson, MacLeod, & Hammond, 2002) or obscures anxiety-related biases (Bradley et al., 1995). In fact, considering the evidence supporting explicit and overgeneral memory bias and the failure to find implicit or subliminal Stroop effects, the pattern of information-processing biases associated with PTSD is in many ways more consistent with depression than with other anxiety disorders. An exception to this statement is the extremely robust effects that are observed in the emotional Stroop task. Whereas Stroop effects have been occasionally found in depressive samples (e.g., Mathews, Ridgeway, & Williamson, 1996), the majority of studies have failed to find evidence of attentional bias in depression (e.g., Mogg, Millar, & Bradley, 2000). The mixed findings for depression stand in stark contrast to the strong emotional Stroop effects observed in PTSD.

Based on a review of extant studies, there are a number of possible future directions for PTSD-related information processing research. As the almost exclusive reliance on verbal stimuli may not provide a fair test of possible bias associated with enhanced perceptual processing of trauma-relevant information, inclusion of nonverbal stimuli, including masked photographic or pictorial stimuli, would permit assessment of possible threat-related bias in attention and judgment (e.g., Ohman & Soares, 1994). Secondly, although there is ample documentation of emotional Stroop effects in PTSD samples, the mechanism for this effect is not well understood. Because the emotional Stroop effect is much larger in PTSD than other anxiety disorders, it is likely that different or additional mechanisms contribute to attentional bias effects in PTSD as compared with other anxiety disorders (Williams et al., 1996). Therefore, incorporation of paradigms that allow further analysis of why attentional bias occurs may help explain attentional changes associated with trauma-related psychopathology (e.g., Yiend & Mathews, 2001). Lastly, increased understanding of trauma memory in PTSD may require use of paradigms that directly motivate trauma recall and simultaneously assess other cognitive processes (e.g., Hellawell & Brewin, 2002). It is possible that only when trauma memories are actively rehearsed do biases in perceptual processes emerge.

In sum, information-processing studies are supportive of clinical descriptions of PTSD as a disorder characterized by difficulty controlling intrusive cognitive phenomena that occur after exposure to trauma cues. A neurocognitive conceptualization might involve PTSD-related dysfunction in regions associated with preattentive processing (i.e., amygdala) as well as in control structures (i.e., prefrontal areas). As described by Rauch et al. (2000), individuals with PTSD show an exaggerated amygdala response when shown masked, angry faces. One functional consequence of this increased amygdaloid activity could be that a mild threat-stimulus is "tagged" as important, thus giving it processing priority during subsequent cognitive operations. This increased priority for mild, trauma-related information could lead to an observed attentional bias for threat words and may lead to increased conscious elaboration of the stimulus. While such a response might be expected for most individuals immediately following a trauma, those with mild dysfunction in control regions (e.g., prefrontal cortex) could show particular difficulty modifying the emotional response to mild trauma information, thus perpetuating attentional and memory biases.

REFERENCES

Amir, N., Coles, M. E., & Foa, E. B. (2002). Automatic and strategic activation and inhibition of threat-related information in posttraumatic stress disorder. *Cognitive Therapy and Research, 26,* 645–655.

Amir, N., McNally, R. J., & Wiegartz, P. S. (1996). Implicit memory bias for threat in posttraumatic stress disorder. *Cognitive Therapy and Research, 26,* 645–655.

Bradley, B. P, Mogg, K., & Williams, R. (1995). Implicit and explicit memory for emotion congruent information in clinical depression and anxiety. *Behaviour Research and Therapy, 33,* 755–770.

Bremner, J. B., Shobe, K. K., & Kihlstrom, J. F. (2000). False memories in women with self-reported childhood sexual abuse: An empirical study. *Psychological Science, 11,* 333–337.

Brewin, C. R. (2001). A cognitive neuroscience account of posttraumatic stress disorder and its treatment. *Behaviour Research and Therapy, 39,* 373–393.

Brewin, C. R., Dalgleish, T., & Joseph, S. (1996). A dual representation of posttraumatic stress disorder. *Psychological Review, 103,* 670–686.

Brewin, C. R., Reynolds, M., & Tata, P. (1999). Autobiographical memory processes and the course of depression. *Journal of Abnormal Psychology, 108,* 511–517.

Brewin, C. R., Watson, M., McCarthy, S., Hyman, P., & Dayson, D. (1998). Intrusive memories and depression in cancer patients. *Behaviour Research and Therapy, 36*, 1131–1142.

Bryant, R. A., & Harvey, A. G. (1995). Processing of threatening information in posttraumatic stress disorder. *Journal of Abnormal Psychology, 104*, 537–541.

Bryant, R. A., & Harvey, A. G. (1997). Attentional bias in posttraumatic stress disorder. *Journal of Traumatic Stress, 10*, 635–644.

Buckley, T. C., Blanchard, E. B., & Hickling, E. J. (2002). Automatic and strategic processing of threat stimuli: A comparison between PTSD, panic disorder, and nonanxiety controls. *Cognitive Therapy and Research, 26*, 97–115.

Buckley, T. C., Blanchard, E. B., & Neill, W. T. (2000). Information processing and PTSD: A review of the empirical literature. *Clinical Psychology Review, 28*, 1041–1065.

Buckley, T. C., Galovski, T., Blanchard, E. B., & Hickling, E. J. (2003). Is the emotional Stroop paradigm sensitive to malingering? A between-groups study with professional actors and actual trauma survivors. *Journal of Traumatic Stress, 16*, 59–66.

Burke, M., & Mathews, A. (1992). Autobiographical memory and clinical anxiety. *Cognition and Emotion, 6*, 23–35.

Bush, G., Whalen, P. J., Rosen, B. R., Jenike, M. A., McInerney, S. C., & Rauch, S. L. (1998). The counting Stroop: An interference task specialized for functional neuroimaging—Validation study with functional MRI. *Human Brain Mapping, 6*, 270–282.

Butler, G., & Mathews, A. M. (1983). Cognitive processes in anxiety. *Advances in Behavior Therapy, 5*, 51–62.

Cassiday, K. L., McNally, R. J., & Zeitlin, S. B. (1992). Cognitive processing of trauma cues in rape victims with post-traumatic stress disorder. *Cognitive Therapy and Research, 16*, 283–295.

Calvo, M. G., Eysenck, M. W., & Estevez, A. (1994). Ego-threat interpretive bias in test anxiety: On-line inferences. *Cognition and Emotion, 8*, 127–146.

Cloitre, M. (1998). Intentional forgetting and the clinical disorders. In J. M. Golding & C. L. MacLeod (Eds.), *Intentional forgetting: Interdisciplinary approaches* (pp. 395–412). Mahwah, NJ: Erlbaum.

Cohen, J. D., Dunbar, K., & McClelland, J. L. (1990). On the control of automatic processes: A parallel distributed processing account of the Stroop effect. *Psychological Review, 97*, 332–361.

Coles, M. E., & Heimberg, R. G. (2002). Memory biases in the anxiety disorders: Current status. *Clinical Psychology Review, 22*, 587–627.

Constans, J. I. (2001). Worry propensity and the perception of risk. *Behaviour Research and Therapy, 39*, 721–729.

Constans, J. I., McCloskey, M., Vasterling, J. J., Brailey, K., & Mathews, A. (2004). Suppression of attentional bias in PTSD. *Journal of Abnormal Psychology, 113*, 315–323.

Constans, J. I., & Mathews, A. M. (1993). Mood and the subjective risk of future events. *Cognition and Emotion, 7*, 545–560.

Constans, J. I., Penn, D. L., Ihen, G., & Hope, D. A. (1999). Interpretive biases for ambiguous stimuli in social anxiety. *Behaviour Research and Therapy, 37*, 643–651.

Dalgleish, T., Taghavi, R., Neshat-Doost, H., Moradi, A., Canterbury, R., & Yule, W. (2003). Patterns of processing bias for emotional information across clinical disorders: A comparison of attention, memory, and prospective cognition in children and adolescents with depression, generalized anxiety, and posttraumatic stress disorder. *Journal of Clinical Child and Adolescent Psychology, 32,* 10–21.

Dalgleish, T., Tchanturia, K., Seerpell, L., Hems, S., Yiend, J., de Silva, P., & Treasure, J. (2003). Self-reported parental abuse relates to autobiographical memory style in patients with eating disorders. *Emotion, 3,* 211–222.

DePrince, A. P., & Freyd, J. J. (2004). Forgetting trauma stimuli. *Psychological Science, 15,* 488–492.

Deese, J. (1959). On the prediction of occurrence of particular verbal intrusions in immediate recall. *Journal of Experimental Psychology, 58,* 17–22.

Drevets, W. C., & Raichle, M. E. (1998). Reciprocal suppression of regional cerebral blood flow during emotional versus higher cognitive processes: Implications for interactions between emotion and cognition. *Cognition and Emotion, 12,* 353–385.

Ehlers, A., & Clark, D. M. (2000). A cognitive model of posttraumatic stress disorder. *Behaviour Research and Therapy, 38,* 319–345.

Eysenck, M. W., MacLeod, C., & Mathews, A. (1987). Cognitive functioning in anxiety. *Psychological Research, 49,* 189–195.

Foa, E. B., Feske, U., Murdock, T. B., Kozak, M. J., & McCarthy, P. R. (1991). Processing of threat-related information in rape victims. *Journal of Abnormal Psychology, 100,* 156–162.

Foa, E. B., Molnar, C., & Cashman, L. (1995). Change in rape narratives during exposure therapy for posttraumatic stress disorder. *Journal of Traumatic Stress, 8,* 675–690.

Fox, E. (1996). Selective processing of threatening words in anxiety: The role of awareness. *Cognition and Emotion, 10,* 449–480.

Golier, J. A., Yehuda, R., Lupien, S. J., & Harvey, P. D. (2003). Memory for trauma-related information in Holocaust survivors with PTSD. *Psychiatry Research, 121,* 133–143.

Harvey, A. G., Bryant, R. A., & Rapee, R. M. (1996). Preconscious processing of threat in posttraumatic stress disorder. *Cognitive Therapy and Research, 20,* 613–623.

Harvey, A. G., Bryant, R. A., & Dang, S. T. (1998). Autobiographical memory in acute stress disorder. *Journal of Consulting and Clinical Psychology, 66,* 500–506.

Hellawell, S. J., & Brewin, C. R. (2002). A comparison of flashbacks and ordinary autobiographical memories of trauma: Cognitive resources and behavioural observations. *Behaviour Research and Therapy, 40,* 1143–1156.

Hermans, D., den Broeck, K. V., Belis, G., Raes, F., Pieters, G., & Eelen, P. (2004). Trauma and autobiographical memory specificity in depressed inpatients. *Behaviour Research and Therapy, 42,* 775–789.

Kaspi, S. P., McNally, R. J., & Amir, N. (1995). Cognitive processing of emotional information in posttraumatic stress disorder. *Cognitive Therapy and Research, 19,* 433–444.

Kimble, M. O., Kaufman, M. L., Leonard, L. L., Nestor, P. G., Riggs, D. S., Kaloupek,

D. G., & Bachrach, P. (2002). Sentence completion test in combat veterans with and without PTSD: Preliminary findings. *Psychiatry Research, 113*, 303–307.

Kuyken, W., & Brewin, C. R. (1995). Autobiographical memory functioning in depression and reports of early abuse. *Journal of Abnormal Psychology, 104*, 585–591.

Lawson, C., MacLeod, C., & Hammond, G. (2002). Interpretation revealed in the blink of an eye: Depressive bias in the resolution of ambiguity. *Journal of Abnormal Psychology, 111*, 321–328.

Litz, B. T., Weathers, F. W., Monaco, V., Herman, D. S., Wulfoshn, M., Marx, B., & Keane, T. M. (1996). Attention, arousal, and memory in posttraumatic stress disorder. *Journal of Traumatic Stress, 9*, 497–519.

Lundh, L. G., Wikstrom, J., Westerlund, J., & Ost, L. G. (1999). Preattentive bias for emotional information in panic disorder with agoraphobia. *Journal of Abnormal Psychology, 108*, 222–232.

MacLeod, C., Mathews, A., & Tata, P. (1986). Attentional bias in emotional disorders. *Journal of Abnormal Psychology, 95*, 15–20.

MacLeod, C., Rutherford, E., Campbell, L., Ebsworthy, G., & Holker, L. (2002). Selective attention and emotional vulnerability: Assessing the causal basis of their association through the experimental manipulation of attentional bias. *Journal of Abnormal Psychology, 111*, 107–123.

MacLeod, C., & Rutherford, E. M. (1992). Anxiety and the selective processing of emotional information: Mediating roles of awareness, trait and state variables, and personal relevance of stimulus materials. *Behaviour Research and Therapy, 30*(5), 479–491.

Mathews, A., & Mackintosh, B. (2000). Induced emotional interpretation bias and anxiety. *Journal of Abnormal Psychology, 109*, 602–615.

Mathews, A., & MacLeod, C. (1994). Cognitive approaches to emotion and emotional disorders. *Annual Review of Psychology, 45*, 25–50.

Mathews, A., & MacLeod, C. (2002). Induced processing biases have causal effects on anxiety. *Cognition and Emotion, 16*, 331–354.

Mathews, A., Ridgeway, V., & Williamson, D. A. (1996). Evidence for attention to threatening stimuli in depression. *Behaviour Research and Therapy, 34*, 695–705.

McKenna, F. P., & Sharma, D. (2004). Reversing the emotional Stroop effect reveals that it is not what it seems: The role of fast and slow components. *Journal of Experimental Psychology: Learning, Memory, and Cognition, 30*, 382–392.

McNally, R. J. (1998). Experimental approaches to cognitive abnormality in posttraumatic stress disorder. *Clinical Psychology Review, 18*, 971–982.

McNally, R. J., & Amir, N. (1996). Perceptual implicit memory for trauma-related information in posttraumatic stress disorder. *Cognition and Emotion, 10*, 551–556.

McNally, R. J., Amir, N., & Lipke, H. J. (1996). Subliminal processing of threat cues in posttraumatic stress disorder. *Journal of Anxiety Disorders, 10*(2), 115–128.

McNally, R. J., English, G. E., & Lipke, H. J. (1993). Assessment of intrusive cognition in PTSD: Use of the modified Stroop paradigm. *Journal of Traumatic Stress, 6*, 33–41.

McNally, R. J., Kaspi, S. P., Riemann, B. C., & Zeitlin, S. B. (1990). Selective processing of threat cues in posttraumatic stress disorder. *Journal of Abnormal Psychology, 99*, 398–402.

McNally, R. J., Lasko, N. B., Macklin, M. L., & Pitman, R. K. (1995). Autobiographical memory disturbance in combat-related posttraumatic stress disorder. *Behaviour Research and Therapy, 33*, 619–630.

McNally, R. J., Litz, B. T., Prassas, A., Shin, L. M., & Weathers, F. (1994). Emotional priming of autobiographical memory in posttraumatic stress disorder. *Cognition and Emotion, 10*, 551–556.

McNally, R. J., Metzger, L. J., Lasko, N. B., Clancy, S. A., & Pitman, R. K. (1998). Directed forgetting of trauma cues in adult survivors of childhood sexual abuse with and without posttraumatic stress disorder. *Journal of Abnormal Psychology, 107*, 596–601.

Metzger, L. J., Orr, S. P., Lasko, N. B., McNally, R. J., & Pitman, R. K. (1997). Seeking the source of the emotional Stroop interference effects in PTSD: A study of P3s to traumatic words. *Integrative Physiological and Behavioral Science, 32*, 43–51.

Mogg, K., & Bradley, B. (1998). A cognitive–motivational analysis of anxiety. *Behaviour Research and Therapy, 36*, 809–848.

Mogg, K., Millar, N., & Bradley, B. P. (2000). Biases in eye movements to threatening facial expressions in generalized anxiety disorder and depressive disorder. *Journal of Abnormal Psychology, 109*, 696–704.

Moulds, M. L., & Bryant, R. A. (2002). Directed forgetting in acute stress disorder. *Journal of Abnormal Psychology, 111*, 175–179.

Myers, L. B., Brewin, C. B., & Power, M. J. (1998). Repressive coping and the directed forgetting of emotional material. *Journal of Abnormal Psychology, 107*, 141–148.

Ohman, A., & Mineka, S. (2001). Fears, phobias, and preparedness: Toward an evolved module of fear and fear learning. *Psychological Review, 108*, 483–522.

Ohman, A., & Soares, J. J. F. (1994). "Unconscious anxiety": Phobic responses to masked stimuli. *Journal of Abnormal Psychology, 103*(2), 231–240.

Paunovic, N., Lundh, L.-G., & Ost, L.-G. (2002). Attentional and memory bias for emotional information in crime victims with acute posttraumatic stress disorder. *Journal of Anxiety Disorders, 16*, 675–692.

Philippot, P., Schaefer, A., & Herbette, G. (2003). Consequences of specific processing of emotional information: Impact of general versus specific autobiographical memory priming on emotion elicitation. *Emotion, 3*, 270–283.

Raes, F., Hermans, D., Decker, A. de, Williams, J. M. G., & Eelen, P. (2003). Autobiographical memory specificity and affect regulation: An experimental approach. *Emotion, 3*, 201–206.

Rauch, S. L., Whalen, P. J., Shin, L. M., McInerney, S. C., Macklin, M. L., Lasko, N. B., Orr, S. P., & Pitman, R. K. (2000). Exaggerated amygdala response to masked facial stimuli in posttraumatic stress disorder: A functional MRI study. *Biological Psychiatry, 47*, 769–776.

Roediger, H. L., & McDermott, K. B. (1995). Creating false memories: Remembering words not presented in lists. *Journal of Experimental Psychology: Learning, Memory, and Cognition, 21*, 803–814.

Shiffrin, R. M., & Schneider, W. (1977). Controlled and automatic human processing: Perceptual learning, automatic attending, and a general theory. *Psychological Review, 84*, 127–190.

Shin, L. M., Whalen, P. J., Pitman, R. K., Bush, G., Macklin, M. L., Lasko, N. B., Orr, S. P., McInerney, S. C., & Rauch, S. L. (2001). An fMRI study of anterior cingulate function in posttraumatic stress disorder. *Biological Psychiatry, 50*, 932–942.

Stroop, J. R. (1935). Studies of interference in serial verbal reactions. *Journal of Experimental Psychology, 18*, 643–662.

Thrasher, S., & Dalgleish, T. (1999). The use of information-processing paradigms to investigate posttraumatic stress disorder: A review of the evidence. In W. Yule (Ed.), *Post-traumatic stress disorder: Concepts and therapy* (pp. 176–192). Chichester, UK: Wiley.

Thrasher, S. M., Dalgleish, T., & Yule, W. (1994). Information processing in posttraumatic stress disorder. *Behaviour Research and Therapy, 32*, 247–254.

Trandel, D. V., & McNally, R. J. (1987). Perception of threat cues in post-traumatic stress disorder: Semantic processing without awareness? *Behaviour Research and Therapy, 25*, 469–476.

Vasterling, J. J., Brailey, K., Constans, J. I., & Sutker, P. B. (1998). Attention and memory dysfunction in posttraumatic stress disorder. *Neuropsychology, 12*, 125–133.

Vrana, S. R., Roodman, A., & Beckman, J. C. (1995). Selective processing of trauma-relevant words in posttraumatic stress disorder. *Journal of Anxiety Disorders, 9*, 515–530.

Warda, G., & Bryant, R. A. (1998). Cognitive bias in acute stress disorder. *Behaviour Research and Therapy, 36*, 1177–1183.

Wessel, I., Merckelbach, H., & Dekkers, T. (2002). Autobiographical memory specificity, intrusive memory, and general memory skills in Dutch–Indonesian survivors of the World War II era. *Journal of Traumatic Stress, 15*, 227–234.

Wilhelm, S., McNally, R. J., Baer, L., & Florin, I. (1997). Autobiographical memory in obsessive–compulsive disorder. *British Journal of Clinical Psychology, 36*, 21–31.

Williams, J. M. G. (1996). In D. C. Rubin (Ed.), *Remembering our past: Studies in autobiographical memory* (pp. 244–267). Cambridge, UK: Cambridge University Press.

Williams, J. M. G., & Broadbent, K. (1986). Autobiographical memory in suicide attempters. *Journal of Abnormal Psychology, 95*, 144–149.

Williams, J. M. G., Mathews, A., & MacLeod, C. (1996). The emotional Stroop task and psychopathology. *Psychological Bulletin, 120*, 3–24.

Williams, J. M. G., Watts, F. N., MacLeod, C., & Mathews, A. (1997). *Cognitive psychology and emotional disorders* (2nd ed.). Chichester, UK: Wiley.

Yiend, J., & Mathews, A. (2001). Anxiety and attention to threatening pictures. *Quarterly Journal of Experimental Psychology, 54A*, 665–681.

Zoellner, L. A., Foa, E. B., Brididi, B., & Przeworski, A. (2000). Are trauma victims susceptible to "false memories?" *Journal of Abnormal Psychology, 109*, 517–524.

Zoellner, L. A., Sacks, M. B., & Foa, E. B. (2003). Directed forgetting following mood induction in chronic posttraumatic stress disorder patients. *Journal of Abnormal Psychology, 112*, 509–514.

CHAPTER 6

Encoding and Retrieval
of Traumatic Memories

CHRIS R. BREWIN

The study of memory for traumatic events has been a persistent source of controversy, and has highlighted the different perspectives of the memory researcher based in the laboratory and the clinician working with actual trauma victims. Typically, clinicians have been impressed by what they see as the unique characteristics of traumatic memory whereas laboratory researchers have been skeptical about the claim that memory for trauma is different from memory for everyday events. On the one hand, critiques of clinical observations based on studies of ordinary memory performance are unconvincing to the clinician, but, on the other hand, clinical claims often appear premature and unwarranted to the laboratory researcher. Despite this potential for misunderstanding, a consensus about what is and is not known about traumatic memory is slowly beginning to emerge. In this chapter I attempt to describe this consensus and make links to the neuropsychology of memory.

EMOTION AND MEMORY IN EVERYDAY LIFE

Studies of "flashbulb memory" in nonclinical participants have provided some of the most striking evidence for the role of emotion in the formation of vivid and persistent memories. In the first and most famous systematic investigation of this phenomenon, participants were asked what they remembered about the circumstances in which they first learned of the death of President John F. Kennedy and of other well-known historical figures (Brown & Kulik, 1977). Information that tended to be recalled included the place participants were in, what they were doing, who the informant was, their own and the informant's emotional reaction, and the aftermath. Brown and Kulik named these "flashbulb memories" because they possessed "a primary, 'live' quality that is almost perceptual. Indeed, it is very like a photograph that indiscriminately preserves the scene in which each of us found himself when the flashbulb was fired" (p. 74). At the same time, Brown and Kulik were clear that this was an imperfect analogy, because flashbulb memories did not record all details indiscriminately and were usually far from complete.

What kinds of events might lead to the formation of a flashbulb memory? Brown and Kulik originally suggested that the three main (and interrelated) characteristics were surprise, level of emotion, and "consequentiality," by which they meant that the event had a lot of direct or indirect consequences for the person, or to put it another way, the event was personally important. Investigations of other public events, such as the assassination of Swedish prime minister Olof Palme, the nuclear accident at Chernobyl, the attempted assassination of President Ronald Reagan, and the loss of the space shuttle *Challenger*, have confirmed that memory for the circumstances in which someone learned about important, emotion-arousing events tends to be persistent and to be associated with vivid visual images (Conway, 1995; Brewer, 1992; Pillemer, 1998). But one of the limitations of these studies is that investigators are totally dependent on their respondents' accounts and have no means of confirming what people say they remember. By collecting memories of the *Challenger* explosion shortly after the event and then following respondents up to check on their recall a year or two later, Neisser and Harsch (1992) showed that a minority of apparent flashbulb memories, even ones in which respondents had high confidence, turned out to be inconsistent.

Subsequent research has indicated that people frequently report vivid memories, but these only rarely concern public events, and are often lacking in any element of surprise or consequentiality (Rubin & Kozin, 1984). Vivid memories are much more likely to concern events that are personally important, and that are associated with strong emotions. These can include positive events such as a romantic attraction, or the first encounter with a person who would prove to be an important influence, or a flash of insight, or a turning point in the person's life (Pillemer, 1998). This suggests that "flashbulb memories" should be regarded as a particular type of emotional memory rather than as a special class of memory in its own right.

To other psychologists the idea that emotion would improve memory appeared unlikely, because of the accompanying narrowing of attention and disruptive effect on mental processing in general. Recall for details has often been found to be worse for emotion-arousing stimuli (e.g., Loftus & Burns, 1982) and by the end of the 1980s there was a general consensus that very high levels of stress would impair the accuracy of memory (Kassin, Ellsworth, & Smith, 1989). A persuasive argument was made that the effect of increased arousal is to increase the accuracy of recall for the central aspects of the event that has been witnessed, while simultaneously decreasing accuracy for its peripheral aspects (Christianson, 1992). Critical objects such as a gun or knife being used in a robbery tend to attract attention, a phenomenon called "weapon focusing," so that while they are well remembered, recall of other aspects of the situation may suffer. Consistent with this, in studies where ordinary people are asked to recall their most traumatic event they typically report remembering more central than peripheral details (Berntsen, 2002; Christianson & Loftus, 1990; Wessel & Merckelbach, 1994).

Comparisons of memory for positive and negative autobiographical events have led to rather inconsistent conclusions. In several studies, it is positive events that appear to be remembered better and in more sensory detail (D'Argembeau, Comblain, & van der Linden, 2003; Destun & Kuiper, 1999; Linton, 1986). Porter and Birt (2001) found that negative memories were associated with fewer taste sensations than positive memories, but included more details overall. Butler and Wolfner (2000) found that negative memories were more likely than positive memories to have a small number of very salient details. The picture is confused because whereas negative memories show an excess of central over peripheral details, this is not true of positive memories (Berntsen, 2002). Thus, studies that explore memory detail may not be comparing like with like. Among other reasons to think that the valence of memories is important is the finding that people recalling positive memories have a "reminiscence bump" with an excess of memories from early adulthood; the same pattern does not hold for negative memories (Berntsen & Rubin, 2002).

Probably a minority of the negative memories in these studies would meet DSM-IV criteria for a traumatic event (e.g., Butler & Wolfner, 2000). Where studies have attempted to isolate extremely stressful memories the results have also been mixed. Porter and Birt (2001) found that memories involving sexual violence were rated as more vivid and containing more sensory components than memories involving other forms of violence. In contrast, Mary Koss and her colleagues (Koss, Figueredo, Bell, Tharan, & Tromp, 1996) found that rape memories, compared to other unpleasant memories, were rated as being less clear and vivid, less likely to occur in a meaningful order, less well-remembered, and were less thought and talked about. Another of the few systematic studies in this area assessed memory in a sample of recent, non-treatment-seeking rape victims (Mechanic, Resick, & Griffin, 1998). Two weeks post-rape, approximately two-thirds of women had a clear memory of the event while one-third had difficulty in remembering at least a few aspects of it. About 10% of the sample said that they were unable to recall many or most aspects of the event. Ten weeks later 82% reported a clear memory, and none of the original 10% with problematic recall were still having problems in remembering the event. Mechanic and colleagues noted that there appeared to be a specific problem in remembering the rape that improved over time.

Investigations of memory for real-life events in normal participants have yielded inconsistent results about the role of emotion. On the one hand, consistent with laboratory studies of experimental materials, emotion tends to be associated with more vivid, detailed recall. Laboratory studies have also indicated that high-arousal and low-arousal events are remembered equally well at short retention intervals, but that memory for high-arousal events increases over time and is superior once time has been allowed to pass after the experiment (e.g., Quevedo et al., 2003). In numerous studies, negative events appear to be recalled overall with less vividness and clarity than positive events, but specific details central to the experience may be retained very well.

Neurobiological studies suggest that increased retention of emotionally arousing material is related to an interaction of arousal at encoding with later modulatory effects of stress hormones such as epinephrine and cortisol (e.g., Cahill, Gorski, & Le, 2003). These effects are at least partly amygdala dependent, and result in enhanced storage for emotional material. Recently it has been shown that the same mechanisms may be responsible both for increased and decreased recall of separate aspects of stimulus material (Strange, Hurlemann, & Dolan, 2003). Under normal conditions, participants presented with a list of words showed increased recall for an unusual emotional word but decreased recall for the immediately preceding (neutral) word. Both effects were blocked by administering propranolol and both were absent in a patient with selective amygdala lesion, suggesting that increased and decreased emotion-dependent recall were both mediated by a beta-adrenergic mechanism influenced by the amygdala.

Almost all of these studies have focused on traditional measures of recall and recognition, and have ignored the tendency for emotional memories to come to mind involuntarily. This is important, because as we will see in the next section, it is involuntary memories that are a particular problem in clinical disorders such as posttraumatic stress disorder (PTSD). Brewin and Saunders (2001), and Holmes, Brewin, and Hennessy (2004) studied voluntary and involuntary memories produced by exposure to a stressful film, and found that measures of recall and recognition were unrelated to the number of involuntary memories reported over the following week. Further progress in understanding the relations between emotion and memory is likely to depend on studies distinguishing more carefully the nature of what is recalled and measuring voluntary and involuntary memories separately.

MEMORY AND PTSD

DSM-IV describes PTSD as characterized by high frequency, distressing, involuntary memories that individuals are unable to forget and make great efforts to prevent coming to mind. Among these is the traumatic "flashback," a type of memory characterized as the spontaneous result of exposure to trauma cues, as being fragmented, as containing prominent perceptual features, and as involving an intense reliving of the event in the present. These characteristics are indeed consistently reported in studies of memory in PTSD patients (Berntsen, Willert, & Rubin, 2003; Bremner et al., 1995; Ehlers et al., 2002; Ehlers & Steil, 1995; van der Kolk & Fisler, 1995), although it should be noted that flashback content sometimes involves not just a literal record but an imaginative extension of what has been experienced (Reynolds & Brewin, 1998). However, few studies have attempted to validate the implied distinction between spontaneous flashbacks and ordinary memories of trauma that may also intrude involuntarily, to measure these separately, or to compare them with deliberately retrievable trauma and nontrauma memories.

One exception was a recent study that focused specifically on involuntary memories, using diary methods, in a small sample of 12 individuals with PTSD (Berntsen, 2001, Study 2). Even when the traumatic event had occurred more than 5 years previously, intrusive trauma memories were more vivid and more likely to be accompanied by physical reactions than were nontrauma memories. Trauma memories were also more likely to have the qualities of flashbacks, although Berntsen reported that some experiences similar to flashbacks occurred in relation to highly positive events.

One possible way of thinking about flashbacks is as involving a breakdown in the everyday process responsible for binding together individual sensory features to form a stable object, episodic memory, or action sequence. Insufficient binding means that objects or memories will be fragmented or incomplete. According to one prominent theory, this binding is brought about by focusing attention on an object or scene, so that the individual features are integrated by virtue of sharing the same location in space (Treisman & Gelade, 1980). During traumatic events attention tends to be restricted and focused on the main source of danger, so that sensory elements from the wider scene will be less effectively bound together. Laboratory research has shown that such unattended patterns or events, provided they are sufficiently novel, produce long-lasting memory traces whose existence can be detected even though they cannot be deliberately retrieved (Treisman & DeSchepper, 1996). A distinct possibility is that flashbacks involve the automatic activation of these memory traces of unattended aspects of the trauma scene.

Controversially, several authors have suggested that some aspects of traumatic events seem to become fixed in the mind, unaltered by the passage of time, being continually reexperienced in the form of images or "video clips" (Ehlers & Steil, 1995; Herman, 1992; van der Kolk & Fisler, 1995). Although this represents PTSD patients' own views of their memories, some systematic studies have found that trauma memories do not invariably remain unaltered over the passage of time (Schwarz, Kowalski, & McNally, 1993; Southwick, Morgan, Nicolaou, & Charney, 1997). Again, the failure to distinguish between flashbacks and ordinary memories, or between voluntary and involuntary memories, means that it is difficult to evaluate whether these claims perhaps apply to one particular type of memory but not the other.

Consistent with research on normal emotional memory, DSM-IV also describes PTSD as being characterized by amnesia for the details of the event. Patients typically remember that the traumatic event happened but describe blanks or periods during which their memory for the details of the event is vague and unclear. In addition to the endorsement of this symptom on diagnostic measures there is some support for the position that memories in traumatized individuals with clinical disorders tend to be disorganized and contain gaps (Foa, Molnar, & Cashman, 1995; Harvey & Bryant, 1999). During psychotherapy it is common for patients to say that these details are returning to them and that they now recall numerous aspects of the event that had been forgotten. The most dramatic examples of memory loss occur when patients describe complete loss of memory for the fact that the event occurred in the first place, followed by recovery of memory. A number of well-documented and independently verified accounts of such recovered memories now exist (Brewin, 2003). How is it possible that the memories of trauma patients are at the same time exceptionally clear and vivid, but also disorganized and fragmented? The two main approaches involve arguing either that these recollections stem from a distorted version of ordinary memories, or reveal the presence of two separate kinds of memory.

Single-Representation Theories

A very influential approach to memory suggests that it can be thought of as a network involving many thousands of nodes with a dense set of interconnections between them. Each node represents a person, an object, a feature such color or shape, a concept, or an emotion. In this theory, the representation consists of the pattern of interconnections between the nodes. Lang (1979, 1985) adapted this theory and proposed that a frightening experience creates a fear network in memory consisting of stimulus information about the traumatic event, response information about emotional and physiological reactions, and meaning information. He suggested that when someone encountered a situation with matching features or cues the original fear memory would be automatically activated, producing the same physiological response and interpretation of being in danger.

Foa and her colleagues (e.g., Foa & Rothbaum, 1998) have developed their emotional processing theory based on these ideas and suggested several ways in which a traumatic event leads to a kind of structure of memory that is different from one created by an everyday frightening experience. One way involved particularly large numbers of potent stimulus–danger interconnections being formed between the relevant nodes, so that their connections to each other became much stronger than their connections to non-trauma-related nodes. They also proposed that the memory structure would contain large numbers of response elements, which might be associated with negative evaluations of the self (such as seeing oneself as weak or vulnerable). Another suggestion was based on the observation that the severity of the event frequently disrupts the cognitive processes of attention and memory at the time of the trauma and produces dissociative states such as out-of-body experiences. Foa and her colleagues argued that this disruption leads to the formation of a disjointed and fragmented fear structure.

In support of this and other memory network theories of PTSD (Chemtob, Roitblat, Hamada, Carlson, & Twentyman, 1988; Creamer, Burgess, & Pattison, 1992), Foa et al. (1995) analyzed the trauma narratives produced by rape victims at the beginning and end of exposure therapy for their PTSD. They found that the percentage of thoughts and feelings increased over the period of therapy, particularly thoughts reflecting attempts to organize the trauma memory. Although a measure of the fragmentation of the narrative did not change over this period, reductions in fragmentation were associated with better treatment outcome. More recently, evidence has been collected supporting the prediction that higher levels of fragmentation in the trauma narrative are related to the occurrence of dissociative responses at the time the event occurred (Murray, Ehlers, & Mayou, 2002).

Some of the main objections to the associative network approach to emotional disorders are theoretical ones, and have been discussed by Teasdale and Barnard (1993). They pointed out that in the original form of the network model there was only one node for each emotion, so that for example, simply talking about fear would necessarily have the effect of arousing some degree of fearful feelings. The single level of representation also prevents the model from distinguishing between remembering an event in an emotion-laden, "hot" way and remembering it on another occasion in a more detached, "cool" fashion. Nor can it easily explain why a therapy client might completely agree intellectually with his or her therapist's assertion that he or she is a good person but continue to have a gut feeling that he or she is a bad person.

A more general problem with the network approach is that it cannot represent knowledge at levels of meaning beyond that of the word or sentence, whereas there is every reason for thinking that the meaning of emotional events tends to be complex, multilayered, and often impossible to capture in words (Dalgleish, 2004). Other objections to the network approach are more specific to PTSD. It is unclear how network models would explain the special characteristics of flashbacks, such as the perceptual detail, the exclusively automatic retrieval, and the distortion in the sense of time, and how some trauma memories take the form of flashbacks while others appear like ordinary memories.

A more recent version of the single-representation approach has been put forward by Conway and Pleydell-Pearce (2000). These cognitive psychologists argued that memories for autobiographical events consist of a hierarchy of information, ranging from the very general (e.g., how the event relates to life periods and life themes) to the very specific (e.g., perceptual details of how things look or feel, which they refer to as event-specific knowledge or ESK). Like Foa, they argued that under extreme stress the representations would be fragmented and that ESK would be poorly integrated with the rest of the trauma memory. These conditions might make it easier for specific reminders that matched the ESK in the trauma memory to automatically activate the representation in the form of a flashback. At other times more general information about the event could be utilized to provide a narrative account to family and friends. This approach meets many of the deficiencies of network theories, but suggests that there is an important distinction in memory between higher-level information about traumas and the largely perceptual ESK.

Multiple-Representation Theories

Brown and Kulik (1977) had suggested that their flashbulb memory findings could be accounted for by a special type of memory system that was brought into play when a person encountered a surprising, consequential, and emotion-arousing event. Unlike an ordinary memory, which is quickly forgotten, the memory record created by the event remained fixed for a long period of time. They speculated that the memory was not of a verbal or narrative form, but might consist of an image. Pillemer and White (1989) also argued for the existence of two separate memory systems: One system "is present from birth and operational throughout life. . . . The memories are expressed through images, behaviors, or emotions." A second memory system "emerges during the preschool years. . . . Event representations entering the higher-order system are actively thought about or mentally processed and thus are encoded in narrative form" (p. 326).

The idea that there is a fundamentally distinct type of memory for traumatic events dates back at least as far as Pierre Janet (1904), the French neurologist who distinguished traumatic memory from ordinary or narrative memory. Janet proposed that people may be unable to assimilate extremely frightening experiences into their ordinary beliefs, assumptions, and meaning structures, in which case these experiences would be stored in a different form, "dissociated" from conscious awareness and voluntary control. Traumatic memory was inflexible and fixed, in contrast to narrative memory, which was adaptable to current circumstances; traumatic memory involved a constellation of feelings and bodily reactions whereas narrative memory consisted of independent elements that did not invariably coexist; traumatic memory was evoked automatically by reminders of the traumatic situation whereas narrative memory occurred in response to conscious attempts at recollection.

Janet's ideas continue to be influential among leading trauma therapists and researchers (e.g., Terr, 1990; van der Hart & Horst, 1989; van der Kolk & van der Hart, 1991). Less has been written, however, about how flashbacks and ordinary memories coexist. It does not seem to be the case that narrative memory simply stops when the trauma starts and does not resume until it is over. Rather, both the narrative memory system and the special trauma memory system continue to operate alongside each other, but from time to time one may take precedence over the other. The dual-representation theory of PTSD (Brewin, 2001, 2003; Brewin, Dalgleish, & Joseph, 1996) attempted to capture this dynamic relationship between the two memory systems.

Dual-representation theory proposes that narrative memory of a trauma reflects the operation of a "verbally accessible memory" system (or VAM), so called to reflect the fact that the trauma memory is integrated with other autobiographical memories and the fact that it can be deliberately retrieved as and when required. VAM memories of trauma are therefore represented within a complete personal context comprising past, present, and future. They contain information that the individual has attended to before, during, and after the traumatic event, and that received sufficient conscious processing to be transferred to a long-term memory store in a form that can later be deliberately retrieved. These memories are available for verbal communication with others, but the amount of information they contain is restricted because they only record what has been consciously attended to. Diversion of attention to the immediate source of threat and the effects of high levels of arousal greatly restrict the volume of information that can be registered during the event itself.

VAM memories are used to evaluate the trauma both at the time it is happening and afterwards, as the person considers the consequences and implications of the event, and asks themselves how it could have been prevented. Thus the emotions that accompany VAM memories are mainly directed at the past (regret about missed opportunities, anger about careless risks being taken), or at the future (sadness at the loss of cherished plans, hopelessness at the thought of not finding fulfillment). They also include emotions generated by retrospectively evaluating what happened at the time. This might involve guilt or shame over a perceived failure to fight back against an attacker or to help other people who were injured. Brewin and colleagues called these "secondary emotions" because they were not experienced at the time of the trauma itself.

In contrast, the theory proposes that reliving reflects the operation of a "situationally accessible memory" system (or SAM), so called to reflect the fact that flashbacks are only ever triggered involuntarily by situational reminders of the trauma (encountered either in the external environment or in the internal environment of a person's mental processes). The SAM system contains information that has been obtained from more extensive, lower-level perceptual processing of the traumatic scene, such as sights and sounds that were too briefly apprehended to be bound together in a conscious memory and hence did not become recorded in the VAM system. The SAM system also stores information about the person's bodily response to the trauma, such as changes in heart rate, flushing, temperature changes, and pain. This results in flashbacks being more detailed and emotion-laden than ordinary memories.

Because the SAM system does not use a verbal code, these memories are difficult to communicate to others and they do not necessarily interact with and get updated by other autobiographical knowledge. For example, someone could have a flashback of being beaten up in a street fight and experience that as happening in the present while knowing that the person beating him up was at that moment sitting in jail. SAM memories can be difficult to control because people cannot always regulate their exposure to sights, sounds, smells, et cetera, that act as reminders of the trauma. The emotions that accompany SAM memories are restricted to those that were experienced during the trauma or subsequent moments of intense arousal ("primary emotions"). They mainly consist of fear, helplessness, and horror but may less often include other emotions such as shame (Grey, Holmes, & Brewin, 2001). The longer and more drawn-out the trauma, the more opportunity there is for the person to experience a range of emotions, and for these to be coded into a SAM memory.

Essentially, single-representation theories imply that there is one type of trauma memory that gradually changes over time, either in therapy or as the person makes a normal recovery. In contrast, the dual-representation theories predict that two types of trauma memory can be detected in the same individual at the same time. What evidence supports this? Turning first to research with normal participants, Mack and Rock (1998) have argued persuasively that only those objects to which attention is voluntarily directed or that capture attention are consciously perceived. Under even ordinary conditions of attentional diversion, people frequently fail to see highly visible but unexpected objects before their eyes, a phenomenon known as "inattentional blindness." They have shown the equivalent phenomenon in other senses, that is, auditory deafness and tactile insensitivity, and suggest that their results are related to some people's reports of not feeling any pain after a serious injury. Critically, Mack and Rock have also found that the unattended objects or items that are not consciously seen in their experiments are nevertheless encoded and analyzed in considerable detail, and can unconsciously affect participants' responses on tests of indirect memory.

These surprising laboratory findings appear to be very relevant to trauma victims, who may report that they simply failed to hear words that were shouted or shots that were fired in close proximity to them. Just as in Mack and Rock's studies, their attention tends to be captured by the immediate source of threat, so that they fail to notice other salient aspects of the trauma scene. The findings are also consistent with the experiments showing that unattended objects or events can leave long-lasting, unconscious memory traces. New evidence suggests that the perceptual features of these unattended objects are recorded in a set of memory stores. Each individual feature, such as color or location, is encoded in parallel in its own limited-capacity store. Information about how features are bound together into a whole is dependent on attention and is recorded in a separate memory system (Wheeler & Treisman, 2002). These results support the idea that information can be encoded in considerable detail even though not consciously perceived at the time, with the result that there can be alternative memory representations of the same experience that differ significantly in what they contain.

Further evidence for the theory was provided by Holmes et al.'s (2004) study of nonclinical participants. They predicted that involuntary intrusive memories of a stressful film, theoretically underpinned by the SAM system, should be reduced if participants carried out a secondary visuospatial task while watching the film. This task was hypothesized to compete for resources with the SAM system, resulting in an impoverished representation. As expected, compared with a control no-task condition, this task produced a consistent and significant decrease in the number of involuntary memories. Holmes and colleagues also predicted that intrusive memories should increase if a secondary verbal task was performed. This task was hypothesized to compete for resources with the VAM system, again resulting in an impoverished representation that would be less able to inhibit the retrieval of involuntary memories from the SAM system. As expected, compared with a control no-task condition, this task produced a consistent and significant increase in the number of involuntary memories.

Hellawell and Brewin (2002, 2004) conducted the first study to test whether flashbacks and ordinary memories of trauma had the different characteristics predicted by dual-representation theory. They described the difference between flashbacks and ordinary memories to people with PTSD and then had them write a detailed narrative of their traumatic event. At the completion of the narrative, participants retrospectively identified periods during which they experienced the two types of memory. Consistent with prediction, during parts of the narrative involving the experience of reliving they used more words describing seeing, hearing, smelling, tasting, and bodily sensations, as well as more verbs and references to motion. Again in line with predictions, fear, helplessness, horror, and thoughts of death were more prominent during the reliving sections and secondary emotions such as sadness were more prominent during the ordinary memory sections.

Hellawell and Brewin also reasoned that if reliving experiences are based on a memory system that selectively processes lower-level perceptual information, then they should interfere with performance on other tasks that also made demands on this system, but not interfere with unrelated tasks. So, while participants were writing their narratives, they were stopped on two occasions, once when they were in a reliving phase and once when they were in an ordinary memory phase, and made to carry out two tasks. One task, trail-making, involved visuospatial abilities and the other, counting backwards in threes, involved more verbal abilities. The results showed that the trail-making performance was much worse when participants had been halted during a reliving phase of their narrative than when they had been halted during an ordinary memory phase, whereas counting backwards in threes was adversely affected to an equal extent in both phases.

In summary, the Hellawell and Brewin (2002, 2004) study offers preliminary evidence that two types of trauma memory exist simultaneously and can readily be distinguished by individuals with PTSD. As predicted by dual-representation theory, these memory types appear to differ in the information they contain, in the emotions that are associated with them, in the spontaneous movements and facial changes that accompany them, and in their impact on the performance of related tasks. All this evidence is indirect, and in need of confirmation by alternative methods. The next section reviews the literature on memory and brain function to consider whether there is a plausible neural substrate for two types of trauma memory.

A NEURAL SUBSTRATE FOR TRAUMA MEMORIES

Within the declarative memory system, which is concerned with the conscious knowledge of facts and events, the hippocampus appears to be specialized for the learning of context (including temporal context; Kesner, 1998), and for learning relational properties among stimuli. It is thought to be crucial in binding together the separate features or elements of an episode to make a coherent and integrated ensemble. Eichenbaum (1997) proposed that the hippocampus encodes separate stimulus elements and the relations between them such that the representations can be utilized flexibly and accessed in a variety of ways. It has also been suggested that the hippocampal system is particularly associated with memories of conscious experience (Moscovitch, 1995).

From the perspective of dual-representation theory, it would appear that hippocampal processing is likely to be a critical aspect of verbally accessible (narrative) memories that form the basis of deliberate appraisal and communication concerning the trauma. The hippocampus is highly sensitive to stress, being well-supplied with receptors that are occupied by stress hormones. A wealth of animal studies confirm that severe stress impairs hippocampal function and memory performance, and there is a corresponding literature in humans. This demonstrates impaired explicit memory performance associated with raised levels of glucocorticoids, adrenal steroid hormones that are released after stressful experiences, in the context of naturally occurring conditions or experimental treatments (Alderson & Novack, 2002). Recently, acutely elevated levels of glucocorticoids were found to be associated with impaired memory and reduced blood flow in areas of the medial temporal lobe adjacent to the hippocampus (de Quervain et al., 2003). At present it is unclear whether high levels of stress hormones impair the consolidation of memories, their retrieval, or both. They appear to have a number of separate neuroanatomical effects on the hippocampus, including the impairment of synaptic plasticity, the retraction of dendritic processes, reduction in volume, the inhibition of neurogenesis, and ultimately neuronal death (Sapolsky, 2003).

Importantly, studies reveal that mild to moderate levels of stress and severe levels of stress have opposite effects on memory function. This has been related to different levels of occupancy of different types of receptors in the hippocampus. At low levels of stress there is heavy occupancy of mineralocorticoid receptors and low to moderate occupancy of glucocorticoid receptors. Memory impairments appear to be associated with the high levels of occupancy of glucocorticoid receptors that are associated with severe stress (Alderson & Novack, 2002; Kim & Diamond, 2002; Sapolsky, 2003). At present it is unclear whether reduced hippocampal functioning in PTSD is primarily related to the effects of severe stress, to preexisting vulnerabilities, or both.

Whereas explicit memory is associated with the hippocampus, the various forms of implicit memory (e.g., priming, fear conditioning) do not appear to have any particular locus in the brain. The involuntary memories that are characteristic of PTSD may be considered to be related to implicit memory, in that they share the characteristics of being automatically retrieved in a predictable, cue-driven manner, and being hard to control. They are unlike normal examples of implicit memory, however, in that they possess explicit trauma-related content that is immediately recognized by the person experiencing them. In the dual-representation theory of PTSD, both flashbacks and fear conditioning are considered to be products of the SAM system. It is possible for fear-relevant information to reach the amygdala via a number of different routes, independently of the hippocampus. For example, the visual areas of the inferior temporal cortex, which are involved in the late stages of sensory processing, project strongly to the amygdala. The pathway from the thalamus to the amygdala has a less sophisticated processing capacity and would be capable of transmitting lower-level sensory features of frightening situations. Memories formed in these ways would not be open to deliberate recall, but could be accessed automatically by reminders, particularly perceptual features, similar to those recorded in the fear memory.

As noted by several authors, stress appears to have very different effects on the hippocampus and the amygdala. The functioning of the amygdala appears generally to be enhanced as stress increases, consistent with the formation of overly strong implicit memories related to autonomic conditioning, and fear (Sapolsky, 2003; Metcalfe & Jacobs, 1998; Pitman, Shalev, & Orr, 2000). Thus, memories originating in the SAM system (such as flashbacks) could be enhanced at the same time as memories originating in the VAM system (narrative memories) were impaired. Consistent with this, there is preliminary evidence that neuronal morphology in the hippocampus and amygdala are affected by stress in very different ways, with the same stress experience producing dendritic atrophy and debranching in the hippocampus while simultaneously producing enhanced dendritic arborization in the amygdala (Vyas, Bernal, & Chattarji, 2003; Vyas, Mitra, Rao, & Chattarji, 2002).

These memory systems, and the effects of stress upon them, provide a plausible neural basis for the verbally accessible and situationally accessible memories proposed earlier in the chapter, and for the symptoms of PTSD. Verbally accessible memories can be deliberately recalled, and used to consciously evaluate the trauma, to relate it to past and present, and to communicate about it with others. These flexible, declarative memories, subject to modification and change but often vague, disorganized, and full of gaps, strongly suggest a form of representation that is dependent on the hippocampus.

Equally, there are many similarities between the notions of situationally accessible memory and nondeclarative memory, although of course flashback memories are not nondeclarative in the usual sense of this term. As we noted earlier, flashbacks are a highly perceptual form of memory that are elicited automatically and are only under limited conscious control. They have been claimed to be relatively stereotyped and unchanging even after multiple recall episodes, whereas ordinary memories are altered by repeated recall. They are also reexperienced in the present, that is, they do not possess an associated temporal context. All of these features suggest an image-based, nonhippocampally dependent form of memory that is unable to encode information about past versus present (Brewin, 2001, 2003). From a neuroanatomical perspective it is interesting that the amygdala projects strongly to almost all regions of the brain involved in visual processing. The function of these projections is poorly understood, but one possibility is that they could support the experience of flashbacks. Given the highly visual nature of most reexperiencing in PTSD, it is also interesting that the amygdala has many more anatomical connections with visual than with auditory areas of the brain (Amaral, Price, Pitkanen, & Carmichael, 1992).

CONCLUSIONS

The study of traumatic memory is currently benefiting from an unprecedented collaboration between neuroscientists, experimental psychologists, and clinicians, with contributions from numerous disciplines such as neuroanatomy, electrophysiology, cognitive psychology, clinical neuropsychology, and phenomenology. There is a remarkable consensus that emotion has complex effects on memory, both enhancing and impairing it, and it is now possible to relate these apparently paradoxical effects to a plausible neural substrate focused particularly on the interaction between the hippocampal system and the amygdala. It is evident that researchers need to measure traumatic memories in much more sophisticated ways than has usually been the case. Specifically, there is evidence that the overall amount of detail in a memory may be less important than the distribution of detail centrally and peripherally, and the presence of particularly salient individual details. There are also compelling reasons to conclude that the mechanisms underlying standard measures of recall and recognition are distinct from the mechanisms underlying involuntary memories. The nature of flashbacks, and the experience of reliving, are central to PTSD but poorly understood and hard to measure. These insights are already beginning to have an impact on theories of PTSD and have important consequences for how psychotherapy, in its systematic attempt to modify trauma memories, should be conceived.

REFERENCES

Alderson, A. L., & Novack, T. A. (2002). Neurophysiological and clinical aspects of glucocorticoids and memory: A review. *Journal of Clinical and Experimental Neurophysiology, 24,* 335–355.

Amaral, D. G., Price, J. L., Pitkanen, A., & Carmichael, S. T. (1992). Anatomical organization of the primate amygdaloid complex. In J. P. Aggleton (Ed.), *The amygdala: Neurobiological aspects of emotion, memory, and mental dysfunction* (pp. 1–66). New York: Wiley-Liss.

Berntsen, D. (2001). Involuntary memories of emotional events: Do memories of traumas and extremely happy events differ? *Applied Cognitive Psychology, 15,* S135–S158.

Berntsen, D. (2002). Tunnel memories for autobiographical events: Central details are remembered more frequently from shocking than from happy experiences. *Memory and Cognition, 30,* 1010–1020.

Berntsen, D., & Rubin, D. C. (2002). Emotionally charged autobiographical memories across the life span: The recall of happy, sad, traumatic, and involuntary memories. *Psychology and Aging, 17,* 636–652.

Berntsen, D., Willert, M., & Rubin, D. C. (2003). Splintered memories or vivid landmarks? Qualities and organization of traumatic memories with and without PTSD. *Applied Cognitive Psychology, 17,* 675–693.

Bremner, J. D., Krystal, J. H., Southwick, S. M., & Charney, D. S. (1995). Functional neuroanatomical correlates of the effects of stress on memory. *Journal of Traumatic Stress, 8,* 527–553.

Brewer, W. F. (1992). The theoretical and empirical status of the flashbulb memory hypothesis. In E. Winograd & U. Neisser (Eds.), *Affect and accuracy in recall: Studies of flashbulb memories* (pp. 274–305). Cambridge, UK: Cambridge University Press.

Brewin, C. R. (2001). A cognitive neuroscience account of posttraumatic stress disorder and its treatment. *Behaviour Research and Therapy, 39,* 373–393.

Brewin, C. R. (2003). *Posttraumatic stress disorder: Malady or myth?* New Haven, CT: Yale University Press.

Brewin, C. R., Dalgleish, T., & Joseph, S. (1996). A dual representation theory of post traumatic stress disorder. *Psychological Review, 103,* 670–686.

Brewin, C. R., & Saunders, J. (2001). The effect of dissociation at encoding on intrusive memories for a stressful film. *British Journal of Medical Psychology, 74,* 467–472.

Brown, R., & Kulik, J. (1977). Flashbulb memories. *Cognition, 5,* 73–99.

Butler, L. D., & Wolfner, A. L. (2000). Some characteristics of positive and negative ("most traumatic") event memories in a college sample. *Journal of Trauma and Dissociation, 1*, 45–68.

Cahill, L., Gorski, L., & Le, K. (2003). Enhanced human memory consolidation with post-learning stress: Interaction with the degree of arousal at encoding. *Learning and Memory, 10*, 270–274.

Chemtob, C., Roitblat, H. L., Hamada, R. S., Carlson, J. G., & Twentyman, C. T. (1988). A cognitive action theory of post-traumatic stress disorder. *Journal of Anxiety Disorders, 2*, 253–275.

Christianson, S. A. (1992). Emotional stress and eyewitness memory: A critical review. *Psychological Bulletin, 112*, 284–309.

Christianson, S. A., & Loftus, E. F. (1990). Some characteristics of people's traumatic memories. *Bulletin of the Psychonomic Society, 28*, 195–198.

Conway, M. A. (1995). *Flashbulb memories*. Hove, UK: Erlbaum.

Conway, M. A., & Pleydell-Pearce, C. W. (2000). The construction of autobiographical memories in the self-memory system. *Psychological Review, 107*, 261–288.

Creamer, M., Burgess, P., & Pattison, P. (1992). Reaction to trauma: A cognitive processing model. *Journal of Abnormal Psychology, 101*, 452–459.

Dalgleish, T. (2004). Cognitive approaches to posttraumatic stress disorder: The evolution of multirepresentational theorizing. *Psychological Bulletin, 130*, 228–260.

D'Argembeau, A., Comblain, C., & van der Linden, M. (2003). Phenomenal characteristics of autobiographical memories for positive, negative, and neutral events. *Applied Cognitive Psychology, 17*, 281–294.

de Quervain, D. J.-F., Henke, K., Aerni, A., Treyer, V., McGaugh, J.L., Berthold, T., Nitsch, R.M., Buck, A., Roozendaal, B., & Hock, C. (2003). Glucocorticoid-induced impairment of declarative memory retrieval is asociated with reduced blood flow in the medial temporal lobe. *European Journal of Neuroscience, 17*, 1296–1302.

Destun, L. M., & Kuiper, N. A. (1999). Phenomenal characteristics associated with real and imagined events: The effects of event valence and absorption. *Applied Cognitive Psychology, 13*, 175–186.

Ehlers, A., Hackmann, A., Steil, R., Clohessy, S., Wenninger, K, & Winter, H. (2002). The nature of intrusive memories after trauma: The warning signal hypothesis. *Behaviour Research and Therapy, 40*, 995–1002.

Ehlers, A., & Steil, R. (1995). Maintenance of intrusive memories in posttraumatic stress disorder: A cognitive approach. *Behavioural and Cognitive Psychotherapy, 23*, 217–249.

Eichenbaum, H. (1997). Declarative memory: Insights from cognitive neurobiology. *Annual Review of Psychology, 48*, 547–572.

Foa, E. B., & Rothbaum, B. O. (1998). *Treating the trauma of rape: Cognitive-behavioral therapy for PTSD*. New York: Guilford Press.

Foa, E. B., Molnar, C., & Cashman, L. (1995). Change in rape narratives during exposure to therapy for posttraumatic stress disorder. *Journal of Traumatic Stress, 8*, 675–690.

Grey, N., Holmes, E., & Brewin, C. R. (2001). Peritraumatic emotional 'hotspots' in traumatic memory: A case series of patients with posttraumatic stress disorder. *Behavioural and Cognitive Psychotherapy, 29*, 367–372.

Harvey, A. G., & Bryant, R. A. (1999). A qualitative investigation of the organization of traumatic memories. *British Journal of Clinical Psychology, 38*, 401–405.

Hellawell, S. J., & Brewin, C. R. (2002). A comparison of flashbacks and ordinary autobiographical memories of trauma: Cognitive resources and behavioural observations. *Behaviour Research and Therapy, 40*, 1139–1152.

Hellawell, S. J., & Brewin, C. R. (2004). A comparison of flashbacks and ordinary autobiographical memories of trauma: Content and language. *Behaviour Research and Therapy, 42*, 1–12.

Herman, J. L. (1992). *Trauma and recovery.* London: Pandora Books.

Holmes, E., Brewin, C. R., & Hennessy, R. (2004). Trauma films, information processing, and intrusive memory development. *Journal of Experimental Psychology: General, 133*, 3–22.

Janet, P. (1904). L'amnésie et la dissociation des souvenirs par l'emotion. *Journal de Psychologie, 1*, 417–453.

Kassin, S. M., Ellsworth, P. C., & Smith, V. L. (1989). The "general acceptance" of psychological research on eyewitness testimony: A survey of the experts. *American Psychologist, 44*, 1089–1098.

Kesner, R. P. (1998). Neural mediation of memory for time: Role of the hippocampus and medial prefrontal cortex. *Psychonomic Bulletin and Review, 5*, 585–596.

Kim, J. J., & Diamond, D. M. (2002). The stressed hippocampus, synaptic plasticity, and lost memories. *Nature Reviews Neuroscience, 3*, 453–462.

Koss, M. P., Figueredo, A. J., Bell, I., Tharan, M., & Tromp, S. (1996). Traumatic memory characteristics: A cross-validated mediational model of response to rape among employed women. *Journal of Abnormal Psychology, 105*, 421–432.

Lang, P. J. (1979). A bio-informational theory of emotional imagery. *Psychophysiology, 16*, 495–512.

Lang, P. J. (1985). The cognitive psychophysiology of emotion: Fear and anxiety. In A. H. Tuma & J. D. Maser (Eds.), *Anxiety and the anxiety disorders* (pp. 131–170). Hillsdale, NJ: Erlbaum.

Linton, M. (1986). Ways of searching and the contents of memory. In D. C. Rubin (Ed.), *Autobiographical memory* (pp. 50–67). Cambridge, UK: Cambridge University Press.

Loftus, E. F., & Burns, T. (1982). Mental shock can produce retrograde amnesia. *Memory and Cognition, 10*, 318–323.

Mack, A., & Rock, I. (1998). *Inattentional blindness.* Cambridge, MA: MIT Press.

Mechanic, M. B., Resick, P. A., & Griffin, M. G. (1998). A comparison of normal forgetting, psychopathology, and information-processing models of reported amnesia for recent sexual trauma. *Journal of Consulting and Clinical Psychology, 66*, 948–957.

Metcalfe, J., & Jacobs, W. J. (1998). Emotional memory: The effects of stress on "cool" and "hot" memory systems. In D. L. Medin (Ed.), *The psychology of learning and motivation* (Vol. 38, pp. 187–222). New York: Academic Press.

Moscovitch, M. (1995). Recovered consciousness: A hypothesis concerning modularity and episodic memory. *Journal of Clinical and Experimental Neuropsychology, 17*, 276–290.

Murray, J., Ehlers, A., & Mayou, R. (2002). Dissociation and posttraumatic stress disorder: Two prospective studies of motor vehicle accident survivors. *British Journal of Psychiatry, 180*, 363–368.

Neisser, U., & Harsch, N. (1992). Phantom flashbulbs: False recollections of hearing the news about *Challenger*. In E. Winograd & U. Neisser (Eds.), *Affect and accuracy in recall: Studies of flashbulb memories* (pp. 9–31). Cambridge, UK: Cambridge University Press.

Pillemer, D. B. (1998). *Momentous events, vivid memories*. Cambridge, MA: Harvard University Press.

Pillemer, D. B., & White, S. H. (1989). Childhood events recalled by children and adults. In H. W. Reese (Ed.), *Advances in child development and behavior* (Vol. 21, pp. 297–340). Orlando, FL: Academic Press.

Pitman, R. L., Shalev, A. Y., & Orr, S. P. (2000). Posttraumatic stress disorder: Emotion, conditioning, and memory. In M. S. Gazzaniga (Ed.), *The new cognitive neurosciences* (2nd ed., pp. 1133–1147). Cambridge, MA: MIT Press.

Porter, S., & Birt, A. R. (2001). Is traumatic memory special? A comparison of traumatic memory characteristics with memory for other emotional life experiences. *Applied Cognitive Psychology, 15*, S101–S117.

Quevedo, J., Sant'Anna, M. K., Madruga, M., Lovato, I., de-Paris, F., Kapczinski, F., Izquierdo, I., & Cahill, L. (2003). Differential effects of emotional arousal in short- and long-term memory in healthy adults. *Neurobiology of Learning and Memory, 79*, 132–135.

Reynolds, M., & Brewin, C. R. (1998). Intrusive cognitions, coping strategies and emotional responses in depression, post-traumatic stress disorder, and a nonclinical population. *Behaviour Research and Therapy, 36*, 135–147.

Rubin, D. C., & Kozin, M. (1984). Vivid memories. *Cognition, 16*, 81–95.

Sapolsky, R. M. (2003). Stress and plasticity in the limbic system. *Neurochemical Research, 28*, 1735–1742.

Schwarz, E. D., Kowalski, J. M., & McNally, R. J. (1993). Malignant memories: Posttraumatic changes in memory in adults after a school shooting. *Journal of Traumatic Stress, 6*, 545–553.

Southwick, S. M., Morgan, A. C., Nicolaou, A. L., & Charney, D.S. (1997). Consistency of memory for combat-related traumatic events in veterans of operation desert storm. *American Journal of Psychiatry, 154*, 173–177.

Strange, B. A., Hurlemann, R., & Dolan, R. J. (2003). An emotion-induced retrograde amnesia in humans is amygdala- and beta-adrenergic-dependent. *Proceedings of the National Academy of Sciences of the United States of America, 100*, 13626–13631.

Teasdale, J. D., & Barnard, P. J. (1993). *Affect, cognition, and change*. Hove, UK: Erlbaum.

Terr, L. (1990). *Too scared to cry*. New York: Basic Books.

Treisman, A., & DeSchepper, B. (1996). Object tokens, attention, and visual memory. In T. Inui & J. L. McClelland (Eds.), *Attention and performance XVI: Information integration in perception and communication* (pp. 15–46). Cambridge, MA: MIT Press.

Treisman, A., & Gelade, G. (1980). A feature integration theory of attention. *Cognitive Psychology, 12*, 97–136.

van der Hart, O., & Horst, R. (1989). The dissociation theory of pierre janet. *Journal of Traumatic Stress, 2*, 397–412.

van der Kolk, B. A., & Fisler, R. (1995). Dissociation and the fragmentary nature of traumatic memories: Overview and exploratory study. *Journal of Traumatic Stress, 8,* 505–525.

van der Kolk, B. A., & van der Hart, O. (1991). The intrusive past: The flexibility of memory and the engraving of trauma. *American Imago, 48,* 425–454.

Vyas, A., Mitra, R., Rao, B. S. S., & Chattarji, S. (2002). Chronic stress induces contrasting patterns of dendritic remodeling in hippocampal and amygdaloid neurons. *Journal of Neuroscience, 22,* 6810–6818.

Vyas, A., Bernal, S., & Chattarji, S. (2003). Effects of chronic stress on dendritic arborization in the central and extended amygdala. *Brain Research, 965,* 290–294.

Wessel, I., & Merckelbach, H. (1994). Characteristics of traumatic memories in normal subjects. *Behavioural and Cognitive Psychotherapy, 22,* 315–324.

Wheeler, M. E., & Treisman, A. M. (2002). Binding in short-term visual memory. *Journal of Experimental Psychology: General, 131,* 48–64.

PART IV

Developmental and Population-Specific Perspectives

CHAPTER 7

Early Trauma Exposure and the Brain

MICHAEL D. DE BELLIS, STEPHEN R. HOOPER,
and JENNIFER L. SAPIA

Early trauma exposure is a serious problem with consequences for the individual and society. Children who are victims of maltreatment may experience chronic and multiple forms of abuse including neglect and physical, sexual, or emotional abuse (Kaufman, Jones, Stieglitz, Vitulano, & Mannarino, 1994; Levy, Markovic, Chaudry, Ahart, & Torres, 1995; McGee, Wolfe, Yuen, Wilson, & Carnochan, 1995; Widom, 1989). Witnessing domestic and/or community violence also are common causes of emotional, behavioral, and developmental difficulties in children (Buka, Stichick, Birdthistle, & Earls, 2001; Kitzmann, Gaylord, Holt, & Kenny, 2003). These traumatic experiences likely produce a chronic stress response that can affect the child's neurobiological, emotional, behavioral, cognitive, and interpersonal development (Cicchetti & Carlson, 1989; De Bellis, 2001; Perry & Pollard, 1998; Rutter & Plomin, 1997). This process may have adverse effects on childhood brain development contributing to posttraumatic stress disorder (PTSD), cognitive–learning problems, and comorbid mental illness. Significant advances have been made in characterizing neurobiological reactions to traumatic stress in adults, particularly with respect to PTSD, but findings with children are only beginning to emerge. The primary focus of this chapter is to review the available literature on the effects of early stress on the developing brain, with particular emphasis on the neurobiology inherent in this relationship. In addition, we present available findings related to neurostructural and neuropsychological–cognitive abnormalities in children with PTSD.

CHILDHOOD MALTREATMENT AND PTSD

Childhood maltreatment may be the single most preventable and inter-venable contributor to child and adult mental illness. Adults with child maltreatment histories are more likely to manifest multiple health risk be-haviors, serious medical illnesses (Felitti et al., 1998), and greater need and utilization of psychiatric and general health care services (Walker et al., 1999) than adults without maltreatment histories. Furthermore, trauma in childhood may be more detrimental than trauma experienced in adulthood because of the interactions between trauma, psychological, and neuro-developmental processes (De Bellis, 2001; De Bellis & Putnam, 1994). Mal-treatment in children and adolescents may cause developmental delays and/ or deficits in the developmental attainment of motor, language, cognitive, emotional, behavioral, and social skills (Beers & De Bellis, 2002; Cicchetti & Lynch, 1995; Perez & Widom, 1994; Trickett & McBride-Chang, 1995). More specifically, maltreated children and adolescents with mood and anx-iety disorders, particularly symptoms of PTSD and depression, evidence al-terations of chemical mediators of stress and adverse brain and cognitive (prefrontal) development (De Bellis, Keshavan, Baum, et al., 1999; De Bellis, Keshavan, Clark, et al., 1999; De Bellis, Keshavan, Shifflett, Iyengar, Beers, et al., 2002; De Bellis, Keshavan, Spencer, & Hall, 2000). Earlier age of onset of abuse, longer duration of abuse, and greater severity of PTSD symptoms are associated with smaller brain volumes (De Bellis, Keshavan, Baum, et al., 1999; De Bellis, Keshavan, Clark, et al., 1999; De Bellis & Keshavan, 2003).

The few epidemiological studies regarding PTSD in children or adoles-cents suggest that PTSD lifetime prevalence rates for children and adoles-cents are similar to, or even higher than, those of adults and are compara-ble to those of adults traumatized by war and sexual assault (for review see DeBellis, 2001). Children are more likely to be diagnosed with PTSD after a traumatic event than their adult counterparts (Fletcher, 1996). Moreover, even in the absence of PTSD diagnosis, partial PTSD responses commonly develop and contribute to substantial functional impairment and distress (Carrion, Weems, Ray, & Reiss, 2001). Adverse childhood experiences such as abuse and neglect also increase the risk for adult PTSD (Bremner, Southwick, Johnson, Yehuda, & Charney, 1993; Widom, 1999) and non-PTSD psychiatric illnesses (Dube, Felitti, Dong, Giles, & Anda, 2003). As an interpersonal trauma (i.e., the cause of the trauma is of human design), childhood maltreatment may override any genetic, constitutional, social, or psychological resilience factors, thus heightening the risk for PTSD and its associated impairments in the majority of victims (for review see DeBellis, 2001).

Whereas the diagnostic picture of PTSD in children may be similar to adults (De Bellis, 1997), that is not the case in children younger than 4 years of age. Very young children can develop symptomatology characteristic of PTSD (Scheeringa, Zeanah, Drell, & Larrieu, 1995), but a significant gap exists in our ability to accurately identify these symptoms, which may be partly attributable to the diagnostic criteria utilized. Detecting the presence of characteristic symptoms, such as hyperarousal, reexperiencing, and avoidance, may be more arduous in preverbal children. Using more developmentally sensitive, behavior-based criteria in young children, Scheeringa, Zeanah, Myers, and Putnam (2003) found a PTSD diagnosis rate of 26%, which was more consistent with PTSD rates of traumatized adults and older children, in contrast to a rate of 0% when they used DSM-IV criteria. Thus, another important factor when considering PTSD in children is that clinical and biological findings in children who meet fewer than three clusters of symptoms may be equivalent to those who meet full PTSD criteria.

NEUROBIOLOGICAL FOUNDATIONS IN CHILDHOOD PTSD

Neurochemical Systems

Results of clinical studies evaluating the neurobiological effects of early trauma exposure have suggested that the overwhelming stress of traumatic experiences in childhood is associated with alterations of biological stress response systems and subsequent adverse influences on brain development (De Bellis, 2001). Multiple, densely interconnected neurobiological systems, including both neurotransmitter systems and the neuroendocrine system, are impacted by the acute and chronic stressors associated with early life stress (see Southwick, Rasmusson, Barron, & Arnsten, Chapter 2, this volume). PTSD symptoms are thought to arise from dysregulation of these biological stress systems. In this section, we will focus on neurochemical systems and their relationship to the neurobiology of PTSD in children and adolescents.

Catecholamines

A traumatic experience is perceived through the five senses in the form of intense fear. From a neurobiological viewpoint, early and prolonged exposure to stress leads individuals to display enhanced stress responsiveness. This stress response is characterized by elevation in levels of catecholamines and cortisol levels, which likely adversely affect brain development. Catecholamines contribute to dilation of the pupils, diaphoresis, renal inhibition, and decrease in peripheral blood flow. Activation of the locus coeruleus–sympathetic nervous system (SNS)–catecholamine system and cortiocotropin-releasing hormone (CRH) and factor (CRF) results in animal behaviors consistent with anxiety, hyperarousal, and hypervigilance (i.e., the core symptoms of PTSD).

In adult PTSD, it is hypothesized that the locus coeruleus–SNS–catecholamine system and limbic–hypothalamic–pituitary–adrenal (LHPA) axis responses to stress become maladaptive, causing long-term negative consequences (Southwick, Yehuda, & Morgan, 1995). Results from adult combat-related PTSD studies suggest that there is increased sensitivity of the locus coeruleus–SNS–catecholamine system, most clearly evident under experimental conditions of stress or challenge, and that these biological responses are more pronounced among PTSD-diagnosed combat veterans, as compared to healthy combat or noncombat controls. However, the limited data relevant to traumatized children suggest that the locus coeruleus–SNS–catecholamine system is dysregulated in traumatized children who may suffer from depressive and PTSD symptoms but who may or may not have a diagnosis of PTSD. Findings of elevated baseline 24-hour urinary catecholamine concentrations were seen in (1) male children who suffered from severe clinical depression and had a history of parental neglect (Queiroz et al., 1991); (2) sexually abused girls, 58% of whom had histories of severely depressed mood with suicidal behavior (but only one of whom had PTSD) (De Bellis, Lefter, Trickett, & Putnam, 1994); and (3) male and female children with abuse-related PTSD (De Bellis, Baum, et al., 1999). Furthermore, decreased platelet alpha$_2$-adrenergic receptors and increased heart rate following orthostatic challenge were found in physically and sexually abused children with PTSD, suggesting an enhancement of SNS tone in childhood PTSD (Perry, 1994). Evidence for increased baseline activity of the locus coeruleus–SNS–catecholamine system in childhood PTSD is also provided by two separate, open-label treatment trials of the medications clonidine (a central alpha$_2$-adrenergic partial agonist) and propranolol (a beta-adrenergic antagonist), both of which dampen catecholamine transmission. Clonidine treatment was associated with general clinical improvement and decreases in PTSD arousal symptoms and basal heart rate (Perry, 1994). Propranolol treatment was associated with decreases in aggressive behaviors and insomnia (Famularo, Kinsherff, & Fenton, 1988).

Serotonergic Neurotransmitter System

The serotonin neurotransmitter system is a stress response system. Serotonin, regarded as a master control neurotransmitter of complex neuronal communication (Lesch & Moessner, 1998), plays important roles in compulsive behaviors and the regulation of emotions (mood) and behavior (aggression, impulsive dysregulation). As such, it is implicated in major depression, impulsivity, and suicidal behaviors. Interaction with CRH and the noradrenergic system suggests that dysregulation of serotonin increases the risk for comorbid major depression in PTSD. In maltreated children, dysregulation of serotonin may not only play a major role in PTSD symptom development, but it may also increase the risk for comorbid major depression and aggression. Breslau, Davis, Peterson, and Schultz (2000) showed that onset of major depression is markedly increased for trauma-exposed persons who suffer from PTSD but not in trauma-exposed persons who do not suffer from PTSD. These findings suggest that PTSD may lead to major depression, with both PTSD and depression influenced by common genetic vulnerabilities to serotonin dysregulation and trauma-related factors, as discussed above. Recently, clinical studies have demonstrated strong support for the efficacy of the serotonin reuptake inhibitor antidepressant and anti-obsessive–compulsive disorder medications, sertraline (Brady et al., 2000) and fluoxetine (van der Kolk et al., 1994) in adult PTSD. However, very little is known about serotonin and trauma in children.

Limbic-Hypothalamic-Pituitary-Adrenal Axis

The LHPA axis, the major neuroendocrine stress response system, has also been implicated in the pathophysiology of PTSD. Elevated levels of CRH or CRF have been consistently reported in traumatized individuals (Southwick, Yehuda, & Wang, 1998). Adults with PTSD, maltreated children with symptoms of mood and anxiety disorders, and pediatric patients with maltreatment-related PTSD evidence this dysregulation (for review, see De Bellis, 2001). However, as summarized below, the findings of studies of trauma-exposed adults and children differ regarding cortisol levels.

Whereas increased cortisol levels are typically found in traumatized young and latency-age children, most adult studies have shown the opposite pattern (for review, see De Bellis, 2003). For example, higher morning serial plasma cortisol levels were found in sexually abused girls, ages 6–15 years, within 6 months of disclosure as compared to nonabused sociodemographically matched controls (Putnam, Trickett, Helmers, Dorn, & Everett, 1991). Similarly, Gunnar, Morison, Chisholm, and Schuder (2001) showed elevated salivary cortisol in 6- to 12-year-old children raised in Romanian orphanages for more than 8 months of their lives, as compared to early adopted and Canadian-born children 6½ years after adoption. DeBellis, Baum, et al. (1999) likewise showed elevated 24-hour urine free cortisol in prepubertal maltreated children with PTSD. Elevated salivary cortisol has also been described in maltreated children with depression (Hart, Gunnar, & Cicchetti, 1996) and in maltreated children with threshold and subthreshold PTSD symptoms (Carrion et al., 2002). In contrast, Goenjian et al. (1996) found that Armenian adolescents who lived close to ground zero of the 1988 earthquake, with a greater threat to life, showed more PTSD and depressive symptoms, and lower nonstimulated mean salivary cortisol levels, and greater afternoon suppression of cortisol by dexamethasone, 5 years *after exposure* compared to adolescents 20 miles away from the epicenter. These results are similar to the LHPA axis findings in adult PTSD and suggest that age is one factor that may explain the developmental neurobiological differences in LHPA axis regulation seen between prepubertal children and adults with PTSD.

Chronic compensatory adaptation of the LHPA axis is seen in children with past trauma. Attenuated plasma ACTH responses to ovine CRH in sexually abused girls were found several years after abuse disclosure (De Bellis, Chrousos, et al., 1994). The abused girls exhibited reduced evening basal, ovine CRH-stimulated, and time-integrated total plasma ACTH concentrations compared with controls. Plasma total and free cortisol responses to ovine CRH stimulation did not differ between the two groups. Thus, sexually abused girls manifested a dysregulatory disorder of the LHPA axis associated with hyporesponsiveness of the pituitary to exogenous CRH, but normal overall cortisol secretion to CRH challenge. CRH hypersecretion may have led to an adaptive down regulation of CRH receptors in the anterior pituitary, which is similar to the mechanism suggested in adult PTSD (Baker et al., 1999; Bremner et al., 1997).

Thomas and De Bellis (2004) showed a significant age-by-group effect in which pituitary volumes were significantly larger in pubertal/postpubertal maltreated pediatric subjects with PTSD than control subjects, but were similar in prepubertal maltreated subjects with PTSD and controls. Age of abuse onset correlated with pituitary volume in all subjects but differed in the direction of association for prepubertal and pubertal/postpubertal subjects. In the prepubertal group, duration of abuse correlated positively with pituitary volume; in the pubertal/postpubertal group (Tanner stages II–V), duration of abuse correlated negatively with pituitary volume. These findings support the hypothesis that adaptive mechanisms and developmental factors influence pituitary size in traumatized children. Endogenous CRH hypersecretion likely occurs with the onset of trauma. Thus, children exposed to trauma may experience chronically elevated CRH during pituitary development. Elevated CRH may lead to pituitary hypertrophy, which may be most pronounced during puberty, possibly due to trophic factors. Chronic exposure to CRH, in turn, may result in down-regulation of pituitary CRH receptors over time. This down-regulation may be an adaptive mechanism that regulates pituitary hypertrophy. If down-regulation of CRH receptors does not occur in response to elevated CRH, resultant high cortisol levels would lead to medical illness and damage to brain structures. Such a mechanism could explain the complex phenomena of low ACTH but elevated cortisol levels seen in studies of traumatized prepubertal and latency-age children, and the normal and low cortisol levels, but elevated central CRH levels, exhibited in many studies of traumatized adolescents and adults. In support of this idea, low urinary cortisol secretion has been found in adult holocaust survivors with PTSD (Yehuda et al., 1995).

However, the LHPA axis functions in a complex manner in children with a history of trauma who are currently experiencing stress. Increased ACTH response to human CRH, but normal cortisol secretion, were reported in maltreated, prepubertal, depressed children undergoing current psychosocial adversity compared to depressed children with prior histories of maltreatment, depressed nonabused children, and healthy children (Kaufman et al., 1997). This finding may be related to "priming" or sensitization in which responses to repeated stress increase in magnitude. A possible long-term consequence of the trauma experience may be to prime the LHPA axis so that ACTH and cortisol secretion are set at lower 24-hour levels (De Bellis, Baum, et al., 1999). Priming may occur as a reflection of chronic compensatory adaptation of the LHPA axis long after trauma exposure. LHPA axis regulation is affected by other hormones that are stress mediated such as arginine, vasopressin and the catecholamines, both of which act synergistically with CRH (Chrousos & Gold, 1992). A "primed system" "hyper"-responds during acute stress. Thus, when a new emotional stressor is experienced, LHPA axis functioning is enhanced (i.e., higher ACTH and higher 24-hour urinary free cortisol concentrations in response to stress). This "hyper" response was also seen in women who experienced abuse and suffered from major depression (Heim et al., 2002).

Neglect and Biological Stress Systems

Several neurobiological consequences of early life stress have been identified, including dysregulation of biological stress systems, smaller intracranial and cerebral volumes, and reduced size of the corpus callosum. The seminal studies of Harlow and colleagues demonstrated the profound effects of neglect in primates (Harlow, Harlow, & Suomi, 1971). Although child neglect is not abuse, neglect often coexists with abuse, and it can be argued that childhood neglect may be perceived by the child as traumatic. Animal models demonstrate that maternal deprivation and maternal stress can alter the development of the LHPA axis of the affected offspring, the effects of which may endure into adulthood (for review, see Caldji et al., 2001). Even brief maternal separations or trauma exposure during infancy have been shown to affect the functioning of the LHPA axis and glucocorticoid receptor gene expression in the hippocampus and frontal cortex in rats (Francis & Meaney, 1999; Meaney et al., 1996). Individual differences in the mothering of rat pups affect their catecholamine regulation and fear response (Caldji et al., 1998), although environmental enrichment reverses some of the effects of maternal separation on stress reactivity (Francis, Diorio, Plotsky, & Meaney, 2002). Similarly, primates that are subjected to prolonged periods of maternal and social deprivation have altered glucocorticoid (Lyons, Yang, Mobley, Nickerson, & Schatzberg, 2000) and catecholamine (Martin, Sackett, Gunderson, & Goodlin-Jones, 1988) function and impaired immune function (Lubach, Coe, & Erhler, 1995). Using a variable foraging demand paradigm, Rosenblum and Andrews (1994) demonstrated that reduced time spent by bonnet macque mothers responding to their infants' solicitations for contact and attention resulted in insecure patterns of attachment behaviors among the infants and corresponding persistent elevations in cerebrospinal fluid levels of CRF when infants were again tested as adults (Coplan et al., 1996). Similar to the elevations in cerebrospinal fluid concentrations of CRF seen in adults with PTSD, cerebrospinal fluid concentrations of serotonin, dopamine and norepinephrine metabolites were also elevated in these monkeys (Coplan et al., 1998). Thus, early neglect in animals appears to exert lasting neurobiological alterations similar to those described in trauma-exposed humans.

Studies of Brain Development in Traumatized Children

Functional neuroimaging studies in adults suggest that the medial prefrontal regions are hyporesponsive and the amygdala is hyperresponsive in PTSD (Bremner, Narayan, et al., 1999; Bremner, Staib, et al., 1999; Lanius et al., 2002; Shin et al., 1999; Shin et al., 2004; Shin et al., 2001). The medial prefrontal cortex and amygdala are thought to be reciprocally related (Hamner, Lorberbaum, & George, 1999; Stefanacci & Amaral, 2002), and exposure to mild to moderate uncontrollable stress impairs prefrontal cortical function in studies of humans and animals (Arnsten, 1998). However, many of the studies in adult PTSD involved radiation using positron emission tomography (PET) scanning, a technique that is not feasible in children. Since there are no published functional magnetic resonance imaging (fMRI) of traumatized children to date, little is known about functional activation patterns in children. The following sections will focus on published studies using structural magnetic resonance imaging (MRI) and magnetic resonance spectroscopy (MRS).

Structural Magnetic Resonance Imaging Studies

In adults, PTSD is associated with specific neurostructural anomalies such as a smaller hippocampus in most (Sapolsky, 2000) but not all studies (Bonne et al., 2001). However, pediatric PTSD was not associated with the predicted decrease in hippocampal volume in cross-sectional (Carrion, Weems, Eliez, et al., 2001; De Bellis, Keshavan, Clark, et al., 1999; De

Bellis, Keshavan, Shifflett, Iyengar, Beers, et al., 2002) or longitudinal studies (De Bellis, Hall, Boring, Frustaci, & Moritz, 2001). Birth to adulthood is marked by progressive physical, behavioral, cognitive, and emotional development. Paralleling these stages are changes in brain maturation. In the developing brain, elevated levels of catecholamines and cortisol may lead to adverse brain development through the mechanisms of accelerated loss (or metabolism) of neurons (Edwards, Harkins, Wright, & Menn, 1990; Sapolsky, 2000; Simantov et al., 1996; Smythies, 1997), delays in myelination (Dunlop, Archer, Quinlivan, Beazley, & Newnham, 1997), abnormalities in developmentally appropriate pruning (Lauder, 1988; Todd, 1992), and/or the inhibition of neurogenesis (Gould, McEwen, Tanapat, Galea, & Fuchs, 1997; Gould, Tanapat, & Cameron, 1997; Gould, Tanapat, McEwen, Flugge, & Fuchs, 1998; Tanapat, Galea, & Gould, 1998). Furthermore, stress decreases brain-derived neurotrophic factor expression (Smith, Makino, Kvetnansky, & Post, 1995). Thus, the overwhelming stress of child maltreatment experiences may have adverse influences on a child's brain maturation. We will next review evidence of adverse brain development (i.e., smaller cerebral volumes and corpus callosum areas) in maltreated children and adolescents with abused-related PTSD. Trauma in childhood may be associated with global brain differences resulting from the experience of chronic stress at this critical developmental period and differences associated with brain structures (e.g., medial prefrontal regions) that are thought to be responsible for PTSD.

Myelinated areas of the brain appear particularly susceptible to the effects of early exposure to significant levels of stress hormones. MRI and related imaging procedures have allowed a noninvasive, safe method to compare the gray and white matter brain structures of healthy children to those exposed to trauma such as abuse and neglect. Neuroimaging is a relatively new area of study for this population of children, and a handful of studies have been published with results that indicate adverse brain structure and development as a consequence of abuse and neglect resulting in PTSD or subthreshold symptoms of PTSD. Teicher et al. (1997) provided the initial evidence that early childhood trauma has deleterious effects on the development of the corpus callosum, finding that the size of the corpus callosum was affected by early adverse experience, and that this effect was gender dependent. These researchers found a reduction in the middle portion of the corpus callosum in children who were hospitalized at psychiatric facilities with a documented history of trauma, which included abuse or neglect, as compared to psychiatric controls. These effects were gender dependent in that males showed more extreme differences. Sanchez, Hearn, Do, Rilling, and Herndon (1998) likewise found that rhesus monkeys that were separated from their mothers at 2 months of age and singly reared until age 12 months had a reduction in the midsagittal size of the corpus callosum, a decrease in white (but not gray) matter volume in the prefrontal and parietal cortices, and corresponding decreases in cognitive performance.

In a study of 44 maltreated children and adolescents with PTSD and 61 matched controls, De Bellis, Keshavan, et al. (1999) extended these findings by demonstrating decreased total midsagittal area of the corpus callosum and enlarged right, left, and total lateral ventricles in PTSD-diagnosed subjects compared to controls. Male children with PTSD had smaller measurements of the corpus callosum and a trend for smaller total brain volume than female children with PTSD, although adverse effects were found regardless of gender. Earlier onset and longer duration of abuse were associated with smaller intracranial volume. Additionally, intracranial volume was decreased by 7%, and total brain volume by 8%, in PTSD subjects compared to controls. Intrusive, avoidance, hyperarousal, and dissociation symptoms correlated positively with ventricular volume and negatively with intracranial volume and total corpus callosum area. These findings suggested disrupted brain development in patients with maltreatment-related PTSD and indicated that adverse effects may be greater with exposure to trauma in early childhood. The association of smaller intracranial volume with longer duration of abuse also suggested that recurrent and chronic abuse may have a cumulative, harmful effect on brain development.

Carrion, Weems, Eliez, et al. (2001) reported that children with PTSD or subthreshold PTSD showed smaller total brain and cerebral volumes when compared to healthy age- and gender-matched archival controls. In addition, findings indicated attenuation of frontal lobe asymmetry in children with maltreatment-related PTSD. Although this study did not match for IQ or for socioeconomic factors, which also influence brain volume, findings were consistent with those of DeBellis, Keshavan, Clark, et al. (1999).

A study of 28 psychotropic naïve children and adolescents with maltreatment-related PTSD showed smaller intracranial, cerebral cortex, prefrontal cortex, prefrontal cortical white matter, and right temporal lobe volumes in comparison to 66 sociodemographically matched healthy controls (De Bellis, Keshavan, Shifflett, Iyengar, Beers, et al., 2002). Subjects with PTSD showed decreased areas of the corpus callosum and subregions 2, 4, 5, 6, and 7, and larger frontal lobe cerebrospinal fluid volumes than controls, even after adjustment for total cerebral volume. Again, total brain volume correlated positively with age of onset of trauma-causing PTSD (i.e., smaller volumes with earlier onset of trauma), and negatively with duration of abuse (i.e., longer duration of abuse with smaller volumes). Another significant gender-by-group interaction was found in which maltreated males with PTSD had larger ventricular volumes than maltreated females with PTSD.

In a secondary analyses of sex differences in the published data of DeBellis and his colleagues (De Bellis, Keshavan, Clark, et al., 1999; De Bellis, Keshavan, Shifflett, Iyengar, Beers, et al., 2002), larger prefrontal lobe cerebrospinal fluid volumes and smaller midsagittal area of the corpus callosum subregion 7 (splenium) were seen in both boys and girls with maltreatment-related PTSD relative to gender-matched comparison subjects (De Bellis & Keshavan, 2003). These findings suggest prefrontal abnormalities in maltreated children with PTSD, a finding similar to functional imaging and neurocognitive findings in adult PTSD. Child subjects with PTSD did not show the normal age-related increases in the area of the total corpus callosum and its region 7 (splenium) compared to nonmaltreated subjects, indicating deficits in myelination in these traumatized children. This later finding is similar to the work in nonhuman primates. Interestingly, the failure to find normal age-related increases in the area of the corpus callosum was more prominent in males with PTSD. Significant sex-by-group effects demonstrated smaller cerebral volumes and corpus callosum regions 1 (rostrum) and 6 (isthmus) in PTSD males and greater lateral ventricular volume increases in maltreated males with PTSD than maltreated females with PTSD, suggesting more adverse brain maturation of boys compared with girls with maltreatment-related PTSD (De Bellis & Keshavan, 2003).

As described above, hippocampal differences were not seen in studies of pediatric PTSD. A suggestion for the discrepancy between the adult and child findings is that PTSD exerts a gradual adverse effect on the structure of the hippocampus such that it may not yet be manifest in developing children. That is, stress-induced hippocampal damage may not be evident until postpubertal development, or it may be an inherent vulnerability for chronic PTSD that persists into adulthood (Gilbertson et al., 2002). It may also be that the higher rate of alcohol and substance abuse/dependence in adults explains the finding of decreased hippocampal volume in adults but not children. This hypothesis has been supported by research indicating decreased hippocampal volumes related to adolescent onset alcohol abuse (De Bellis, Clark, et al., 2000). A final suggestion for the differences in hippocampal findings between children and adults with PTSD is the capacity for primate neurogenesis in the hippocampus and frontal cortex (Gould, McEwen, et al., 1997; Gould et al., 1998). Disclosure of abuse, separation from the perpetrator, and therapeutic interventions may enhance hippocampal neurogenesis. Thus, neurodevelopmental plasticity and normal developmental increases in the hippocampus may "mask" any effects of traumatic stress in maltreated children with PTSD. As such, longitudinal research of chronically stressed children, with a particular focus on hippocampal neurogenesis, is critical to understanding the complex interactions between hippocampal maturation, stress, and PTSD.

As adverse effects on brain structure are observed in children with

PTSD symptoms secondary to abuse and neglect, findings of decreased intracranial and cerebral volumes in maltreated children with PTSD are worthy of further exploration. Because traumatized subjects without PTSD have not been studied in the imaging literature, it will be particularly important to dissociate the effects of early life stress from those specifically associated with PTSD diagnosis.

Magnetic Resonance Spectroscopy Studies

MRS is a safe approach to measuring neuronal integrity in children. N-Acetylaspartate (NAA), considered to be a marker of neuronal health or integrity, is measured by MRS via the N-acetyl signal in the proton (^{1}H) spectrum. Low levels of NAA are associated with neuronal damage or loss (Prichard, 1996). A study of 11 children with maltreatment-related PTSD suggested that maltreated children and adolescents with PTSD have lower NAA–creatine ratios compared to controls matched for age, race, socioeconomic status, and IQ (De Bellis, Keshavan, et al., 2000). These findings specifically suggested loss of neuronal integrity in the anterior cingulate region of the medial prefrontal cortex. Unlike structural imaging findings, no sex differences were seen. In terms of implications, effective PTSD treatment may improve anterior cingulate functioning and alleviate PTSD symptoms by removing the stress mediated inhibition on the rate of medial prefrontal neurogenesis. PTSD remission may be associated with enhanced medial prefrontal neurogenesis (increase in posttreatment NAA from baseline), cognitive improvement, and down regulation of cortisol and catecholamine activity. In a case study of a 7-year-old boy, treatment with clonidine, an antihypertensive that centrally down regulates the catecholamine activity of the locus coeruleus, was associated with remission of PTSD, improvement of sleep efficiency, and increased anterior cingulate NAA–creatine ratio from baseline (De Bellis, Keshavan, & Harenski, 2001). This case illustrates how this novel proton MRS approach can be used in treatment research to track brain maturation of specific regions of interest during treatment of pediatric PTSD.

CHILDHOOD TRAUMA AND THEORY OF MIND

The neural basis of our ability to interpret others' behavior in terms of mental states (e.g., thoughts, intentions, desires, beliefs) is called theory of mind or social intelligence (Brothers, 1990). Because of the interpersonal nature of most childhood trauma events, the essential symptoms of pediatric PTSD are social worries and associated autonomic hyperarousal. Trauma reminders in maltreated children are interpersonal in nature (e.g., raising or lowering the tone of voice, facial expressions), and such social cues may trigger PTSD symptoms of hypervigilance. The amygdala, a brain region involved in fear and fear-related behaviors in animals, and its projections to the superior temporal gyrus (STG), thalamus, and prefrontal cortex are thought to comprise the neural basis of theory of mind (Brothers, 1990). The STG and amygdala are involved in processing social information (Baron-Cohen et al., 1999). The STG in particular has been associated with the performance of social intelligence tasks in humans (Brother, 1990) and facial expression identification tasks in primates (Desimone, 1991; Hasselmo, Rolls, & Baylis, 1989). In studies of experimental conditioning, the STG is thought to be involved in higher cognitive processing of the fear experience and modulation of amygdala activity (Quirk, Armony, & LeDoux, 1997).

It is of interest that maltreated subjects with PTSD had significantly larger mainly right-sided STG grey matter volumes than nonmaltreated controls (De Bellis, Keshavan, Frustaci, et al., 2002). These findings suggested a more pronounced right > left asymmetry in total and posterior STG volumes, but a less pronounced left > right asymmetry in total, anterior, and posterior STG grey matter volumes (because of the relative increase in overall STG grey matter) in maltreated subjects with PTSD compared to controls. Similarly, a study of healthy adult subjects with high-trait anxiety showed greater right > left ratios of cerebral metabolism than healthy subjects with low-trait anxiety (Stapleton et al., 1997). Adults with social phobia (Davidson, Marshall, Tomarken, & Henriques, 2000) and with PTSD (Metzger et al., 2004) demonstrated increased right-sided EEG activation compared to controls. These results are interesting in light of a preliminary report of greater left hemispheric EEG coherence suggesting diminished left hemispheric differentiation in abused children (Teicher et al., 1997). The finding of a relatively larger STG in maltreated children and adolescents with PTSD, who had previously reported findings of smaller intracranial, cerebral, and corpus callosum structures, is also notable. Specifically, larger STG grey matter volumes in maltreated children with PTSD may reflect a trauma-related increase in sensitivity to conditioned auditory stimuli during development, resulting in compensatory synaptic increase of the STG.

On the other hand, larger STG grey matter may be the result of decreased developmentally related input from other brain areas such as the frontal cortex resulting in decreased STG pruning (Arnsten, 1998). A preliminary investigation found that maltreated children and adolescents with PTSD have lower NAA–creatine ratios, suggestive of neuronal loss in the anterior cingulate region of the medial prefrontal cortex, compared to sociodemographically matched controls (De Bellis, Keshavan, et al., 2000). One may speculate that these findings are due to a "traumatic-interference" with the developmental trajectory of the STG in pediatric PTSD. That is, the larger STG in pediatric PTSD may be related to the presence of specific anxiety symptoms.

In support of this idea, compared to healthy controls, larger STG volumes and a more pronounced right > left asymmetry were also found in a preliminary study of children and adolescents with pediatric generalized anxiety disorder who had no history of trauma, maltreatment, or PTSD (De Bellis, Keshavan, Shifflett, Iyengar, Dahl, et al., 2002). Thus, a relatively larger STG may be a preexisting, neuroanatomical risk factor for tendencies to manifest anxiety symptoms in response to anxiety provoking social triggers. However, the nature of the STG differed in that PTSD-diagnosed children showed larger volumes of STG grey matter, whereas children diagnosed with generalized anxiety disorder showed a more pronounced right > left asymmetry in total and white matter STG volumes. These findings indicate that anxious children without trauma histories may have an inherent propensity for larger right amygdala volumes and "connectivity" to larger STG volumes, resulting in predispositional traits such as increased sensitivity to social cues with anxious arousal (De Bellis, Casey, et al., 2000; De Bellis, Keshavan, Shifflett, Iyengar, Dahl, et al., 2002). In contrast, maltreated children may be "conditioned" to be more fearful of social cues (De Bellis, Keshavan, Frustaci, et al., 2002).

NEUROCOGNITIVE FINDINGS IN TRAUMATIZED CHILDREN

Impairments in the cognitive abilities of individuals diagnosed with PTSD have been reported in adults with PTSD, particularly in the areas of learning, memory, and concentration (see Vasterling & Brailey, Chapter 8, this volume). Consistent with these findings, a mounting body of literature has documented the deleterious effects of early exposure to extreme stress on children's neurocognitive development, including intellectual impairment, verbal deficiencies, and poor school performance. Although most studies report temporal stability of intelligence in various pediatric populations including handicapped children (Atkinson et al., 1990; Elliot & Boeve, 1987), a literature review suggests that compromised intellectual ability, as reflected by IQ scores, may be a consequence of child maltreatment.

A variety of intellectual and academic impairments, with resultant poor school performance, have been consistently reported in abused children not evaluated for PTSD (Augoustinos, 1987; Azar, Barnes, & Twentyman, 1988; Kolko, 1992; National Research Council, 1993; Trickett & McBride-Chang, 1995). Carrey, Butter, Persinger, and Bialik (1995) noted a negative correlation between Verbal IQ score and severity of abuse. Perez and Widom (1994) reported lower IQ and reading ability in a large sample of adult survivors of child maltreatment who were followed in a long-term, well-controlled prospective study of early-onset (i.e., before age 11 years) abuse or neglect. Other investigations indicated changes in IQ in high-risk samples that were related to the quantity of parent–child interactions and the home environment and to the degree of maternal depression (Money, Annecillo, & Kelly, 1983; Pianta, Egeland, & Erickson, 1989). In one case–control study, persistent impairments of IQ were associated with abuse disclosure, while IQ elevations were positively correlated with duration of "rescue" (in years) from an abusive upbringing (Money et al., 1983). However, cognitive function as indexed by performance on standardized neuropsychological instruments has not been extensively evaluated in children with PTSD. It is critical to characterize these deficits as they are likely to have broad ramifications across domains of development and general functioning.

In one of the few neuropsychological studies conducted with children with PTSD, Beers and De Bellis (2002) found that 14 children with maltreatment-related PTSD showed more deficits in attention and abstract reasoning/executive functions than a group of sociodemographically matched controls. Compared to controls, children with PTSD demonstrated deficits on measures of frontal executive functioning (e.g., card sorting and word-list generation tasks), were more susceptible to distraction, showed higher rates of impulsivity, and exhibited greater problems with sustained attention. Although based on a small number of subjects, findings were consistent with neuroimaging studies indicating CNS changes in the frontal cortex in individuals with PTSD. Relatedly, Moradi, Doost, Taghavi, Yule, and Dalgleish (1999) found general memory deficits in children with PTSD. Further research is necessary to ascertain how psychiatric symptoms interact with neuropsychological deficits.

Evidence for biological mechanisms underlying the association between family violence and IQ, such as cortisol-induced neuronal loss, was reported by De Bellis and colleagues (De Bellis, Keshavan, Clark, et al., 1999). Using MRI procedures, these investigators found that maltreated children with PTSD had smaller intracranial and cerebral volumes, as well as a smaller midsaggital area of the corpus callosum, than nonmaltreated children. Additionally, IQ was positively correlated with intracranial volume and negatively correlated with duration of maltreatment. Specifically, Verbal IQ, Performance IQ, and Full Scale IQ correlated negatively with duration of the abuse that led to PTSD in maltreated children.

Koenen, Moffit, Caspi, Taylor, and Purcell (2003) extended these findings by focusing on the relationship between domestic violence and cognitive–intellectual ability as measured by IQ. Limitations of previous studies included the inability to partial out potential genetic effects on the domestic violence–IQ association. This large-scale twin study, which utilized 1,116 monozygotic and dizygotic 5-year-old twin pairs, aimed at assessing whether domestic violence had environmentally mediated effects on young children's intelligence. Domestic violence was associated with delayed intellectual development, showing a dose–response relationship. On average, children exposed to high levels of domestic violence had IQ scores eight points lower than children who were not exposed. This effect did not differ by gender. This is a revolutionary study as it revealed that domestic violence is linked to an environmental effect on suppression of children's IQ that is independent of possible confounding genetic effects. Moreover, this environmental effect was speculated to be specific to domestic violence as it persisted even after controlling for maltreatment, which is the larger source of extreme childhood stress. The impact of domestic violence on more specific cognitive functions in children will require further investigation.

SUMMARY AND CONCLUSIONS

As can be seen from this chapter, early trauma clearly can affect the brain and brain development in a negative fashion. These abnormalities may play a causal role in cognitive and developmental deficits, as well as in the emotional and behavioral problems that many traumatized children with PTSD symptoms express. The results of various studies provide indirect evidence that PTSD in maltreated children may be regarded as a complex environmentally induced developmental disorder (De Bellis, 2001), with much of the neurochemical literature being particularly compelling. The need for further studies of the causes, psychobiologic consequences, sequelae, prognosis, and treatment of child maltreatment and related PTSD cannot be overstated. An important task for future research in developmental traumatology is the pursuit of longitudinal studies that may begin to identify the pathway from trauma exposure to abnormalities of brain structure. Further, because comorbidity is not the exception with PTSD but, rather, the rule, focusing exclusively on PTSD symptoms may inhibit the comprehensive assessment and treatment of typical accompanying disorders such as major depression, anxiety, and substance use. Thus, increasing our understanding of the relationship between maltreatment and comorbid psychiatric illness may inform research on the psychobiology of these disorders. Finally, increased linkages across neurochemical, neurostructural, and neuropsychological data will increase our understanding of the effects of early trauma on the developing brain. This increased knowledge should guide treatment efforts to improve the quality of life for these children and adolescents, particularly as they move into the challenges of adulthood.

ACKNOWLEDGMENTS

This chapter was completed with support from Grant Nos. NIMH RO1-MH63407, NIMH/NINDS RO1-MH61744, and NIAAA RO1-AA12479 (to Michael D. De Bellis).

REFERENCES

Arnsten, A. F. T. (1998). The biology of being frazzled. *Science, 280*, 1711–1712.

Atkinson, L., Bowman, T. G., Dickens, S., Blackwell, J., Vasarhelyi, J., Szep, P., Dunleavy, B., MacIntyre, R., & Bury, A. (1990). Stability of Wechsler Adult Intelligence Scale—Revised factor scores across time. *Psychological Assessment, 2*, 447–450.

Augoustinos, M. (1987). Developmental effects of child abuse: A number of recent findings. *Child Abuse and Neglect, 11*, 15–27.

Azar, S. T., Barnes, K. T., & Twentyman, C. T. (1988). Developmental outcomes in abused children: Consequences of parental abuse or a more general breakdown in caregiver behavior? *Behavior Therapist, 11*, 27–32.

Baker, D. G., West, S. A., Nicholson, W. E., Ekhator, N. N., Kasckow, J. W., Hill, K. K., Bruce, A. B., Orth, D. N., & Geracioti, Jr., T. D. (1999). Serial CSF corticotropin-releasing hormone levels and adrenocortical activity in combat veterans with posttraumatic stress disorder. *American Journal of Psychiatry, 156*, 585–588.

Baron-Cohen, S., Ring, H. A., Wheelwright, S., Bullmore, E. T., Brammer, M. J., Simmons, A., & Williams, S. C. R. (1999). Social intelligence in the normal and autistic brain: An fMRI study. *European Journal of Neuroscience, 11*, 1891–1898.

Beers, S. R., & De Bellis, M. D. (2002). Neuropsychological function in children with maltreatment-related posttraumatic stress disorder. *American Journal of Psychiatry, 159*, 483–486.

Bonne, O., Brandes, D., Gilboa, A., Gomori, J. M., Shenton, M. E., Pitman, R. K., & Shalev, A. Y. (2001). Longitudinal MRI study of hippocampal volume in trauma survivors with PTSD. *American Journal of Psychiatry, 158*, 1248–1251.

Brady, K., Pearlstein, T., Asnis, G. M., Baker, D., Rothbaum, B., Sikes, C. R., & Farfel, G. M. (2000). Efficacy and safety of sertraline treatment of posttraumatic stress disorder: A randomized controlled trial. *Journal of the American Medical Association, 283*, 1837–1844.

Bremner, J. D., Licinio, J., Darnell, A., Krystal, J. H., Owens, M. J., Southwick, S. M., Nemeroff, C. B., & Charney, D. S. (1997). Elevated CSF corticotropin-releasing factor concentrations in posttraumatic stress disorder. *American Journal of Psychiatry, 154*, 624–629.

Bremner, J. D., Narayan, M., Staib, L., Southwick, S. M., McGlashan, T., & Charney, D. S. (1999). Neural correlates of memories of childhood sexual abuse in women with and without posttraumatic stress disorder. *American Journal of Psychiatry, 156*, 1787–1795.

Bremner, J. D., Southwick, S. M., Johnson, D. R., Yehuda, R., & Charney, D. S.

(1993). Childhood physical abuse and combat-related posttraumatic stress disorder in Vietnam Veterans. *American Journal of Psychiatry, 150,* 235–239.

Bremner, J. D., Staib, L., Kaloupek, D., Southwick, S. M., Soufer, R., & Charney, D. S. (1999). Neural correlates of exposure to traumatic pictures and sound in Vietnam combat veterans with and without posttraumatic stress disorder: A positron emission tomography study. *Biological Psychiatry, 45,* 806–816.

Breslau, N., Davis, G. C., Peterson, E., & Schultz, L. R. (2000). A second look at comorbidity in victims of trauma: The posttraumatic stress disorder–major depression connection. *Biological Psychiatry, 48,* 902–909.

Brothers, L. (1990). The social brain: A project for integrating primate behavior and neurophysiology in a new domain. *Concepts in Neuroscience, 1,* 27–51.

Buka, S. L., Stichick, T. L., Birdthistle, I., & Earls, F. J. (2001). Youth exposure to violence: Prevalence, risks, and consequences. *American Journal of Orthopsychiatry, 71,* 298–310.

Caldji, C., Liu, D., Sharma, S., Diorio, J., Francis, D. D., Meaney, M. J., & Plotsky, P. M. (2001). Development of individual differences in behavioral and endocrine responses to stress: Role of the postnatal environment. In B. S. McEwen (Ed.), *Handbook of physiology: Coping with the environment* (pp. 271–292). New York: Oxford University Press.

Caldji, C., Tannenbaum, B., Sharma, S., Francis, D., Plotsky, P. M., & Meaney, M. J. (1998). Maternal care during infancy regulates the development of neural systems mediating the expression of fearfulness in the rat. *Proceedings of the National Academy of Sciences of the United States of America, 95,* 5335–5340.

Carrey, N. J., Butter, H. J., Persinger, M. A., & Bialik, R. J. (1995). Physiological and cognitive correlates of child abuse. *Journal of the American Academy of Child and Adolescent Psychiatry, 34,* 1067–1075.

Carrion, V. G., Weems, C. F., Eliez, S., Patwardhan, A., Brown, W., Ray, R. D., & Reiss, A. L. (2001). Attenuation of frontal asymmetry in pediatric posttraumatic stress disorder. *Biological Psychiatry, 50,* 943–951.

Carrion, V. G., Weems, C. F., Ray, R. D., Glaser, B., Hessl, D., & Reiss, A. L. (2002). Diurnal salivary cortisol in pediatric posttraumatic stress disorder. *Biological Psychiatry, 51,* 575–582.

Carrion, V. G., Weems, C. F., Ray, R. D., & Reiss, A. L. (2001). Toward an empirical definition of pediatric PTSD: The phenomenology of PTSD symptoms in youth. *Journal of the American Academy of Child and Adolescent Psychiatry, 41,* 166–173.

Chrousos, G. P., & Gold, P. W. (1992). The concepts of stress and stress system disorders: Overview of physical and behavioral homeostasis. *Journal of the American Medical Association, 267,* 1244–1252.

Cicchetti, D., & Carlson, V. (Eds.). (1989). *Child maltreatment: Theory and research on the causes and consequences of child abuse and neglect.* New York: Cambridge University Press.

Cicchetti, D., & Lynch, M. (1995). Failures in the expectable environment and their impact on individual development: The case of child maltreatment. In D. Cicchetti & D. J. Cohen (Eds.), *Developmental psychopathology* (pp. 32–71). New York: Wiley.

Coplan, J. D., Andrews, M. W., Rosenblum, L. A., Friedman, S., Owens, M. J.,

Gorman, J. M., & Nemeroff, C. B. (1996). Persistent elevations of cerebrospinal fluid concentrations of corticotropin-releasing factor in adults nonhuman primates exposed to early-life stressors: Implications for the pathophysiology of mood and anxiety disorders. *Proceedings of the National Academy of Sciences of the United States of America, 93,* 1619–1623.

Coplan, J. D., Trost, R. C., Owens, M. J., Cooper, T. B., Gorman, J. M., Nemeroff, C. B., & Rosenblum, L. A. (1998). Cerebrospinal fluid concentrations of somatostatin and biogenic amines in grown primates reared by mothers exposed to manipulated foraging conditions. *Archives of General Psychiatry, 55,* 473–477.

Davidson, R. J., Marshall, J. R., Tomarken, A. J., & Henriques, J. B. (2000). While a phobic waits: Regional brain electrical and autonomic activity in social phobics during anticipation of public speaking. *Biological Psychiatry, 47,* 85–95.

De Bellis, M. D. (1997). Posttraumatic stress disorder and acute stress disorder. In R. T. Ammerman & M. Hersen (Eds.), *Handbook of prevention and treatment with children and adolescents* (pp. 455–494). New York: Wiley.

De Bellis, M. D. (2001). Developmental traumatology: The psychobiological development of maltreated children and its implications for research, treatment, and policy. *Development and Psychopathology, 13,* 537–561.

De Bellis, M. D. (2003). The neurobiology of posttraumatic stress disorder across the life cycle. In J. C. Soares & S. Gershon (Eds.), *The handbook of medical psychiatry* (pp. 449–466). New York: Dekker.

De Bellis, M. D., Baum, A., Birmaher, B., Keshavan, M., Eccard, C. H., Boring, A. M., Jenkins, F. J., & Ryan, N. D. (1999). A. E. Bennett Research Award. Developmental traumatology: Part I: Biological stress systems. *Biological Psychiatry, 45,* 1259–1270.

De Bellis, M. D., Casey, B. J., Dahl, R., Birmaher, B., Williamson, D., Thomas, K. M., Axelson, D. A., Frustaci, K., Boring, A. M., Hall, J., & Ryan, N. (2000). A pilot study of amygdala volumes in pediatric generalized anxiety disorder. *Biological Psychiatry, 48,* 51–57.

De Bellis, M. D., Chrousos, G. P., Dorn, L. D., Burke, L., Helmers, K., Kling, M. A., Trickett, P. K., & Putnam, F. W. (1994). Hypothalamic–pituitary–adrenal axis dysregulation in sexually abused girls. *Journal of Clinical Endocrinology and Metabolism, 78,* 249–255.

De Bellis, M. D., Clark, D. B., Beers, S. R., Soloff, P., Boring, A. M., Hall, J., Kersh, A., & Keshavan, M. S. (2000). Hippocampal volume in adolescent onset alcohol use disorders. *American Journal of Psychiatry, 157,* 737–744.

De Bellis, M. D., Hall, J., Boring, A. M., Frustaci, K., & Moritz, G. (2001). A pilot longitudinal study of hippocampal volumes in pediatric maltreatment-related posttraumatic stress disorder. *Biological Psychiatry, 50,* 305–309.

De Bellis, M. D., & Keshavan, M. S. (2003). Sex differences in brain maturation in maltreatment-related pediatric posttraumatic stress disorder. *Special Edition of Neurosciences and Biobehavioral Reviews: Brain development, sex differences, and stress: Implications for psychopathology, 27,* 103–117.

De Bellis, M. D., Keshavan, M., Baum, A., Birmaher, B., Clark, D. B., Casey, B. J., Giedd, J., Boring, A. M., Frustaci, K., & Ryan, N. D. (1999). A. E. Bennett Research Award. Developmental traumatology, Part I & II: Biological stress systems and brain development. *Biological Psychiatry, 45,* 1259–1284.

De Bellis, M. D., Keshavan, M., Clark, D. B., Casey, B. J., Giedd, J., Boring, A. M., Frustaci, K., & Ryan, N. D. (1999). A. E. Bennett Research Award. Developmental traumatology, Part II: Brain development. *Biological Psychiatry, 45,* 1271–1284.

De Bellis, M. D., Keshavan, M., Frustaci, K., Shifflett, H., Iyengar, S., Beers, S. R., & Hall, J. (2002). Superior temporal gyrus volumes in maltreated children and adolescents with PTSD. *Biological Psychiatry, 51,* 544–552.

De Bellis, M. D., Keshavan, M. S., & Harenski, K. A. (2001). Case study: Anterior cingulate N-acetylaspartate concentrations during treatment in a maltreated child with PTSD. *Journal of Child and Adolescent Psychopharmacology, 11,* 311–316.

De Bellis, M. D., Keshavan, M., Shifflett, H., Iyengar, S., Beers, S. R., Hall, J., & Moritz, G. (2002). Brain structures in pediatric maltreatment-related PTSD: A sociodemographically matched study. *Biological Psychiatry, 52,* 1066–1078.

De Bellis, M. D., Keshavan, M., Shifflett, H., Iyengar, S., Dahl, R., Axelson, D. A., Birmaher, B., Hall, J., Moritz, G., & Ryan, N. (2002). Superior temporal gyrus volumes in pediatric generalized anxiety disorder. *Biological Psychiatry, 51,* 553–562.

De Bellis, M. D., Keshavan, M. S., Spencer, S., & Hall, J. (2000). N-acetylaspartate concentration in the anterior cingulate in maltreated children and adolescents with PTSD. *American Journal of Psychiatry, 157,* 1175–1177.

De Bellis, M. D., Lefter, L., Trickett, P. K., & Putnam, F. W. (1994). Urinary catecholamine excretion in sexually abused girls. *Journal of the American Academy of Child and Adolescent Psychiatry, 33,* 320–327.

De Bellis, M. D., & Putnam, F. W. (1994). The psychobiology of childhood maltreatment. *Child and Adolescent Psychiatric Clinics of North America, 3,* 663–677.

Desimone, R. (1991). Face-selective cells in the temporal cortex of monkeys. *Journal of Cognitive Neuroscience, 3,* 1–8.

Dube, S. R., Felitti, V. J., Dong, M., Giles, W. H., & Anda, R. F. (2003). The impact of adverse childhood experiences on health problems: Evidence from four birth cohorts dating back to 1900. *Preventive Medicine, 37,* 268–277.

Dunlop, S. A., Archer, M. A., Quinlivan, J. A., Beazley, L. D., & Newnham, J. P. (1997). Repeated prenatal corticosteroids delay myelination in the ovine central nervous system. *Journal of Maternal-Fetal Medicine, 6,* 309–313.

Edwards, E., Harkins, K., Wright, G., & Menn, F. (1990). Effects of bilateral adrenalectomy on the induction of learned helplessness. *Behavioral Neuropsychopharmacology, 3,* 109–114.

Elliot, S. N., & Boeve, K. (1987). Stability of WISC–R IQs: An investigation of ethnic differences over time. *Educational and Psychological Measurement, 47,* 461–465.

Famularo, R., Kinsherff, R., & Fenton, T. (1988). Propranolol treatment for childhood posttraumatic stress disorder, acute type. *American Journal of the Diseases of Children, 142,* 1244–1247.

Felitti, V. J., Anda, R. F., Nordenberg, D., Williamson, D. F., Spitz, A. M., Edwards, V., Koss, M. P., & Marks, J. S. (1998). Relationship of childhood abuse and household dysfunction to many of the leading causes of death in adults: The Adverse Childhood Experiences (ACE) Study. *American Journal of Preventive Medicine, 14,* 245–258.

Fletcher, K. E. (1996). Childhood posttraumatic stress disorder. In E. J. Mash & R. A. Barkley (Eds.), *Child psychopathology* (pp. 242–276). New York: Guilford Press.

Francis, D. D., Diorio, J., Plotsky, P. M., & Meaney, M. J. (2002). Environmental enrichment reverses the effects of maternal separation on stress reactivity. *Journal of Neuroscience, 22*, 7840–7843.

Francis, D. D., & Meaney, M. J. (1999). Maternal care and the development of stress responses. *Current Opinion in Neurobiology, 9*, 128–134.

Gilbertson, M. W., Shenton, M. E., Ciszewski, A., Kasai, K., Lasko, N. B., Orr, S. P., & Pitman, R. K. (2002). Smaller hippocampal volume predicts pathologic vulnerability to psychological trauma. *Nature Neuroscience, 5*, 1242–1247.

Goenjian, A. K., Yehuda, R., Pynoos, R. S., Steinberg, A. M., Tashjian, M., Yang, R. K., Najarian, L. M., & Fairbanks, L. A. (1996). Basal cortisol, dexamethasone suppression of cortisol, and MHPG in adolescents after the 1988 earthquake in Armenia. *American Journal of Psychiatry, 153*, 929–934.

Gould, E., McEwen, B. S., Tanapat, P., Galea, L. A., & Fuchs, E. (1997). Neurogenesis in the dentate gyrus of the adult tree shrew is regulated by psychosocial stress and NMDA receptor activation. *Journal of Neuroscience, 17*, 2492–2498.

Gould, E., Tanapat, P., & Cameron, H. A. (1997). Adrenal steroids suppress granule cell death in the developing dentate gyrus through an NMDA receptor-dependent mechanism. *Developmental Brain Research, 103*, 91–93.

Gould, E., Tanapat, P., McEwen, B. S., Flugge, G., & Fuchs, E. (1998). Proliferation of granule cell precursors in the dentate gyrus of adult monkeys is diminished by stress. *Proceedings of the National Academy of Sciences of the United States of America, 95*, 3168–3171.

Gunnar, M. R., Morison, S. J., Chisholm, K., & Schuder, M. (2001). Salivary cortisol levels in children adopted from Romanian orphanages. *Development and Psychopathology, 13*, 611–628.

Hamner, M. B., Lorberbaum, J. P., & George, M. S. (1999). Potential role of the anterior cingulate cortex in PTSD: Review and hypothesis. *Depression and Anxiety, 9*, 1–14.

Harlow, H. F., Harlow, M. K., & Suomi, S. J. (1971). From thought to therapy: Lessons from a primate laboratory. *American Scientist, 59*, 538–549.

Hart, J., Gunnar, M., & Cicchetti, D. (1996). Altered neuroendocrine activity in maltreated children related to symptoms of depression. *Development and Psychopathology, 8*, 201–214.

Hasselmo, M. E., Rolls, E. T., & Baylis, G. C. (1989). The role of expression and identity in the face-selective responses of neurons in the temporal visual cortex of the monkey. *Behavioural Brain Research, 32*, 203–218.

Heim, C., Newport, D. J., Wagner, D., Wilcox, M. M., Miller, A. H., & Nemeroff, C. B. (2002). The role of early adverse experience and adulthood stress in the prediction of neuroendocrine stress reactivity in women: A multiple regression analysis. *Depression and Anxiety, 15*, 117–125.

Kaufman, J., Birmaher, B., Perel, J., Dahl, R. E., Moreci, P., Nelson, B., Wells, W., & Ryan, N. (1997). The corticotropin-releasing hormone challenge in depressed abused, depressed nonabused, and normal control children. *Biological Psychiatry, 42*, 669–679.

Kaufman, J., Jones, B., Stieglitz, E., Vitulano, l., & Mannarino, A. (1994). The use of multiple informants to assess children's maltreatment experiences. *Journal of Family Violence, 9,* 227–248.

Kitzmann, K. M., Gaylord, N. K., Holt, A. R., & Kenny, E. D. (2003). Child witnesses to domestic violence: A meta-analytic review. *Journal of Consulting and Clinical Psychology, 71,* 339–352.

Koenen, K. C., Moffitt, T. E., Caspi, A., Taylor, A., & Purcell, S. (2003). Domestic violence is associated with environmental suppression of IQ in young children. *Development and Psychopathology, 15,* 297–311.

Kolko, D. (1992). Characteristics of child victims of physical violence: Research findings and clinical implications. *Journal of Interpersonal Violence, 7,* 244–276.

Lanius, R. A., Williamson, P. C., Boksman, K., Densmore, M., Gupta, M., Neufeld, R. W., Gati, J. S., & Menon, R. S. (2002). Brain activation during script-driven imagery induced dissociative responses in PTSD: A functional magnetic resonance imaging investigation. *Biological Psychiatry, 52,* 305–311.

Lauder, J. M. (1988). Neurotransmitters as morphogens. *Progress in Brain Research, 73,* 365–388.

Lesch, K. P., & Moessner, R. (1998). Genetically driven variation in serotonin update: Is there a link to affective spectrum, neurodevelopmental and neurodegenerative disorders? *Biological Psychiatry, 44,* 179–192.

Levy, H. B., Markovic, J., Chaudry, U., Ahart, S., & Torres, H. (1995). Reabuse rates in a sample of children followed for 5 years after discharge from a child abuse inpatient assessment program. *Child Abuse and Neglect, 11,* 1363–1377.

Lubach, G. R., Coe, C. L., & Erhler, W. B. (1995). Effects of early rearing environment on immune responses of infant rhesus monkeys. *Brain, Behavior, and Immunity, 9,* 31–46.

Lyons, D. M., Yang, C., Mobley, B. W., Nickerson, J. T., & Schatzberg, A. (2000). Early environment regulation of glucocorticoid feedback sensitivity in young adult monkeys. *Journal of Neuroendocrinology, 12,* 723–728.

Martin, L. J., Sackett, G. P., Gunderson, V. M., & Goodlin-Jones, B. M. (1988). Auditory evoked heart rate responses in pigtailed macaques raised in isolation. *Developmental Psychobiology, 22,* 251–260.

McGee, R., Wolfe, D., Yuen, S., Wilson, S., & Carnochan, J. (1995). The measurement of maltreatment: A comparison of approaches. *Child Abuse and Neglect, 19,* 233–249.

Meaney, M. J., Diorio, J., Francis, D., Widdowson, J., LaPlante, P., Caldji, C., Sharma, S., Seckl, J. R., & Plotsky, P. M. (1996). Early environmental regulation of forebrain glucocorticoid receptor gene expression: Implications for adrenocortical responses to stress. *Developmental Neuroscience, 18,* 49–72.

Metzger, L. J., Paige, S. R., Carson, M. A., Lasko, N. B., Paulus, L. A., Pitman, R. K., & Orr, S. P. (2004). PTSD arousal and depression symptoms associated with increased right-sided parietal asymmetry. *Journal of Abnormal Psychology, 113,* 324–329.

Money, J., Annecillo, C., & Kelly, J. F. (1983). Abuse–dwarfism syndrome: After rescue, statural and intellectual catchup growth correlate. *Journal of Clinical Child Psychology, 12,* 279–283.

Moradi, A. R., Doost, H. T. N., Taghavi, M. R., Yule, W., & Dalgleish, T. (1999). Everyday memory deficits in children and adolescents with PTSD: Performance on the Rivermead Behavioral Memory test. *Journal of Child Psychology and Psychiatry, 40,* 357–361.

National Research Council. (1993). *Understanding child abuse and neglect.* Washington, DC: National Academies Press.

Perez, C., & Widom, C. S. (1994). Childhood victimization and long-term intellectual and academic outcomes. *Child Abuse and Neglect, 18,* 617–633.

Perry, B. D. (Ed.). (1994). *Neurobiological sequelae of childhood trauma: PTSD in children.* Washington, DC: American Psychiatric Press, Inc.

Perry, B. D., & Pollard, R. (1998). Homeostasis, stress, trauma and adaptation. A neurodevelopmental view of childhood trauma. *Child and Adolescent Psychiatric Clinics of North America, 7,* 33–51.

Pianta, R., Egeland, B., & Erickson, M. F. (1989). Results of the mother–child interaction research project. In D. Cicchetti & V. Carlson (Eds.), *Child maltreatment: Theory and research on the causes and consequences of child abuse and neglect* (pp. 203–253). New York: Cambridge University Press.

Prichard, J. W. (1996). MRS of the brain—Prospects for clinical application. In I. R. Young & H. C. Charles (Eds.), *MR spectroscopy: Clinical applications and techniques* (pp. 1–25). London: Livery House.

Putnam, F. W., Trickett, P. K., Helmers, K., Dorn, L., & Everett, B. (1991). *Cortisol abnormalities in sexually abused girls.* Paper presented at the 144th Annual Meeting of the American Psychiatric Association, Washington, DC.

Queiroz, E. A., Lombardi, A. B., Santos Furtado, C. R. H., Peixoto, C. C. D., Soares, T. A., Fabre, Z. L., Basques, J. C., Fernandes, M.L.M., & Lippi, J. R. S. (1991). Biochemical correlate of depression in children. *Arq Neuro-Psiquiat, 49,* 418–425.

Quirk, G. J., Armony, J. L., & LeDoux, J. E. (1997). Fear conditioning enhances different temporal components of tone-evoked spike trains in auditory cortex and lateral amygdala. *Neuron, 19,* 613–624.

Rosenblum, L. A., & Andrews, M. W. (1994). Influences of environmental demand on maternal behavior and infant development. *Acta Paediatrica, 397*(Suppl.), 57–63.

Rutter, M., & Plomin, R. (1997). Opportunities for psychiatry from genetic findings. *British Journal of Psychiatry, 171,* 209–219.

Sanchez, M. M., Hearn, E. F., Do, D., Rilling, J. K., & Herndon, J. G. (1998). Differential rearing affects corpus callosum size and cognitive function of rhesus monkeys. *Brain Research, 812,* 38–49.

Sapolsky, R. M. (2000). Glucocorticoids and hippocampal atrophy in neuropsychiatric disorders. *Archives of General Psychiatry, 57,* 925–935.

Scheeringa, M. S., Zeanah, C. H., Drell, M. J., & Larrieu, J. A. (1995). Two approaches to the diagnosis of posttraumatic stress disorder in infancy and early childhood. *Journal of the American Academy of Child and Adolescent Psychiatry, 34,* 191–200.

Scheeringa, M. S., Zeanah, C. H., Myers, L., & Putnam, F. W. (2003). New findings on alternative criteria for PTSD in preschool children. *Journal of the American Academy of Child and Adolescent Psychiatry, 42,* 561–570.

Shin, L. M., McNally, R. J., Kosslyn, S. M., Thompson, W. L., Rauch, S. L., Alpert, N.

M., Metzger, L. J., Lasko, N. B., Orr, S. P., & Pitman, R. K. (1999). Regional cerebral blood flow during script-imagery in childhood sexual abuse-related PTSD: A PET investigation. *American Journal of Psychiatry, 156*, 575–584.

Shin, L. M., Orr, S. P., Carson, M. A., Rauch, S. L., Macklin, M. L., Lasko, N. B., Peters, P. M., Metzger, L. J., Dougherty, D. D., Cannistraro, P. A., Alpert, N. M., Fischman, A. J., & Pitman, R. K. (2004). Regional cerebral blood flow in the amygdala and medial prefrontal cortex during traumatic imagery in male and female Vietnam veterans with PTSD. *Archives of General Psychiatry, 61*, 168–176.

Shin, L. M., Whalen, P. J., Pitman, R. K., Bush, G., Macklin, M. L., Lasko, N. B., Orr, S. P., McInerney, S. C., & Rauch, S. L. (2001). An fMRI study of anterior cingulate function in posttraumatic stress disorder. *Biological Psychiatry, 50*, 932–942.

Simantov, R., Blinder, E., Ratovitski, T., Tauber, M., Gabbay, M., & Porat, S. (1996). Dopamine induced apoptosis in human neuronal cells: Inhibition by nucleic acids antisense to the dopamine transporter. *Neuroscience, 74*, 39–50.

Smith, M. A., Makino, S., Kvetnansky, R., & Post, R. M. (1995). Effects of stress on neurotrophic factor expression in the rat brain. *Annals of the New York Academy of Sciences, 771*, 234–239.

Smythies, J. R. (1997). Oxidative reactions and schizophrenia: A review-discussion. *Schizophrenia Research, 24*, 357–364.

Southwick, S. M., Yehuda, R., & Morgan, C. A. (1995). Clinical studies of neurotransmitter alterations in post-traumatic stress disorder. In M. J. Friedman, D. S. Charney, & A. Y. Deutsch (Eds.), *Neurobiological and clinical consequences of stress: From normal adaptation to post-traumatic stress disorder* (pp. 335–349). Philadelphia: Lippincott-Raven.

Southwick, S. S., Yehuda, R., & Wang, S. (1998). Neuroendocrine alterations in posttraumatic stress disorder. *Psychiatric Annals, 28*, 436–442.

Stapleton, J. M., Morgan, M. J., Liu, X., Yung, B. C., Phillips, R. L., Wong, D. F., Shaya, E. K., Dannals, R. F., & London, E. D. (1997). Cerebral glucose utilization is reduced in second test session. *Journal of Cerebral Blood Flow and Metabolism, 17*, 704–712.

Stefanacci, L., & Amaral, D. G. (2002). Some observations on cortical inputs to the macaque monkey amygdala: An antergade tracing study. *Journal of Comparative Neurology, 451*, 301–323.

Tanapat, P., Galea, L. A., & Gould, E. (1998). Stress inhibits the proliferation of granule cell precursors in the developing dentate gyrus. *Journal of Developmental Neuroscience, 16*, 235–239.

Teicher, M. H., Ito, Y., Glod, C. A., Andersen, S. L., Dumont, N., & Ackerman, E. (Eds.). (1997). *Preliminary evidence for abnormal cortical development in physically and sexually abused children using EEG coherence and MRI* (Vol. 821). New York: Annals of the New York Academy of Sciences.

Thomas, L. A., & De Bellis, M. D. (2004). Pituitary volumes in pediatric maltreatment related PTSD. *Biological Psychiatry, 55*, 752–758.

Todd, R. D. (1992). Neural development is regulated by classical neuro-transmitters: Dopamine D2 receptor stimulation enhances neurite outgrowth. *Biological Psychiatry, 31*, 794–807.

Trickett, P. K., & McBride-Chang, C. (1995). The developmental impact of different forms of child abuse and neglect. *Developmental Review, 15,* 311–337.

van der Kolk, B. A., Dreyfuss, D., Michaels, M., Shera, D., Berkowitz, R., Fisler, R., & Saxe, G. (1994). Fluoxetine in posttraumatic stress disorder. *Journal of Clinical Psychiatry, 55,* 517–522.

Walker, E. A., Unutzer, J., Rutter, C., Gelfand, A., Saunders, K., VonKorff, M., Koss, M. P., & Katon, W. (1999). Costs of health care use by women HMO members with a history of childhood abuse and neglect. *Archives of General Psychiatry, 56,* 609–613.

Widom, C. S. (1989). The cycle of violence. *Science, 244,* 160–166.

Widom, C. S. (1999). Posttraumatic stress disorder in abused and neglected children grown up. *American Journal of Psychiatry, 156,* 1223–1229.

Yehuda, R., Kahana, B., Binder-Brynes, K., Southwick, S., Mason, J. W., & Giller, E. L. (1995). Low urinary cortisol excretion in Holocaust survivors with post-traumatic stress disorder. *American Journal of Psychiatry, 152,* 982–986.

CHAPTER 8

Neuropsychological Findings in Adults with PTSD

JENNIFER J. VASTERLING
and KEVIN BRAILEY

Attention and memory impairments are thought to be integral to post-traumatic stress disorder (PTSD), so much so that they are included as PTSD criteria (C3, D3, and D4) in the fourth edition of the *Diagnostic and Statistical Manual of Mental Disorders* (DSM-IV; American Psychiatric Association, 1994). Complaints of cognitive impairment characterize sizable subsets of patients treated for PTSD (e.g., Burstein, 1985), but subjective complaints do not necessarily accurately gauge objective neuropsychological performance in such patients (Roca & Freeman, 2001). Because of the potential adverse impact of cognitive compromise on daily life activities and the well-established links between brain dysfunction and neuropsychological impairment, researchers have recently begun to examine the extent to which objective neuropsychological deficits accompany PTSD. Documentation of such deficits holds potential to inform both clinical management of PTSD and theoretical conceptualizations relevant to disorder etiology and maintenance.

This chapter focuses primarily on information derived from research examining performance on traditional neuropsychological tasks in adults, whereas Constans (Chapter 5, this volume) focuses on information-processing paradigms. We first summarize the literature according to functional categorizations common to neuropsychological practice, with emphasis on studies that both include comparison samples and report univariate or multivariate comparisons organized by functional domain. We then integrate findings into three possible frameworks relative to PTSD: (1) cognitive dysfunction as a byproduct of reduced motivation or poor concentration; (2) cognitive dysfunction as a feature of neurobiological abnormalities; and (3) neurocognitive integrity as a risk–resilience factor for the development and/or maintenance of PTSD. There is much debate regarding the extent to which neuropsychological deficits accompanying PTSD are reflective of comorbidities, population characteristics, and treatment factors rather than a direct consequence of PTSD (see Duke & Vasterling, Chapter 1, this volume; Danckwerts & Leathem, 2003; Horner & Hamner, 2002 for recent reviews). Therefore, we conclude the chapter by addressing the specificity of neuropsychological abnormalities to PTSD and the potential influence of comorbid psychopathology, somatic factors, and medications on cognitive functioning.

NEUROPSYCHOLOGICAL FINDINGS

Intellectual Functioning

The term "IQ" is somewhat misleading in that, as typically measured, "intelligence" is rarely a unitary or static construct. Discussion of theories of intelligence is beyond the scope of the chapter; however, it is worth noting that conventional intellectual tasks may measure a number of distinct cognitive processes, such as attention, reasoning, and visuospatial processing. Whereas some of the tasks comprising an intellectual assessment are likely sensitive to change (i.e., "fluid" tasks), others are thought to be "crystallized" and thus less likely to be affected by many forms of adult-acquired brain insult or situational factors. This distinction becomes important when trying to make causal inferences regarding PTSD and cognitive compromise.

Few studies have measured intellectual functioning in PTSD, and even fewer have used comprehensive measurement methodologies that address multiple facets of intellectual functioning. Nonetheless, a pattern has emerged in which PTSD diagnosis is associated with lower estimated and omnibus IQ scores (Brandes et al., 2002; Gil, Calev, Greenberg, Kugelmass, & Lerer, 1990; Gilbertson, Gurvits, Lasko, Orr, & Pitman, 2001; Gurvits et al., 1993, 2000; Macklin et al., 1998; Vasterling, Brailey, Constans, Borges, & Sutker, 1997; Vasterling et al., 2002). Although there are too few studies examining intellectual functioning comprehensively to make firm conclusions regarding which aspects of intelligence are impaired in PTSD, Vasterling et al. (1997) found that verbal intellectual performances appeared to be particularly sensitive to PTSD status, and that within verbal tasks, PTSD was associated with performance deficits on both "fluid" and "crystallized" tasks. This pattern was generally consistent with Gil et al.

(1990), in which group differences were largest for verbal tasks. Because many of the studies examining intellectual functioning in PTSD used military veteran samples, it is possible that findings could be explained by military personnel with higher levels of education (correlated with performance on traditional intellectual tasks) being assigned to less combat-intensive war-zone duties than personnel with lower levels of formal academic education. However, when combat exposure (as a proxy for stressor severity) has been controlled statistically, PTSD symptom severity has remained negatively correlated with intellectual performance (Macklin et al., 1998; McNally & Shin, 1995; Vasterling et al., 2002), suggesting that the relationship between intellectual performance and PTSD symptom severity in veteran populations cannot be explained solely on the basis of military personnel with lower IQ being assigned to heavier combat duties.

Attentional and Executive Functioning

Historically, the delineation between attention and executive functioning, which may be viewed as the capacity to exert appropriate attentional control to participate in purposive action and goal-directed behavior (cf. Baddeley, 2002; Lezak, 1995), has been somewhat indistinct. Because of the overlap in the measurement of these constructs, findings relevant to attention and executive functions are reviewed together.

Poor "concentration" is so commonly reported in PTSD that it constitutes a DSM diagnostic symptom criterion within the arousal cluster (D3). Consistent with this observation, PTSD is often accompanied by relative performance deficits on objective, performance-based attentional tasks (e.g., Sachinvala et al., 2000; Sutker, Vasterling, Brailey, & Allain, 1995). However, not all aspects of attention appear to be impaired in PTSD. In a series of studies (Vasterling, Brailey, Constans, & Sutker, 1998; Vasterling et al., 2002) conducted on two distinct military veteran populations (1991 Gulf War and Vietnam War veterans), we used Mirsky, Anthony, Duncan, Ahearn, and Kellam's (1991) model of attention to examine dissociations across attentional domains. The Mirsky model conceptualizes attention as encompassing four components: (1) Focus–Execute—the ability to focus on specific environmental cues from an array and respond appropriately to them; (2) Sustain—the capacity to maintain optimal levels of focused attention or vigilance over time; (3) Shift—the ability to change the focus of attention in an adaptive manner; and (4) Encode—the capacity to register, recall, and mentally manipulate information. We found that, in both veteran cohorts, veterans with PTSD diagnosis performed more poorly than war-zone-exposed veterans without PTSD on tasks requiring sustained attention and tasks requiring encoding capacity but not on tasks within the Focus–Execute or Shift domains. More specifically, PTSD-related impairments were found on continuous performance tasks (Sustain) and on digit repetition and mental arithmetic tasks (Encode) but not on such tasks as letter cancellation (Focus–Execute), the standard Stroop (Focus–Execute), or a card sorting task requiring set shifting (Shift).

These findings generally mirror those of other behavioral studies in which PTSD-related performance deficits were found on "encode," or working memory, tasks (e.g., Beckham, Crawford, & Feldman, 1998; Brandes et al., 2002; Gil et al., 1990; Gilbertson et al., 2001; Gurvits et al., 1993; Jenkins, Langlais, Delis, & Cohen, 2000; Uddo, Vasterling, Brailey, & Sutker, 1993; Vasterling et al., 1997), but not on "shift" tasks such as the Wisconsin Card Sorting Test (WCST; Heaton, 1981) (Barrett, Green, Morris, Giles, & Croft, 1996; Gurvits et al., 1993; Sullivan et al., 2003; Vasterling, Brailey, & Sutker, 2000) or the Posner Visual Selective Attention Task (Posner, Walker, Friedrich, & Rafal, 1984; Jenkins et al., 2000), especially when potentially confounding factors were controlled (e.g., Gilbertson et al., 2001). The absence of PTSD-related deficits on set shifting tasks may not be universal across age groups, as such deficits have been associated with PTSD in elderly former prisoners of war (Sutker et al., 1995). Although some researchers have not documented working memory deficits in select samples restricted to higher educational ranges (Neylan et al., 2004), lower levels of PTSD symptom severity (Pederson et al., 2004), and treatment seekers with and without PTSD (Sullivan et al., 2003), findings of working memory deficits are supported by a growing functional imaging literature suggesting that PTSD is also associated with alterations in neural activation during working memory tasks (see Shin, Rauch, & Pitman, Chapter 3, this volume).

As compared to other attentional domains, replications of sustained attention task performances are less robust, possibly because of differences in task demands (e.g., stimulus duration, interstimulus interval, task duration, response/nonresponse requirements) across studies and/or population differences. Whereas some studies documented deficits on continuous performance tasks similar to those in our work described above (Gil et al., 1990; Jenkins et al., 2000; McFarlane, Weber, & Clark, 1993; Semple et al., 1996), others failed to replicate this finding (Golier et al., 1997; Sullivan et al., 2003; Vasterling, Brailey, et al., 2000).

Although the standard Stroop paradigm, which is comprised of emotionally neutral stimuli, has rarely been employed in PTSD research, studies using this paradigm have not revealed PTSD-related abnormalities in the interference condition (Litz et al., 1996; Sullivan et al., 1993; Vasterling et al., 1998, 2002). However, robust abnormalities suggestive of attentional bias to threat-relevant information occur when the paradigm is altered to include trauma-relevant information (see Constans, Chapter 5, this volume), suggesting that emotional context influences performance and, in this case, the ability to inhibit threat-relevant semantic interference.

The more general failure to inhibit inappropriate responses and to perseverate responses may contribute to impaired performance across cognitive domains. Noting a pattern of disinhibition and commission errors across attention and memory tasks, Vasterling et al. (1998) used commission errors, false positives, and intrusion errors to create a "cognitive intrusion" factor derived from principal components analysis and found that the tendency to make intrusions on emotionally neutral neuropsychological tasks was positively correlated with reexperiencing symptoms and negatively correlated with avoidance/numbing symptoms when controlling for other PTSD symptom clusters. Similarly, Koenen et al. (2001) found that PTSD was associated with perseveration of response on an object-alternation task, which is a comparative neuropsychology task sensitive to dysfunction of the prefrontal cortex and especially of the ventromedial prefrontal region (Freedman, Black, Ebert, & Binns, 1998; Oscar-Berman, McNamara, & Freedman, 1991).

Learning and Memory

Much of the neuropsychological literature in PTSD has focused on explicit, anterograde learning and memory tasks using emotionally neutral stimuli (see Constans, Chapter 5, this volume, for a review of memory tasks using emotionally relevant stimuli). Although there are clear exceptions (cf. Neylan et al., 2004; Pederson et al., 2004; Stein, Hanna, Vaerum, & Koverola, 1999; Stein, Kennedy, & Twamley, 2002; Sullivan et al., 2003; Zalewski, Thompson, & Gottesman, 1994), most studies comparing learning and memory performances between PTSD-diagnosed and non-PTSD-diagnosed participants have documented PTSD-related deficits on one or more learning or memory measures (e.g., Barrett et al., 1996[1]; Bremner et al., 1993; Brandes et al., 2002; Bremner, Randall, Scott, Capelli, et al.,

---

[1]Following adjustment for a number of demographic and military variables, group differences in immediate recall disappeared. Although a covariance strategy has been successfully employed in regression models in a handful of studies in this area, it could be argued that some of the covariates (e.g., military occupational specialty, combat exposure) included by Barrett et al. (1996) were likely to be so highly correlated with PTSD as to remove most of the variance attributable to PTSD, especially with multiple covariates of this type included in the model. Unfortunately, because of the dose–response relationship between stress exposure and PTSD, and the likelihood of some military assignments being associated with greater combat exposure, there is no ideal solution to tease apart stress exposure from PTSD in combat veterans. Even when the comparison sample is combat exposed, the PTSD group is likely as a whole to have experienced more extensive combat.

1995; Bustamante, Mellman, David, & Fins, 2001; Gil et al., 1990; Gilbertson et al., 2001; Golier et al., 2002; Gurvits et al., 1993; Jenkins, Langlais, Delis, & Cohen, 1998; Koenen et al., 2001; Sachinvala et al., 2000; Uddo et al., 1993; Vasterling et al., 1998, 2002; Vasterling, Brailey, et al., 2000; Yehuda, Golier, Halligan, & Harvey, 2004; Yehuda et al., 1995). However, inspection of the findings relevant to specific measures suggests that not all aspects of anterograde memory may be compromised in PTSD. Anterograde memory is not a unitary construct and may instead be broken down into several component processes including, at its most basic level, initial registration of information (measured at immediate recall and during learning trials) and retention of newly learned information over time (measured at delayed recall, relative to immediate recall or learning proficiency).

Taken as a whole, PTSD studies yielding positive findings of memory dysfunction have revealed that initial acquisition is the most pervasively impaired aspect of memory dysfunction associated with PTSD. Although fewer in number, studies employing interference lists to examine proactive interference (i.e., previously learned material interferes with the learning and recall of new information) and retroactive interference (i.e., the interference of newly presented information on recall of previously learned information) have typically revealed that PTSD is also associated with heightened sensitivity to proactive (Uddo et al., 1993) and retroactive (Vasterling et al., 1998, 2002; Yehuda et al., 1995) interference when initial learning is taken into account (see Neylan et al., 2004; Stein et al., 1999, for counterexamples).

The evidence that PTSD is associated with degraded retention of newly learned information over longer delayed intervals is less compelling. The distinction between initial acquisition and memory retention is important, as retention (i.e., "memory savings") has been closely associated with the integrity of the hippocampal system (Eichenbaum, 1994), an area that has received much emphasis in some neurobiological formulations of PTSD. Although a number of studies documented that PTSD-diagnosed participants were impaired on one or more delayed recall measures compared to participants without PTSD (e.g., Brandes et al., 2002; Bremner et al., 1993; Bremner, Randall, Scott, Capelli, et al., 1995; Gilbertson et al., 2001; Jenkins et al., 1998; Vasterling et al., 1998, 2002; Vasterling, Brailey, et al., 2000), relative impairment on delayed recall does not necessarily reflect a loss in retention, especially in disorders such as PTSD in which initial acquisition of new information is impaired. That is, loss in retention implies that recall after a delay is less proficient than earlier recall more proximal to stimulus presentation. Thus, to measure retention, it is useful for interpretation to take into account initial acquisition.

A number of PTSD studies have used savings ratios, percent retention, difference scores, or covariance to adjust for strength of initial acquisition.

However, the findings produced by these studies are mixed. Whereas several studies conducted with civilian (Brandes et al., 2002; Stein et al., 1999; Stein et al., 2002) and military veteran (Sullivan et al., 2003; Vasterling et al., 1998, 2002; Vasterling, Brailey, et al., 2000) samples failed to reveal PTSD-related deficits in memory retention, in other studies, PTSD was associated with less proficient memory retention in samples of Vietnam veterans (Bremner et al., 1993) and adult survivors of childhood abuse (Bremner, Randall, Scott, Capelli, et al., 1995). Although Yehuda et al. (1995) found that delayed recall on a list learning task was degraded relative to recall during learning trials, this decrement appeared to be secondary to retroactive interference, as performance remained stable from recall immediately after an interference list to recall after a 20-minute interval.

A final distinction regarding explicit, anterograde memory tasks can be made between "free," or unstructured, and structured retrieval formats such as cued recall or recognition. Most PTSD studies have typically restricted measurement of memory to free recall formats. The few studies using both structured and unstructured retrieval formats indicated that PTSD and comparison samples did not differ significantly when memory was assessed with cued recall or recognition formats, even when PTSD-related free recall decrements were found during learning and over delayed intervals (Jenkins et al., 1998; Vasterling et al., 1998). Using a directed forgetting paradigm and a mood-induction manipulation, Zoellner, Sacks, and Foa (2003) likewise found that recall was poorer among PTSD-diagnosed sexual assault victims as compared to a nontraumatized control group across experimental conditions but did not find group differences on a recognition task. As with retention versus initial acquisition, the distinction between recognition and free recall is important regarding the underlying neuroanatomical substrates. Namely, hippocampal dysfunction is typically associated with impaired retrieval under both structured and unstructured conditions, whereas performance is typically enhanced with imposed structure (e.g., recognition) in the context of prefrontal dysfunction (Shimamura, 2002).

Implicit memory (i.e., memory without awareness) using neutral stimuli has rarely been examined in PTSD. Golier et al. (2002) found that, as compared to Holocaust survivors without PTSD and age-matched Jewish adults without Holocaust exposure, Holocaust survivors with PTSD did not differ in performance on a word-stem completion task despite performing more poorly on the learning trials of a paired-associates task.

Visuospatial Functioning

As summarized above, visuospatial measures derived from intellectual tasks have not tended to differ between PTSD and comparison samples. Likewise, studies measuring visuospatial functioning with tasks such as mental organization (Sullivan et al., 2003) and figural drawing (Gilbertson et al., 2001; Gurvits et al., 1993; Gurvits, Carson, et al., 2002) have not revealed group differences on most measures. As an exception, Gurvits, Lasko, et al. (2002) found that PTSD-diagnosed participants performed more poorly on a figure-copying task than trauma-exposed participants without PTSD diagnoses, but that these findings were largely explained by pretrauma variables.

Language

Primary language functions have infrequently been examined in PTSD, likely because there is little clinical or theoretical reason to believe that functions such as language production, comprehension, or repetition would be impaired. For example, Gurvits et al. (1993) found no evidence of dysgraphia or dysphasia in either PTSD-diagnosed or non-PTSD combat-exposed veterans. However, verbal fluency, as measured by word-list generation, has been examined in several PTSD studies because of its purported sensitivity to prefrontal cortical dysfunction and to semantic memory loss (see Shimamura, 2002). With rare exception (e.g., Stein et al., 2002), the literature suggests that PTSD is associated with performance decrements in phonemic list generation (i.e., providing words that begin with a target letter; Gil et al., 1990; Bustamante et al., 2001; Koenen et al., 2001), whereas studies examining semantic list generation (i.e., providing words that belong to a target category) have provided mixed results (Gil et al., 1990; Uddo et al., 1993; Stein et al., 2002). Interestingly, although Matsuo et al. (2003) did not find behavioral performance differences during a phonemic list-generation task between PTSD- and non-PTSD-diagnosed victims of the Tokyo subway sarin attack, PTSD was associated with attenuated hemodynamic response in the prefrontal cortex during the task, suggesting that regions not typically associated with word-list generation may have compensated for deficient prefrontal activation during the task.

Motor Functioning

Except on tasks involving "executive" control, there is little evidence of motor dysfunction in PTSD. The one study examining fine motor speed and manual dexterity with formal neuropsychological tests (i.e., finger oscillation and pegboard) did not reveal a group difference between PTSD- and non-PTSD-diagnosed Gulf War veterans (Sullivan et al., 2003). Similarly, in a series of studies assessing neurological soft signs, performance on tests of motor coordination, fine motor movements, and ideomotor praxis did not differentiate between PTSD- and non-PTSD-diagnosed, trauma-exposed participants (Gurvits et al., 1993, 2000; Gurvits, Carson, et al., 2002). However, in two of the three studies in the Gurvits series, motor sequencing, a task thought also to involve executive control (Fama & Sullivan, 2002) was impaired (Gurvits et al., 1993; Gurvits et al., 2000).

NEUROPSYCHOLOGICAL FRAMEWORKS

Cognitive Dysfunction as a Motivational Byproduct

One possible explanation of neurocognitive performance deficits in PTSD is that individuals with PTSD are not sufficiently engaged in the tasks to perform to their full potential. Diminished motivation could be explained by poor concentration associated with psychological distress or intentionally poor performance associated with secondary gain. Although formal tasks of motivation have not typically been included in research examining neuropsychological functioning in PTSD, it is difficult to ascribe motivational or generalized concentration deficits as the salient etiological factors for cognitive dysfunction in these studies for several reasons.

First, although PTSD diagnosis is associated with attentional impairment, most studies examining different aspects of attention have found that only specific attentional processes are impaired, with little evidence of the type of global pattern of impairment that would be expected to occur with a generalized concentration problem or poor effort. In fact, as described in Constans (Chapter 5, this volume), PTSD is instead associated with enhanced attention in specific contexts (i.e., to trauma-relevant information). Second, as described later in this chapter, the emerging pattern of neurocognitive deficits associated with PTSD converges with neurobiological models of PTSD, paralleling findings from neurophysiological, neuroimaging, and electrophysiological research (see Southwick, Rasmusson, Barron, & Arnsten, Chapter 2, this volume; Shin, Rauch, & Pitman, Chapter 3, this volume; and Metzger, Gilbertson, & Orr, Chapter 4, this volume). Third, regarding secondary gain issues, it is noteworthy that neuropsychological deficits have emerged across PTSD populations, including in both treatment-seeking (e.g., Vasterling et al., 2002) and community-recruited, nontreatment and noncompensation-seeking samples (e.g., Vasterling et al., 1998), producing almost identical patterns of results when measurement methodologies have been kept similar. Finally, excepting specific subgroups for whom secondary gain is a particular issue (e.g., compensation seekers, litigants), there is not compelling evidence that individuals with PTSD are likely to deliver a deliberately poor performance. Even when financial compensation is a consideration, cognitive performance is often not as central or face valid to the issue of PTSD compensation as are psychological symptoms. Supporting this contention, Beckham et al. (1998) demonstrated that

PTSD-related performance deficits on the Trail Making Test remained among Vietnam theater veterans when subgroup analyses were conducted in which those receiving compensation were removed from the analyses.

Nonetheless, the field would benefit from direct assessment of motivation, either through experimental manipulation or with cognitive tasks designed specifically to detect inadequate effort. A particularly fruitful area of research may be the experimental examination of initiative processes in PTSD. As is the case with depression (see Hertel, 2000, for a review), apparent motivational limitations in PTSD may instead reflect basic deficits in cognitive initiation, possibly reflective of prefrontal dysfunction. Such deficits are characterized by failures to access optimal strategic cognitive processes spontaneously when learning new information in contrast to the successful use of such strategies when specifically directed to use them.

Cognitive Dysfunction as a Feature of Neurobiological Abnormalities

As discussed in Part II of this volume, functional and/or structural abnormalities in several brain regions, including the prefrontal cortex, amygdala, and hippocampus, may account for much of the neuropsychological dysfunction associated with PTSD. Whereas hyperactivation of the amygdala is likely most relevant to information processing biases associated with emotionally relevant information (see Constans, Chapter 5, this volume; Brewin, Chapter 6, this volume), performance deficits on emotionally neutral tasks may be explained more directly by dysfunction of the prefrontal cortex and/or hippocampus. Early neurobiological conceptualizations of PTSD focused heavily on dysfunction within the hippocampus (Bremner, 2001), hypothesized to be a result of HPA-axis alterations and associated glucocorticoid abnormalities (Bremner, 1999; Golier & Yehuda, 1998); however, more recent conceptualizations have included a broader range of neurobiological systems and neuroanatomical loci (see Southwick, Rasmusson, Barron, & Arnsten, Chapter 2, this volume).

A survey of the neuropsychological literature supports the view that neural dysfunction in PTSD is not limited to the hippocampus but extends to other limbic and paralimbic regions. Similar to findings produced by neuroradiological studies, neuropsychological studies have produced mixed results on measures purported to be sensitive to hippocampal system, or medial temporal, dysfunction. As summarized above, the most consistently impaired learning and memory indices have been those (e.g., initial acquisition, sensitivity to interference) that are often associated with frontal system dysfunction (Shimamura, 1996). Findings on measures of memory savings, an index more sensitive to medial temporal dysfunction (Butters & Delis, 1995), have been somewhat less robust. The interdependency of the hippocampus and prefrontal cortex in supporting certain cognitive functions (e.g., new learning) precludes statements regarding specific localizations (Tulving, Markowitsch, Craik, Habib, & Houle, 1996). However, neuropsychological performance patterns can address the relative involvement of frontal versus medial temporal systems.

We hypothesize that, whereas there may be subtle cognitive performance deficits reflective of hippocampal dysfunction, much of the cognitive impairment observed on emotionally neutral tasks in PTSD is likely attributable to dysfunction in regions (e.g., prefrontal cortex) more sensitive to abnormalities in neurotransmitter systems (e.g., noradrenergic and serotonergic systems) involved in the regulation of arousal. For example, the findings of Koenen et al. (2001) using comparative neuropsychological tasks (described earlier in this chapter) pointed to the disruption of both dorsolateral and ventral (orbitofrontal) prefrontal regions in PTSD. We have also found that PTSD diagnosis is associated with relative performance deficits in olfactory identification (Vasterling, Brailey, et al., 2000), a function linked to orbitofrontal integrity (Savic, Bookheimer, Fried, & Engel, 1997). Disruption of the orbitofrontal region may be particularly relevant to PTSD, as it is richly connected with both the hippocampus and amygdala (Freedman et al., 1998; Goldman-Rakic, Ranagashi, & Bruce, 1990).

Similar to the neuroanatomical models discussed in Chapters 2 and 3 of this volume, we hypothesize that PTSD is associated in particular with diminished prefrontal inhibitory functions. From a neuropsychological perspective, decreased cognitive inhibition would be expected to lead to difficulty avoiding distraction from extraneous information. We documented a tendency across tasks for PTSD-diagnosed individuals to make more errors of commission (Vasterling et al., 1998), a finding associated with induced arousal states in animals (Robbins & Everitt, 1996). Working memory deficits are also frequently found in PTSD. Although also potentially linked to hippocampal integrity, working memory is thought to be strongly related to prefrontal dysfunction in humans (Baddeley, 1986; Smith & Jonides, 1996) and, of relevance to PTSD, has been theorized to reflect a failure to inhibit information not central to the task (Shimamura, 1996). Our own work (Vasterling et al., 1998) suggested that failure to inhibit information on neutral neurocognitive tasks is associated with reexperiencing symptoms, which could be conceptualized as a failure to inhibit unwanted emotional memories. Interestingly, antiadrenergic agents such as clonidine, which have been found to be helpful in reducing arousal-based symptoms of PTSD in humans (see Morgan, Krystal, & Southwick, 2003, for a review), have been noted to improve prefrontal cortical functioning at the level of alpha$_2$ receptors in animals. Specifically, Arnsten and Goldman-Rakic (1998) found that administration of clonidine improved performance on working memory tasks via facilitation of inhibition of irrelevant and potentially distracting stimuli.

Whether or not neural dysfunction in PTSD is lateralized to one cerebral hemisphere to a greater extent than the other, as some theories of hemispheric specialization of emotion might predict, remains unclear. Taken as a whole, findings generated by the neuropsychological literature suggest bilateral cerebral involvement. However, the degree to which neural abnormalities in PTSD occur to the same extent across the right and left cerebral hemispheres is less certain. Although neuroimaging studies have generally revealed unilateral findings indicating greater activation of the right hemisphere and smaller left hemisphere volumes in PTSD participants compared to controls (e.g., Bremner et al., 2003; Shaw et al., 2002; Villarreal et al., 2002), this pattern of results is not universal (cf. Bremner, Randall, Scott, Bronen, et al., 1995). Bolstering the neuroimaging literature, Metzger et al. (2004) used electrophysiological methods to examine cerebral asymmetry in PTSD and found that PTSD arousal symptoms were associated with increased right-sided parietal activation. Likewise, we have documented evidence of relative right hemisphere advantage on behavioral tasks. Using a block design construction task, PTSD was associated with an error pattern (i.e., minor rotations in right hemispace) suggestive of relative left hemisphere hypoactivation (Vasterling, Rogers, & Kaplan, 2000). Similarly, on a visual attention task, PTSD-diagnosed combat veterans responded more slowly than a no-disorders comparison sample to local, but not global, targets, a finding consistent with relative right hemisphere advantage (Vasterling, Duke, Tomlin, Lowery, & Kaplan, 2004). These findings are consistent with research demonstrating that PTSD is associated with reduced right lateral preference (Chemtob & Taylor, 2003; Spivak, Segal, Mester, & Weizman, 1998). However, further evidence using convergent methodologies is warranted.

Cognitive Dysfunction: Cause or Effect?

The supposition that neuropsychological performance decrements are related to neurobiological abnormalities associated with PTSD does not address whether biological and neuropsychological abnormalities are a consequence of PTSD, represent a risk–resilience factor for PTSD, or both. As discussed in Southwick, Rasmusson, Barron, and Arnsten (Chapter 2, this volume), the association between exposure to life-threatening events and physiological response (e.g., the "fight or flight" response) has long been documented in both animals and humans. However, whether biological responses and associated psychopathology endure or dissipate after removal of threat is not uniform across individuals. Thus, it is not clear whether individuals with PTSD and associated neurobiological (and neuropsychological) abnormalities (1) suffer greater neurobiological/neuropsychological sequelae of PTSD, (2) developed PTSD because they were at greater neurobiological/neuropsychological risk prior to trauma exposure, and/or (3) maintain the disorder longer because of neurobiological and neuropsychological factors present either prior to trauma and/or early in the course of the disorder.

The most direct evidence that stress exposure leads to neurobiological and behavioral alterations comes from animal research. Animal studies in which stress was induced have suggested that stress exposure may lead to both neurobiological alterations and changes in behavior, including performance decrements on prefrontal working memory tasks (e.g., Arnsten & Goldman-Rakic, 1998; Birnbaum, Gobeske, Auerbach, Taylor, & Arnsten, 1999; Shansky et al., 2004) and hippocampally mediated learning and memory tasks (e.g., Ohl, Michaelis, Vollman-Honsdorf, Kirschbaum, & Fuchs, 2000). In humans, because ethical considerations prohibit manipulating exposure to trauma, the most direct examination of causation would incorporate prospective pretrauma assessment. However, to date no published studies exist in which individuals at high risk for trauma exposure were examined prospectively on neuropsychological tasks.[2]

Four alternate methodological approaches examining neuropsychological integrity as a risk–resilience factor for PTSD development or maintenance have provided evidence that at least some aspects of cognitive functioning may be viewed as risk–resilience factors. First, several studies using retrospective estimates of pretrauma cognitive functioning (e.g., vocabulary, fund of information, and verbal IQ screening tasks) have found that less proficient performance was associated with PTSD on these measures (e.g., Gurvits et al., 2000; McNally & Shin, 1995; Vasterling et al., 1998), even when performance on more situationally sensitive tasks was controlled statistically (Vasterling et al., 2002). Second, with one exception (Crowell, Kieffer, Siders, & Vanderploeg, 2002), studies using archival data have indicated that PTSD diagnosis was associated with fewer intellectual resources, as measured by indirect estimates of intellectual functioning measured prior to trauma exposure such as military aptitude test results (Centers for Disease Control Vietnam Experiences Study, 1988; Macklin et al., 1998; Pitman, Orr, Lowenhagen, Macklin, & Altman, 1991), educational achievement (Green, Grace, Lindy, Gleser, & Leonard, 1990; Harel, Kahana, & Kahana, 1988; Kulka et al., 1990), and military rank (Sutker, Bugg, & Allain, 1990). Third, Bustamante et al. (2001) assessed neuropsychological functioning longitudinally in 38 participants with physically in-

---

[2]Prospective work by our group that may help address causal directionality is underway.

duced traumatic injuries. Findings indicated that, whereas PTSD symptom severity and neuropsychological performances measured shortly after trauma exposure were not correlated, learning, memory, and verbal fluency performances measured shortly after trauma exposure were negatively correlated with PTSD symptom severity measured 6 weeks later. That is, early neuropsychological performance predicted later PTSD symptom severity, suggesting that the degree of neuropsychological integrity following trauma exposure may be a risk–resilience factor for the subsequent course of psychopathology development and maintenance.

Finally, Gilbertson and his colleagues (M. W. Gilbertson, personal communication, July 14, 2004) studied monozygotic twin pairs who were discordant for combat exposure and found that the identical co-twins of PTSD combat veterans, who had neither combat exposure nor PTSD themselves, showed nearly the same pattern of cognitive results as their PTSD brothers in the areas of IQ, verbal memory, and executive function. These combat-unexposed co-twins of PTSD combat veterans also performed less proficiently than the unexposed co-twins of combat veterans who never developed PTSD, suggesting that the most frequently observed neurocognitive differences in PTSD represent a familial predisposition factor.

While speculative, there are several possible mechanisms by which neuropsychological integrity could serve as a risk–resilience factor. It may be that neurobiological factors confer risk, or resilience, via central nervous system vulnerability to stress (e.g., Morgan et al., 2000), and that neuropsychological functioning is simply a byproduct of these biological alterations. Findings of increased psychological symptomatology in trauma survivors with acquired history of brain injury as compared to trauma survivors without history of brain injury provide indirect support for this possibility (Chemtob et al., 1998; Mollica, Henderson, & Tor, 2002; Vasterling, Constans, & Hanna-Pladdy, 2000). However, neuropsychological functioning may in and of itself confer risk or enhance resilience. For example, increased executive and inhibitory control of emotions, trauma memories, and impulses would be expected to result in better psychosocial outcome. Heightened cognitive and intellectual proficiency may also be expected to lead to increased attainment of personal resources, including higher education, enhanced occupational functioning, and higher socioeconomic levels, all of which appear to buffer stress impact (Hobfoll, 1989; Sutker & Allain, 1995; Ursano, Wheatley, Sledge, Rahe, & Carlson, 1986). Conversely, cognitive impairment would be expected to disrupt educational, occupational, and social endeavors, potentially resulting in increased financial and daily life stress. Finally, more proficient neuropsychological and intellectual skills may also lead to more effective and active use of coping techniques, such as the establishment of more extensive social support networks (Cohen & Willis, 1985) and formation of narratives in assimilation of traumatic memories and emotions (Harber & Pennebaker, 1992) into accessible forms (Brewin, 2001, 2003).

As suggested by the results of Vasterling et al. (2002), which indicated that estimated premorbid functioning and measures of attention and learning were independently associated with PTSD diagnosis, it may be that neurocognitive dysfunction may represent both a risk factor for the development and maintenance of PTSD and a consequence of PTSD. It could be speculated that a downward spiral (Hobfoll, 1989) exists in which neurocognitive dysfunction leads to increased risk of PTSD via ineffective coping or resource diminishment and the development of PTSD leads to greater cognitive dysfunction, which in turn leads to further exacerbation of PTSD symptoms. However, only prospective research will allow adequate examination of this hypothesis.

ARE NEUROPSYCHOLOGICAL IMPAIRMENTS FOLLOWING TRAUMA EXPOSURE SPECIFIC TO PTSD?

Although there is converging evidence that PTSD is associated with less proficient neuropsychological performance, the degree to which performance decrements are specific to PTSD has been the subject of much recent debate. As summarized in Duke and Vasterling (Chapter 1, this volume), PTSD does not occur in a vacuum and is associated with psychiatric comorbidities, adverse health consequences, and somatic insult at the time of traumatization, each of which could potentially exert adverse consequences on neuropsychological functioning. Moreover, it is possible that either trauma exposure, impacting independently of psychological sequelae, or centrally acting medications could also lead to neuropsychological impairment. Each of these categories of possible contributing factors is considered below.

Trauma Exposure

In studies comparing PTSD-diagnosed individuals to healthy, non-trauma-exposed individuals or to a combined group of non-trauma-exposed and trauma-exposed individuals, it is difficult to parcel out the effects of trauma exposure from the psychological sequelae of exposure (i.e., PTSD). However, studies comparing trauma-exposed participants with PTSD to those without PTSD have typically indicated that PTSD is associated with neuropsychological or intellectual deficits above and beyond trauma exposure alone (e.g., Barrett et al., 1996; Beckham et al., 1998; Brandes et al.,

2002; Gilbertson et al., 2001; Gurvits et al., 2000; Gurvits et al., 1993; Jenkins et al., 1998, 2000; Kivling-Boden & Sundbom, 2003; Koenen et al., 2001; Vasterling et al., 1997, 1998, 2002; Vasterling, Brailey, et al., 2000; Vasterling, Rogers, et al., 2000), although this finding is not uniform (Neylan et al., 2004; Sullivan et al., 2003).

Fewer studies have examined both healthy trauma-exposed and non-trauma-exposed comparison samples, allowing for direct examination of the association of trauma exposure without PTSD to neuropsychological performance deficits. Studies comparing trauma-exposed and non-trauma-exposed healthy comparison samples have not revealed differences on neuropsychological measures between psychopathology-free Vietnam combat theater and nondeployed Vietnam-era veterans (Vasterling, Brailey, et al., 2000), rape victims without mental disorders and age- and education-matched nontraumatized individuals (Jenkins et al., 1998, 2000), or healthy Holocaust survivors and age-matched Jewish adults not exposed to the Holocaust (Golier et al., 2002), whereas in each of these studies PTSD-diagnosed individuals showed relative cognitive impairment. Although Pederson et al. (2004) did not find differences in cognitive performance among trauma-exposed and non-trauma-exposed participants, results likewise revealed no evidence of significant differences between adult survivors of childhood abuse with PTSD and those without PTSD.

The use of covariance procedures to demonstrate unique relationships between PTSD and cognitive performance in some ways is a particularly stringent test, given that PTSD and trauma exposure severity tend to be highly correlated (Foy, Osato, Houskamp, & Neumann, 1992) and it might be expected that much of the variance in PTSD would be eliminated once variance shared with trauma severity is removed. However, studies attempting to control statistically for trauma severity have provided evidence that PTSD is associated with cognitive performance above and beyond trauma exposure, particularly on measures of intellectual functioning (e.g., Gilbertson et al., 2001; Macklin et al., 1998; McNally & Shin, 1995; Vasterling et al., 2002). Supporting these findings with a subgroup analysis approach, Beckham et al. (1998) demonstrated that among both the total sample of Vietnam veterans included in the study, as well as in a subsample of veterans with relatively lower levels of combat exposure, those with PTSD diagnoses showed greater relative impairment on Trails B, a visuomotor tracking task requiring alternation of alphabetical and numerical sequences. In contrast, Barrett et al. (1996) found that covarying for combat exposure and a number of other military and sociodemographic variables eliminated a significant group difference in verbal immediate recall performance. Likewise, Nixon, Nishith, and Resick (2004) found that magnitude of trauma exposure but not PTSD symptom severity predicted verbal immediate recall. Thus, it may be that some neurocognitive measures (e.g., immediate recall) are more sensitive to trauma exposure than others.

Psychiatric Comorbidities

As summarized in Duke and Vasterling (Chapter 1, this volume), the prevalence of psychiatric comorbidities in PTSD, including mood, substance use, and anxiety disorders, is high (e.g., Kulka et al., 1990). In some respects, because certain disorders (e.g., depression) are sufficiently common in PTSD to be considered variants of PTSD (Breslau, Davis, Peterson, & Schultz, 2000), the relative contribution to neuropsychological dysfunction of such comorbid disorders may have only minimal relevance to decisions regarding clinical care. However, we would argue that there is considerable clinical benefit to understanding under which circumstances PTSD is associated with the most pronounced neuropsychological deficits. Overlap in the neuropsychological profile of different emotional disorders would not be surprising, given that the limbic system is thought to be a common substrate of a range of emotions. However, using as an analogy the relationship of different language components to subregions within the left cerebral hemisphere, it would also be expected that neuroanatomical substrates within limbic and paralimbic networks would vary in their relative importance to the specific behaviors associated with different emotional disorders. Thus, identification of the unique associations of PTSD with particular neuropsychological functions potentially allows more refined dissociations of brain–behavior relationships within the limbic system and associated regions.

A number of studies have suggested that PTSD contributes above and beyond lifetime or current psychiatric comorbidities to at least some aspects of neuropsychological dysfunction; however, findings have been sufficiently mixed that this question remains unresolved. Some studies documenting PTSD-related cognitive deficits (e.g., Jenkins et al., 2000; Vasterling et al., 1998) approached this problem through establishment of more stringent eligibility criteria that excluded on the basis of comorbid conditions. Though this approach reflects scientific rigor and is an important first step, such exclusion criteria have typically been limited to current substance use disorders, psychotic disorders, and lifetime bipolar disorders, with more common comorbidities (e.g., depression, past substance use) included. Although it could be argued that exclusion of more commonly occurring comorbidities would lead to "clean" variants of PTSD sufficiently unusual that it would be difficult to generalize to the broader PTSD population, it is noteworthy that when participants have been restricted to those with more advanced educational backgrounds and without current psychiatric comorbidity, there was no evidence of PTSD-related deficits (Neylan et al., 2004). In contrast, Jenkins et al. (2000) documented PTSD-related attentional deficits, even after excluding on the basis of neurological, anxiety, affective, schizophrenia, and substance-use disorders and matching PTSD positive and PTSD negative groups on age and education. Other studies (Jenkins et al., 1998) have equated PTSD and comparison samples on key continuous variables (most commonly lifetime and current indices of alcohol use) but have been limited in the types of variables that can be equated across groups.

In addition to strategies pertaining to sampling, researchers have examined the influence of psychiatric comorbidities more directly with three approaches: (1) inclusion of symptom severity indices (e.g., depression severity) as covariates in statistical analyses or in correlational analyses with cognitive performance measures; (2) examination of subgroups with and without comorbid disorders; and (3) inclusion of non-PTSD psychiatric comparison samples. Using a covariate approach, Brandes et al. (2002) found that group differences between PTSD-diagnosed and comparison samples in attention and immediate recall of figural information could not be explained by anxiety or dissociation, but that these differences disappeared when depression was included as a covariate. Gilbertson et al. (2001) found that although group differences on executive, visual copy, and select memory tasks did not remain significant after depression severity and past alcohol history were included as covariates, significant differences on measures of attention and immediate recall/learning index persisted. Likewise, Bremner et al. (1993) found that alcohol abuse exerted no significant effect as a covariate on learning and memory performances; Jenkins et al. (1998) found that depression severity as a covariate exerted no significant influence on learning and memory performances; and Gurvits et al. (1993) found that inclusion of indices of historical use of alcohol and substances as a covariate had no effect on neurological soft signs observed to differ between PTSD-diagnosed and comparison samples. Similarly, several studies have revealed no evidence of significant correlations between neuropsychological performance measures and substance use variables (e.g., Vasterling, Brailey, et al., 2000) or depression (e.g., Golier et al., 2002; Stein et al., 2002) in PTSD samples. Sachinvala et al. (2000) found that although depression severity was negatively correlated with performance on a memory index, depression and attentional performance were not correlated.

Studies examining subgroups of PTSD participants failed to reveal differences between depressed and nondepressed PTSD subsets on block construction errors (Vasterling, Rogers, et al., 2000) or attention and learning measures (Vasterling et al., 2002) that were found to differ between the overall PTSD and comparison samples. Vasterling et al. (2002) found a similar pattern of results examining subgroups of PTSD participants with and without lifetime history of alcohol use disorders. Although subsamples were relatively small in size, inspection of F and p values suggested that statistical power was unlikely to factor prominently in failing to find differences between groups with and without psychiatric comorbidity. Using a related approach, Beckham at al. (1998) found that significant group differences observed between the overall PTSD and comparison samples remained on Trail Making (a visuomotor tracking task) when subsets without anxiety disorders, history of major depressive disorder, and history of substance use disorders were created.

Several studies addressed the specificity of neurocognitive deficits to PTSD through comparison of PTSD-diagnosed samples to non-PTSD psychiatric samples, finding that PTSD diagnosis, especially in the absence of comorbidities, confers only minimal, if any, additional risk for neuropsychological dysfunction over that posed by mood or non-PTSD anxiety disorders (Barrett et al., 1996; Crowell et al., 2002; Gil et al., 1990; Zalewski et al., 1994). Using small sample sizes ($n = 12$ per group), Gil et al. (1990) found that the PTSD group did not differ from a mixed psychiatric comparison sample on most measures, although PTSD was associated with less proficient performance on measures of verbal fluency, verbal abstraction, and nonverbal memory. Using a larger sample (with increased statistical power) derived from archival data from the Centers for Disease Control Vietnam Experience Study, Barrett et al. (1996), Zalewski et al. (1994), and Crowell et al. (2002) all found a similar pattern of minimal association of PTSD diagnosis with neuropsychological measures. However, there appears to be significant sample overlap and almost total overlap in the neuropsychological measures among the three studies, likely leading to nonindependent findings.

Somatic Factors

PTSD is often associated with externally induced (i.e., not inherent to neurobiological alterations within the organism associated with stress exposure) neurological insult or development of health conditions affecting the central nervous system. By virtue of the very nature of life-threatening events, trauma exposure is not uncommonly associated with neurological insult (Horton, 1995; Knight, 1997; Wolfe & Charney, 1991). For example, war-zone exposure brings with it the risk of penetrating and nonpenetrating traumatic brain injury from such events as explosions, motor vehicle accidents, falls, bullet and other high-velocity missile wounds, falls, and neurotoxicant exposures. Political and war prisoners may suffer from beatings or other forms of torture (e.g., suffocation, malnutrition, electrocution). Similarly, interpersonal violence, natural disasters, motor vehicle accidents, and other civilian accidents may be associated with head injury. In addition to neurological insult at the time of trauma, it is also becoming increasingly apparent that chronic PTSD confers the risk of health problems (see Schnurr & Green, 2003) potentially associated with the development of neurological disease (e.g., stroke, anoxia secondary to myocardial infarction) later in the course of PTSD. Such trauma- or health-related somatic factors would be expected to be associated with cognitive dysfunction and thus may contribute to the cognitive impairment associated with PTSD.

The most recent studies documenting cognitive dysfunction in individuals diagnosed with PTSD exclude cases in which frank neurological insult is present, suggesting that cognitive impairment may be associated with PTSD in the absence of neurological insult. However, the combination of physical and psychological insult appears to be particularly detrimental to cognitive functioning (e.g., Bryant & Harvey, 1999; Goldfeld, Mollica, Pesavento, & Faraone, 1988; Levy, 1988; McGrath, 1997; Sutker, Galina, West, & Allain, 1990). Studies that have attempted to examine the relative influences of neurological insult and psychological trauma suggest that the severity of impairment that occurs when both are present may reflect that each contributes to cognitive dysfunction. Examining a former prisoner of war sample in which extreme captivity weight loss was associated with both malnourishment and high levels of psychological traumatization, Sutker et al. (1995) found that captivity weight loss contributed uniquely to learning and memory performance whereas PTSD symptom severity contributed uniquely to executive and attentional performance. Similarly, Lindem et al. (2003) found that PTSD symptom severity and self-reported exposure to chemical–biological warfare agents contributed independently to cognitive dysfunction in non-treatment-seeking Gulf War veterans.

When viewed from the perspective of emotional outcome, a pattern emerges in which neurological insult confers risk of poorer psychological outcome among trauma survivors. For example, case studies have suggested that Guillain-Barré syndrome (Chemtob & Herriott, 1994), cerebrovascular accident (Cassiday & Lyons, 1992), and late-life dementia onset (Johnston, 2000; van Achterberg, Rohrbaugh, & Southwick, 2001) exacerbate or lead to the new onset of PTSD symptoms, sometimes years after trauma exposure. Studying a large sample of Cambodian refugee survivors of mass violence, Mollica et al. (2002) found that traumatic brain injury explained 20% of the variance in depression scores and 8% of the variance in PTSD symptom scores. Likewise, history of head injury in combat veterans was associated with more severe depression (Vasterling, Constans, et al., 2000) and PTSD symptomatology, even with combat exposure controlled for statistically (Chemtob et al., 1998). It is likely that neurological insult adversely affects psychological functioning following trauma exposure both directly via neurotransmitter dysfunction and other brain alterations and indirectly via psychosocial sequelae that lead to increased risk of reactive emotional distress. As suggested by Cassiday and Lyons (1992), it may also be that brain trauma involving frontal inhibitory systems adversely affects coping and emotional control. Although some have speculated that if neurological insult at the time of trauma is severe enough to preclude formation of trauma memories, it is not possible to develop PTSD, the development of PTSD following co-occurrence of psychological trauma and neurological insult remains controversial (see Harvey, Kopelman, & Brewin, Chapter 10, this volume).

Medications

Similar to strategies used to either control for, or examine, the influence of psychiatric comorbidities, the impact of psychotropic medication has been addressed via sampling strategies, subgroup analysis, covariance procedures, and correlational analysis. In general, these approaches have suggested that PTSD remains associated with neurocognitive abnormalities, even when medications are taken into consideration. For example, PTSD-related deficits were found in studies that excluded on the basis of psychotropic medication use or that required medication "wash outs" prior to participation (e.g., Gilbertson et al., 2001; Stein et al., 2002). Similarly, studies conducting subgroup analyses between PTSD participants taking psychotropic medications and those not taking psychotropic medications (e.g., Vasterling, Brailey, et al., 2000; Vasterling, Rogers, et al., 2000; Vasterling et al., 2002) found no significant differences among PTSD subgroups. Following exclusion of participants with antianxiety, antidepressant, and cardiac medications, Beckham et al. (1998) found that the PTSD group continued to perform more poorly on Trails B than did the comparison sample, although group differences on the less attentionally demanding Trails A disappeared following removal of participants with anxiety and cardiac medications. Neither Golier et al. (2002) nor Nixon et al. (2004) found a relationship between memory performance and use of psychotropic medications. Interestingly, although concerns related to medications have tended to focus on adverse CNS effects, Vermetten, Vythilingam, Southwick, Charney, and Bremner (2003) demonstrated significant performance improvements on a range of verbal declarative memory measures among 23 PTSD-diagnosed men and women who were treated with paroxetine, a selective serotonin reuptake inhibitor. In a subset of this sample (n = 20) who underwent magnetic resonance imaging, participants showed a corresponding 4.6% increase in hippocampal volume following treatment. Although this was not a controlled trial, this study provides preliminary evidence suggesting that medications may exert a positive influence on neuropsychological functioning (see Friedman, Chapter 13, this volume).

SUMMARY AND CONCLUSIONS

Several themes have emerged from the recently burgeoning literature addressing neuropsychological concomitants of PTSD. First, cognitive abnormalities associated with PTSD are not limited to tasks using emotional stimuli but are also found on traditional neuropsychological tasks using emotionally neutral stimuli. Second, cognitive deficits are not global but are instead limited to specific domains, in particular, attention and memory functions. Within these domains, aspects of attention and memory dependent on executive control (inhibition, working memory, initial acquisition, freedom from sensitivity to distraction and interference) appear to be especially vulnerable in PTSD. The emerging pattern of deficits is closely aligned with specific neural abnormalities involving limbic and paralimbic regions, perhaps most prominently, prefrontal cortical regions subserving arousal regulation and inhibitory functions.

However, many questions remain, one of the more interesting being whether cognitive deficits represent a vulnerability to PTSD development and maintenance, a consequence of trauma exposure and associated stress-related psychopathology, or both. Another question related to disorder course is whether neuropsychological impairment is yoked to PTSD symptom presentation or persists independently of any natural recovery of PTSD or in response to psychological or pharmacological interventions. Additionally, although the nonglobal nature of neuropsychological deficits found in PTSD suggests that performance deficits are not the result of conscious control of responses, the extent to which cognitive deficits, especially those involving mnemonic functions, represent a cognitive initiation failure similar to that seen in depressive disorders is unknown. Finally, although there is growing support for the notion that clinical concomitants of PTSD (e.g., differences in trauma exposure, comorbidities, or medication regimens) do not account entirely for the neuropsychological deficits associated with PTSD, the degree to which associated clinical features of PTSD contribute to the cognitive impairment observed in PTSD is far from resolved.

Careful replications across populations using similar measurement methodologies, experimental evaluation of motivation and cognitive initiation, linkage to convergent measures of neural integrity (e.g., electrophysiological and functional imaging measurements), and longitudinal research, including prospective assessment in at-risk samples, hold promise in addressing the remaining questions. However, regardless of the etiological issues, the current literature suggests that attention to neuropsychological impairment is paramount in clinical settings.

REFERENCES

American Psychiatric Association. (1994). *Diagnostic and statistical manual of mental disorders* (4th ed.). Washington, DC: Author.

Arnsten, A. F., & Goldman-Rakic, P. S. (1998). Noise stress impairs prefrontal cortical cognitive function in monkeys: Evidence for a hyperdopaminergic mechanism. *Archives of General Psychiatry, 55,* 362–368.

Baddeley, A. (1986). *Working memory.* Oxford, England: Oxford University Press.

Baddeley, A. (2002). Fractionating the central executive. In D. T. Stuss & R. T. Knight (eds.), *Principles of frontal lobe functioning* (pp. 246–260). New York: Oxford University Press.

Barrett, D. H., Green, M. L., Morris, R., Giles, W. H., & Croft, J. B. (1996). Cognitive functioning and posttraumatic stress disorder. *American Journal of Psychiatry, 259,* 2701–2707.

Beckham, J. C., Crawford, A. L., & Feldman, M. E. (1998). Trail Making Test performance in Vietnam combat veterans with and without posttraumatic stress disorder. *Journal of Traumatic Stress, 11,* 811–819.

Birnbaum, S., Gobeske, K. T., Auerbach, J., Taylor, J. R., & Arnsten, A. F. (1999). A role for norepinephrine in stress-induced cognitive deficits: Alpha-1-adrenoceptor mediation in the prefrontal cortex. *Biological Psychiatry, 46,* 1266–1274.

Brandes, D., Ben-Schachar, G., Gilboa, A., Bonne, O., Freedman, S., & Shalev, A. Y. (2002). PTSD symptoms and cognitive performance in recent trauma survivors. *Psychiatry Research, 110,* 231–238.

Bremner, J. D. (1999). Does stress damage the brain? *Biological Psychiatry, 45,* 797–805.

Bremner, J. D. (2001). Hypotheses and controversies related to effects of stress on the hippocampus: An argument for stress-induced damage to the hippocampus in patients with posttraumatic stress disorder. *Hippocampus, 11,* 75–81.

Bremner, J. D., Randall, P., Scott, T. M., Bronen, R. A., Seibyl, J. P., Southwick, S. M., Delaney, R. C., McCarthy, G., Charney, D. S., & Innis, R. B. (1995). MRI-based measurement of hippocampal volume in patients with combat-related posttraumatic stress disorder. *American Journal of Psychiatry, 152,* 973–981.

Bremner, J. D., Randall, P., Scott, T. M., Capelli, S., Delaney, R., McCarthy, G., & Charney, D. S. (1995). Deficits in short-term memory in adult survivors of childhood abuse. *Psychiatry Research, 59,* 97–107.

Bremner, J. D., Scott, T. M., Delaney, R. C., Southwick, S. M., Mason, J. W., Johnson, D. R., Innis, R. B., McCarthy, G., & Charney, D. S. (1993). Deficits in short-term memory in posttraumatic stress disorder. *American Journal of Psychiatry, 150,* 1015–1019.

Bremner, J. D., Vythilingam, M., Vermetten, E., Southwick, S. M., McGlashan, T., Nazeer, A., Khan, S., Vaccarino, L. V., Soufer, R., & Garg, P. K. (2003). MRI and

PET study of deficits in hippocampal structure and function in women with childhood sexual abuse and posttraumatic stress disorder. *American Journal of Psychiatry, 160,* 924–932.

Breslau, N., Davis, G. C., Peterson, E. L., & Schultz, L. R. (2000). A second look at comorbidity in victims of trauma: The posttraumatic stress disorder–major depression connection. *Biological Psychiatry, 48,* 902–909.

Brewin, C. R. (2001). A cognitive neuroscience of posttraumatic stress disorder and its treatment. *Behaviour Research and Therapy, 39,* 373–393.

Brewin, C. R. (2003). *Posttraumatic stress disorder: Malady or myth?* New Haven, CN: Yale.

Bryant, R. A., & Harvey, A. G. (1999). Postconcussive syndrome and posttraumatic stress disorder after mild traumatic brain injury. *Journal of Nervous and Mental Disease, 187,* 302–305.

Burstein, A. (1985). Post-traumatic flashbacks, dream disturbance, and mental imagery. *Journal of Clinical Psychiatry, 46,* 374–378.

Bustamante, V., Mellman, T. A., David, D., & Fins, A. I. (2001). Cognitive functioning and the early development of PTSD. *Journal of Traumatic Stress, 14,* 791–797.

Butters, N., & Delis, D. C. (1995). Clinical assessment of memory disorders in amnesia and dementia. *Annual Review of Psychology, 46,* 494–523.

Cassiday, K. L., & Lyons, J. A. (1992). Recall of traumatic memories following cerebral vascular accident. *Journal of Traumatic Stress, 5,* 627–631.

Centers for Disease Control Vietnam Experiences Study (1988). Health status of Vietnam veterans I: Psychosocial characteristics. *Journal of the American Medical Association, 259,* 2701–2707.

Chemtob, C. M., & Herriott, M. G. (1994). Posttraumatic stress disorder as a sequela of Guillain-Barré syndrome. *Journal of Traumatic Stress, 7,* 705–711.

Chemtob, C. M., Muraoka, M. Y., Wu-Holt, P., Fairbank, J. A., Hamada, R. S., & Keane, T. M. (1998). Head injury and combat-related posttraumatic stress disorder. *Journal of Nervous and Mental Disease, 186,* 701–708.

Chemtob, C. M., & Taylor, K. B. (2003). Mixed lateral preference and parental left-handedness: Possible markers of risk for PTSD. *Journal of Nervous and Mental Disease, 191,* 332–338.

Cohen, S., & Willis, T. A. (1985). Stress, social support, and the buffering hypothesis. *Psychological Bulletin, 98,* 310–357.

Crowell, T. A., Kieffer, K. M., Siders, C. A., & Vanderploeg, R. D. (2002). Neuropsychological findings in combat-related posttraumatic stress disorder. *The Clinical Neuropsychologist, 16,* 310–321.

Danckwerts, A., & Leathem, J. (2003). Questioning the link between PTSD and cognitive dysfunction. *Neuropsychology Review, 13,* 221–235.

Eichenbaum, H. (1994). The hippocampal system and declarative memory in humans and animals: Experimental analysis and historical origins. In D. S. Schacter & E. Tulving (Eds.), *Memory systems* (pp. 147–201). Cambridge, MA: Allyn & Bacon.

Fama, R., & Sullivan, E. V. (2002). Motor sequencing in Parkinson's disease: Relationship to executive function and motor rigidity. *Cortex, 38,* 753–767.

Foy, D.W., Osato, S.S., Houskamp, B.M., & Neumann, D.A. (1992). Etiology of posttraumatic stress disorder. In P.A. Saigh (Ed.), *Posttraumatic stress disorder* (pp. 29–49). Boston: Allyn & Bacon.

Freedman, M., Black, S., Ebert, P., & Binns, M. (1998). Orbitofrontal function, object alternation, and perseveration. *Cerebral Cortex, 8,* 18–27.

Gil, T., Calev, A., Greenberg, D., Kugelmass, S., & Lerer, B. (1990). Cognitive functioning in post-traumatic stress disorder. *Journal of Traumatic Stress, 3,* 29–45.

Gilbertson, M. W., Gurvits, T. V., Lasko, N. B., Orr, S. P., & Pitman, R. K. (2001). Multivariate assessment of explicit memory function in combat veterans with posttraumatic stress disorder. *Journal of Traumatic Stress, 14,* 413–432.

Goldfeld, A. E., Mollica, R. F., Pesavento, B. H., & Faraone, S. V. (1988). The physical and psychological effects of torture: Symptomatology and diagnosis. *Journal of the American Medical Association, 259,* 2725–2729.

Goldman-Rakic, P., Runagashi, S., & Bruce, C. J. (1990). Neocortical memory circuits. *Cold Spring Harbor Symposia on Quantitative Biology, 55,* 1025–1038.

Golier, J., & Yehuda, R. (1998). Neuroendocrine activity and memory-related impairments in posttraumatic stress disorder. *Development and Psychopathology, 10,* 857–869.

Golier, J., Yehuda, R., Cornblatt, B., Harvey, P., Gerber, D., & Levengood, R. (1997). Sustained attention in combat-related posttraumatic stress disorder. *Integrative Physiological and Behavioral Science, 32,* 52–61.

Golier, J. A., Yehuda, R., Lupien, S. J., Harvey, P. D., Grossman, R., & Elkin, A. (2002). Memory performance in Holocaust survivors with posttraumatic stress disorder. *American Journal of Psychiatry, 159,* 1682–1688.

Green, B. L., Grace, M. C., Lindy, J. D., Gleser, G. C., & Leonard, A. (1990). Risk factors for PTSD and other diagnoses in a general sample of Vietnam veterans. *American Journal of Psychiatry, 147,* 729–733.

Gurvits, T. V., Carson, M. A., Metzger, L., Croteau, H. B., Lasko, N. B., Orr, S. P., & Pitman, R. K. (2002). Absence of selected neurological soft signs in Vietnam nurse veterans with post-traumatic stress disorder. *Psychiatry Research, 110,* 81–85.

Gurvits, T. V., Gilbertson, M. W., Lasko, N. B., Tarhan, A. S., Simeon, D., Macklin, M. L., Orr, S. P., & Pitman, R. K. (2000). Neurologic soft signs in chronic posttraumatic stress disorder. *Archives of General Psychiatry, 57,* 181–186.

Gurvits, T. V., Lasko, N. B., Repak, A. L., Metzger, L. J., Orr, S. P., & Pitman, R. K. (2002). Performance on visuospatial copying tasks in individuals with chronic posttraumatic stress disorder. *Psychiatry Research, 112,* 263–268.

Gurvits, T. V., Lasko, N. B., Schacter, S. C., Kuhne, A. A., Orr, S. P., & Pitman, R. K. (1993). Neurological status of Vietnam veterans with chronic posttraumatic stress disorder. *Journal of Neuropsychiatry and Clinical Neurosciences, 5,* 183–188.

Harber, K. D., & Pennebaker, J. W. (1992). Overcoming traumatic memories. In S. A. Christianson (Ed.), *The handbook of emotion and memory: Research and theory* (pp. 359–387). Hillsdale, NJ: Erlbaum.

Harel, Z., Kahana, B., & Kahana, E. (1988). Psychological well-being among Holocaust survivors and immigrants in Israel. *Journal of Traumatic Stress, 1,* 413–429.

Heaton, R. K. (1981). *Wisconsin Card Sorting Test manual.* Odessa, FL: Psychological Assessment Resources.

Hertel, P. T. (2000). The cognitive initiative account of depression-related impairments in memory. In D. L. Medin (Ed.), *The psychology of learning and motivation* (Vol. 39, pp. 47–71). New York: Academic Press.

Hobfoll, S. E. (1989). Conservation of resources: A new attempt at conceptualizing stress. *American Psychologist, 44,* 513–524.

Horner, M. D., & Hamner, M. B. (2002). Neurocognitive functioning in posttraumatic stress disorder. *Neuropsychology Review, 12,* 15–30.

Horton, A. M. (1995). Neuropsychology of PTSD: Problems, prospects, and promises. In G. S. Everly & J. M. Lating (Eds.), *Psychotraumatology: Key papers and core concepts in post-traumatic stress* (pp. 147–156). New York: Plenum Press.

Jenkins, M. A., Langlais, P. J., Delis, D., & Cohen, R. (1998). Learning and memory in rape victims with posttraumatic stress disorder. *American Journal of Psychiatry, 155,* 278–279.

Jenkins, M. A., Langlais, P. J., Delis, D., & Cohen, R. A. (2000). Attentional dysfunction associated with posttraumatic stress disorder among rape survivors. *The Clinical Neuropsychologist, 14,* 7–12.

Johnston, D. (2000). A series of cases of dementia presenting with PTSD symptoms in World War II combat veterans. *Journal of the American Geriatrics Society, 48,* 70–72.

Kivling-Boden, G., & Sundbom, E. (2003). Cognitive abilities related to post-traumatic symptoms among refugees from the former Yugoslavia in psychiatric treatment. *Nordic Journal of Psychiatry, 57,* 191–198.

Knight, J. A. (1997). Neuropsychological assessment in posttraumatic stress disorder. In J. P. Wilson & T. M. Keane (Eds.), *Assessing psychological trauma and PTSD* (pp. 448–492). New York: Guilford Press.

Koenen, K. C., Driver, K. L., Oscar-Berman, M., Wolfe, J., Folsom, S., Huang, M. T., & Schlesinger, L. (2001). Measures of prefrontal system dysfunction in posttraumatic stress disorder. *Brain and Cognition, 45,* 64–78.

Kulka, R. A., Schlenger, W. E., Fairbank, J. A., Hough, R. L., Jordan, B. K., Marmar, C. R., & Weiss, D. S. (1990). *Trauma and the Vietnam War generation: Report of findings from the National Vietnam Veterans Readjustment Study.* New York: Brunner/Mazel.

Levy, C. L. (1988). Agent orange exposure and posttraumatic stress disorder. *The Journal of Nervous and Mental Disease, 176,* 242–245.

Lezak, M. (1995). *Neuropsychological assessment* (3rd ed.). New York: Oxford University Press.

Lindem, K., Heeren, T., White, R. F., Proctor, S. P., Krengel, M., Vasterling, J., Sutker, P. B., Wolfe, J., & Keane, T. M. (2003). Neuropsychological performance in Gulf War era veterans: Traumatic stress symptomatology and exposure to chemical–biological warfare agents. *Journal of Psychopathology and Behavioral Assessment, 25,* 105–119.

Litz, B. T., Weathers, F. W., Monaco, V., Herman, D. S., Wulfsohn, M., Marx, B., & Keane, T. M. (1996). Attention, arousal, and memory in posttraumatic stress disorder. *Journal of Traumatic Stress, 9,* 497–520.

Macklin, M. L., Metzger, L. J., Litz, B. T., McNally, R. J., Lasko, N. B., Orr, S. P., &

Pitman, R. K. (1998). Lower precombat intelligence is a risk factor for post-traumatic stress disorder. *Journal of Consulting and Clinical Psychology, 66,* 323–326.

Matsuo, K., Taneichi, K., Matsumoto, A., Ohtani, T., Yamasue, H., Sakano, Y., Sasaki, T., Sadamatsu, M., Kasai, K., Iwanami, A., Asukai, N., Kato, N., & Kato, T. (2003). Hypoactivation of the prefrontal cortex during verbal fluency test in PTSD: A near-infrared spectroscopy study. *Psychiatry Research: Neuroimaging, 124,* 1–10.

McFarlane, A. C., Weber, D. L., & Clark, C. R. (1993). Abnormal stimulus processing in post-traumatic stress disorder. *Biological Psychiatry, 5,* 817–826.

McGrath, J. (1997). Cognitive impairment associated with post-traumatic stress disorder and minor head injury: A case report. *Neuropsychological Rehabilitation, 7,* 231–239.

McNally, R. J., & Shin, L. M. (1995). Association of intelligence with severity of posttraumatic stress disorder symptoms in Vietnam combat veterans. *American Journal of Psychiatry, 152,* 936–938.

Metzger, L. J., Paige, S. R., Carson, M. A., Lasko, N. B., Paulus, L. A., Pitman, R. K., & Orr, S. P. (2004). PTSD arousal and depression symptoms associated with increased right-sided parietal EEG asymmetry. *Journal of Abnormal Psychology, 113,* 324–329.

Mirsky, A. F., Anthony, B. J., Duncan, C. C., Ahearn, M. B., & Kellam, S. G. (1991). Analysis of the elements of attention: A neuropsychological approach. *Neuropsychology Review, 2,* 109–145.

Mollica, R. F., Henderson, D. C., & Tor, S. (2002). Psychiatric effects of traumatic brain injury events in Cambodian survivors of mass violence. *British Journal of Psychiatry, 181,* 339–347.

Morgan, C. A., Krystal, J. H., & Southwick, S. M. (2003). Toward early pharmacological posttraumatic stress intervention. *Biological Psychiatry, 53,* 834–843.

Morgan, C. A., Wang, S., Southwick, S. M., Rasmusson, A., Hazlett, G., Hauger, R. L., & Charney, D. S. (2000). Plasma neuropeptide-Y concentrations in humans exposed to military survival training. *Biological Psychiatry, 47,* 902–909.

Neylan, T. C., Lenoci, M., Rothlind, J., Metzler, T. J., Schuff, N., Franklin, K. W., Weiss, D. S., Weiner, M. W., & Marmar, C. R. (2004). Attention, learning, and memory in posttraumatic stress disorder. *Journal of Traumatic Stress, 17,* 41–46.

Nixon, R. D. V., Nishith, P., & Resick, P. A. (2004). The accumulative effect of trauma exposure on short-term and delayed verbal memory in a treatment-seeking sample of female rape victims. *Journal of Traumatic Stress, 17,* 31–35.

Ohl, F., Michaelis, T., Vollman-Honsdorf, G. K., Kirschbaum, C., & Fuchs, E. (2000). Effect of chronic psychosocial stress and long-term cortisol treatment on hippocampus-mediated memory and hippocampal volume: A pilot study in tree shrews. *Psychoneuroendocrinology, 25,* 357–363.

Oscar-Berman, M., McNamara, P., & Freedman, M. (1991). Delayed-response tasks: Parallels between experimental ablation studies and findings in patients with frontal lesions. In H. S. Levin, H. M., Eisenberg, & A. L. Benton (Eds.), *Frontal lobe function and dysfunction* (pp. 230–255). New York: Oxford University Press.

Pederson, C. L., Maurer, S. H., Kaminski, P. L., Zander, K. A., Peters, C. M., Stokes-Crowe, L. A., & Osborn, R. E. (2004). Hippocampal volume and memory performance in a community-based sample of women with posttraumatic stress disorder secondary to child abuse. *Journal of Traumatic Stress, 17*, 37–40.

Pitman, R. K., Orr, S. P., Lowenhagen, M. J., Macklin, J. L., & Altman, B. (1991). Pre-Vietnam contents of posttraumatic disorder veterans' service medical and personnel records. *Comprehensive Psychiatry, 32*, 416–422.

Posner, M. I., Walker, J. A., Friedrich, R. J., & Rafal, R. D. (1984). Effects of parietal injury on covert orienting of attention. *Journal of Neuroscience, 4*, 1863–1874.

Roca, V., & Freeman, T. W. (2001). Complaints of impaired memory in veterans with PTSD. *American Journal of Psychiatry, 158*, 1738–1739.

Robbins, T. W., & Everitt, B. J. (1996). Arousal systems and attention. In M. S. Gazzaniga (Ed.), *The cognitive neurosciences* (pp. 703–720). Cambridge, MA: MIT Press.

Sachinvala, N., von Scotti, H., McGuire, M., Fairbanks, L., Bakst, K., McGuire, M., & Brown, N. (2000). Memory, attention, function, and mood among patients with chronic posttraumatic stress disorder. *Journal of Nervous and Mental Disease, 188*, 818–823.

Savic, I., Bookheimer, S. Y., Fried, I., & Engel, J., Jr. (1997). Olfactory bedside test: A simple approach to identify temporo-orbitofrontal dysfunction. *Archives of Neurology, 54*, 162–168.

Schnurr, P. P., & Green, B. L. (2003). *Trauma and health: Physical consequences of exposure to extreme stress.* Washington, DC: American Psychological Association.

Semple, W. E., Goyer, P. F., McCormick, R., Compton-Toth, B., Morris, E., Donovan, B., Muswick, G., Nelson, D., Garnett, M. L., Sharkoff, J., Leisure, G., Miraldi, F., & Schulz, S. C. (1996). Attention and regional cerebral blood flow in posttraumatic stress disorder patients with substance abuse histories. *Psychiatry Research: Neuroimaging, 67*, 17–28.

Shansky, R. M., Glavis-Bloom, C., Lerman, D., McRae, P., Benson, C., Miller, K., Cosand, L., Horvath, T. L., & Arnsten, A. F. (2004). Estrogen mediates sex differences in stress-induced prefrontal cortex dysfunction. *Molecular Psychiatry, 9*, 531–538.

Shaw, M. E., Strother, S. C., McFarlane, A. C., Morris, P., Anderson, J., Clark, C. R., & Egan, G. F. (2002). Abnormal functional connectivity in posttraumatic stress disorder. *Neuroimage, 15*, 661–674.

Shimamura, A. P. (1996). Memory and frontal lobe function. In M. S. Gazzaniga (Ed.), *The cognitive neurosciences* (pp. 803–814). Cambridge, MA: MIT Press.

Shimamura, A. P. (2002). Memory retrieval and executive control processes. In D. T. Stuss & R. T. Knight (Eds.), *Principles of frontal lobe function* (pp. 210–220). New York: Oxford University Press.

Smith, E. E., & Jonides, J. (1996). Working memory in humans: Neuropsychological evidence. In M. S. Gazzaniga (Ed.), *The cognitive neurosciences* (pp. 1009–1020). Cambridge, MA: MIT Press.

Spivak, B., Segal, M., Mester, R., & Weizman, A. (1998). Lateral preference in posttraumatic stress disorder. *Psychological Medicine, 28*, 229–232.

Stein, M. B., Hanna, C., Vaerum, V., & Koverola, C. (1999). Memory functioning in adult women traumatized by childhood sexual abuse. *Journal of Traumatic Stress, 12*, 527–534.

Stein, M. B., Kennedy, C. M., & Twamley, E. W. (2002). Neuropsychological function in female victims of intimate partner violence with and without posttraumatic stress disorder. *Biological Psychiatry, 52*, 1079–1088.

Sullivan, K., Krengel, M., Proctor, S. P., Devine, S., Heeren, T., & White, R. F. (2003). Cognitive functioning in treatment-seeking Gulf War veterans: Pyridostigmine bromide use and PTSD. *Journal of Psychopathology and Behavioral Assessment, 25*, 95–103.

Sutker, P. B., & Allain, A. N. (1995). Psychological assessment of aviators captured in World War II. *Psychological Assessment, 7*, 66–68.

Sutker, P. B., Bugg, F., & Allain, A. N. (1990). Person and situation correlates of posttraumatic stress disorder among POW survivors. *Psychological Reports, 66*, 912–914.

Sutker, P. B., Galina, Z. H., West, J. A., & Allain, A. N. (1990). Trauma-induced weight loss and cognitive deficits among former prisoners of war. *Journal of Consulting and Clinical Psychology, 58*, 323–328.

Sutker, P. B., Vasterling, J. J., Brailey, K., & Allain, A. N. (1995). Memory, attention, and executive deficits in POW survivors: Contributing biological and psychological factors. *Neuropsychology, 9*, 118–125.

Tulving, E., Markowitsch, H. J., Craik, F. I. M., Habib, R., & Houle, S. (1996). Novelty and familiarity in PET studies of memory encoding and retrieval. *Cerebral Cortex, 6*, 71–79.

Uddo, M., Vasterling, J. J., Brailey, K., & Sutker, P. B. (1993). Memory and attention in combat-related post-traumatic stress disorder (PTSD). *Journal of Psychopathology and Behavioral Assessment, 15*, 43–52.

Ursano, R. J., Wheatley, R., Sledge, W., Rahe, A., & Carlson, E. (1986). Coping and recovery styles in Vietnam era prisoners of war. *Journal of Nervous and Mental Disease, 174*, 707–714.

Vasterling, J. J., Brailey, K., Constans, J. I., Borges, A., & Sutker, P. B. (1997). Assessment of intellectual resources in Gulf War veterans: Relationship to PTSD. *Assessment, 4*, 51–59.

Vasterling, J. J., Brailey, K., Constans, J. I., & Sutker, P. B. (1998). Attention and memory dysfunction in posttraumatic stress disorder. *Neuropsychology, 12*, 125–133.

Vasterling, J. J., Brailey, K., & Sutker, P. B. (2000). Olfactory identification in combat-related posttraumatic stress disorder. *Journal of Traumatic Stress, 13*, 241–253.

Vasterling, J. J., Constans, J. I., & Hanna-Pladdy, B. (2000). Head injury as a predictor of psychological outcome in combat veterans. *Journal of Traumatic Stress, 13*, 441–451.

Vasterling, J. J., Duke, L. M., Brailey, K., Constans, J. I., Allain, A. N., Jr., & Sutker, P. B. (2002). Attention, learning, and memory performances and intellectual resources in Vietnam veterans: PTSD and no disorder comparisons. *Neuropsychology, 16*, 5–14.

Vasterling, J. J., Duke, L. M., Tomlin, H., Lowery, N., & Kaplan, E. (2004). Global-local visual processing in posttraumatic stress disorder. *Journal of the International Neuropsychological Society, 10*, 709–718.

Vasterling, J. J., Rogers, C., & Kaplan, E. (2000). Qualitative Block Design analysis in posttraumatic stress disorder. *Assessment, 7,* 217–226.

van Achterberg, M. E., Rohrbaugh, R. M., & Southwick, S. M. (2001). Emergence of PTSD in trauma survivors with dementia. *Journal of Clinical Psychiatry, 62,* 206–207.

Vermetten, E., Vythilingam, M., Southwick, S. M., Charney, D. S., & Bremner, J. D. (2003). Long-term treatment with paroxetine increases verbal declarative memory and hippocampal volume in posttraumatic stress disorder. *Biological Psychiatry, 54,* 693–702.

Villarreal, G., Petropoulos, H., Hamilton, D. A., Rowland, L. M., Horan, W. P., Griego, J. A., Moreshead, M., Hart, B. L., & Brooks, W. M. (2002). Proton magnetic resonance spectroscopy of the hippocampus and occipital white matter in PTSD: Preliminary results. *Canadian Journal of Psychiatry, 47,* 666–670.

Yehuda, R., Golier, J. A., Halligan, S. L., & Harvey, P. D. (2004). Learning and memory in Holocaust survivors with posttraumatic stress disorder. *Biological Psychiatry, 55,* 291–295.

Yehuda, R., Keefe, R. S. E., Harvey, P. D., Levengood, R. A., Gerber, D. K., Geni, J., & Siever, L. J. (1995). Learning and memory in combat veterans with posttraumatic stress disorder. *American Journal of Psychiatry, 152,* 137–139.

Wechsler, D. (1981). *Manual for the Wechsler Adult Intelligence Scale-Revised*. New York: Psychological Corporation.

Wolfe, J., & Charney, D. S. (1991). Use of neuropsychological assessment in posttraumatic stress disorder. *Psychological Assessment: A Journal of Consulting and Clinical Psychology, 3,* 573–580.

Zalewski, C., Thompson, W., & Gottesman, I. (1994). Comparison of neuropsychological test performance in PTSD, generalized anxiety disorder, and control Vietnam veterans. *Assessment, 1,* 133–142.

Zoellner, L. A., Sacks, M. B., & Foa, E. B. (2003). Directed forgetting following mood induction in chronic posttraumatic stress disorder patients. *Journal of Abnormal Psychology, 112,* 508–514.

CHAPTER 9

Learning and Memory in Aging Trauma Survivors with PTSD

RACHEL YEHUDA, KARINA STAVITSKY, LISA TISCHLER,
JULIA A. GOLIER, *and* PHILIP D. HARVEY

Although considerable work exists examining neuropsychological functioning in nonelderly adults, and new information addressing the neurobiological and neuropsychological consequences of trauma exposure in early life is now emerging (see De Bellis, Hooper, & Sapia, Chapter 7, this volume; Vasterling & Brailey, Chapter 8, this volume), the literature does not yet portray a complete picture of neuropsychological correlates of posttraumatic stress disorder (PTSD) throughout the lifespan. Especially lacking are neuropsychological studies of elderly trauma survivors.

Much of the existing research examining neuropsychological functioning in elderly trauma-exposed samples is derived from the former prisoner of war (POW) literature. Such studies were among the first efforts to investigate links between trauma exposure and cognitive dysfunction (e.g., Klonoff, McDougall, Clark, Kramer, & Horgan, 1976; Sutker, Allain, & Johnson, 1993; Sutker, Winstead, Galina, & Allain, 1991) and provided evidence that, similar to younger PTSD populations, aging trauma survivors demonstrate cognitive dysfunction. However, POW confinement was often associated with both psychological trauma and biological insults (e.g., semistarvation) linked to cognitive dysfunction (Sutker, Allain, Johnson, & Butters, 1992; Sutker, Galina, West, & Allain, 1990), making it difficult to parcel out the relative contributions of each (cf. Sutker, Vasterling, Brailey, & Allain, 1995).

We have begun studying the neurobiological and neuropsychological correlates of PTSD in aging trauma survivors. Because of the paucity of empirical information regarding PTSD and neuropsychological functioning in aging trauma survivors, this chapter highlights recent work that we have completed examining neuropsychological functioning across the adult lifespan, with particular focus on an empirical reanalysis of data from our lab.

BACKGROUND

Normal aging has been linked to changes in both cognitive (Golomb et al., 1993, 1994, 1996) and neuroendocrine (de Leon et al., 1997, 1998) functioning. In a substantial proportion of the normal elderly, these changes are also associated with neuroanatomical alterations. In particular, hippocampal atrophy has been associated with both cognitive decline and high levels of glucocorticoids (cortisol) (de Leon et al., 1993, 1996, 1997). In PTSD, both smaller hippocampal volume and memory impairments have been described (Bremner et al., 1995; Bremner et al., 1997; Gurvits et al., 1996; Stein, Koverola, Hanna, Torchia, & McClarty, 1997); however, cortisol levels appear to be lower in this disorder than in nonexposed nonpsychiatric (Boscarino, 1996; Golomb et al., 1993; Yehuda et al., 1990) and other psychiatric groups (Mason, Giller, Kosten, Ostroff, & Podd, 1986; Yehuda, Boisoneau, Mason, & Giller, 1993). The coexistence of these hormonal alterations in PTSD imply that there are explanations other than exposure to high levels of circulating glucocorticoids that account for the observed alterations associated with memory impairments in PTSD.

Our recent work in the area of cognitive neuroscience of PTSD, particularly in aging trauma survivors, has been a direct outgrowth of our findings in the neuroendocrinology of PTSD, which have documented a distinct pattern of hypothalamic–pituitary–adrenal (HPA) alterations in elderly trauma survivors. In particular, we have observed that elderly trauma survivors with PTSD show a flattening of the circadian rhythm of cortisol (Yehuda, Golier, & Kaufmann, in press), which is similar to what has been described in normal aging (Deuschle et al., 1997; Dori et al., 1994; Sandyk, Anninos, & Tsagas, 1991; Sherman, Wysham, & Pfohl, 1985). However, unlike findings of increased glucocorticoids in normal aging (de Leon et al., 1993, 1996, 1997), cortisol levels in elderly trauma survivors with PTSD appear to be even lower than in younger combat veterans with PTSD (Yehuda, Teicher, Trestman, Levengood, & Siever, 1996; Yehuda, Golier, & Kaufman, in press). In contrast, other HPA-axis alterations in elderly trauma survivors, such as the percent suppression of cortisol following dexamethasone (DEX) administration (Yehuda, Boisoneau, Lowy, & Giller, 1995), appear to be a stable feature of PTSD regardless of age.

Because the literature has repeatedly linked hippocampal alterations and cognitive decline in both normal aging and PTSD to increased rates of glucocorticoid toxicity (Sapolsky, 1997) and because this link contradicts our observations with respect to cortisol in aging, we embarked on a series of studies to examine neuroendocrine, neuroanatomic and cognitive measures in aging trauma survivors. This chapter reports on our experience evaluating cognitive performance using the California Verbal Learning Test (CVLT) (Delis, Kramer, Kaplan, & Ober, 1987) in two distinct cohorts: Holocaust survivors and aging combat veterans.

The CVLT consists of a multitrial serial learning and delayed memory test that allows for a comprehensive analysis of multiple domains of memory relevant to both PTSD and aging. We initially used this test to identify memory alterations in younger combat veterans. In that study, we reported decrements only in short- and long-delay recall in Vietnam veterans (then in their early 40s) as compared to nonexposed nonpsychiatric volunteers (Yehuda, Keefe, et al., 1995). Interestingly, Holocaust survivors with PTSD demonstrated a completely different profile of impairments. Holocaust survivors with PTSD showed more deficits in measures of attention and learning, particularly as compared to nonexposed subjects, implicating differences in memory capacity and learning rate. They did not, however, show evidence of rapid forgetting, suggesting that their impairments may be specifically related to the ability to encode and consolidate information (Golier et al., 2002), an abnormality that was not observed in younger combat veterans (Yehuda, Keefe, et al., 1995).

The presence of a completely different profile of memory alterations in younger combat veterans and aging Holocaust survivors raised the question of whether either set of alterations observed could be directly attributable to PTSD. In a prior study examining explicit memory (using a cognitive task associated specifically with hippocampal functions), we reported that Holocaust survivors with PTSD showed poorer performance than both Holocaust survivors without PTSD and demographically comparable subjects (Golier et al., 2002). Yet, similar differences were not observed in younger combat veterans with PTSD compared to similar controls in the only other study of paired-associate learning in PTSD (Yehuda, Keefe, et al., 1995). Because memory changes in Holocaust survivors were correlated with age in the paired-associates study and, in fact, PTSD subjects seemed to demonstrate an accelerated age-related decline in performance (based on the cross-sectional correlation between age and performance), it seemed plausible that there might be age-related changes in PTSD that are not present in younger persons with this disorder.

Of course it was more difficult to conceptualize how a circumscribed alteration in memory that might have been present in younger survivors with PTSD (i.e., rapid forgetting, and decrements in retaining previously learned information after presentation of an intervening word list) would not be maintained in the course of aging in PTSD, particularly since cognitive alterations in this disorder are thought to be a reflection of structural brain abnormalities. Accordingly, we speculated that the cognitive alterations we had observed in the younger combat veterans and Holocaust survivors with PTSD were not related to PTSD per se, but rather, another aspect of trauma exposure or individual differences that might be present in one cohort and not the other. Certainly Vietnam veterans and Holocaust survivors appeared to differ in several variables: type and chronicity of the traumatic experience, age at trauma exposure, various sociodemographic risk factors for PTSD, rates and severity of substance abuse, and the duration of PTSD, any or all of which might have been related to memory changes, rather than PTSD.

For this reason, we undertook an investigation of learning and memory performance using the CVLT in elderly combat veterans. Elderly combat veterans are similar to Vietnam veterans with respect to the nature of the trauma, the age at trauma exposure, some of the psychiatric comorbidities, and sociodemographics, but are similar to Holocaust survivors with respect to age. Thus, we reasoned that, to the extent that elderly combat veterans with PTSD would show memory alterations similar to those observed in Holocaust survivors, it would be possible to conclude that such alterations are generically associated with aging in individuals with PTSD. If, on the other hand, elderly combat veterans demonstrated similar cognitive performance as younger combat veterans, this would suggest that cognitive alterations in PTSD are related to either the nature of trauma or other factors related to those exposed to military combat. In any event, we believe that our strategy of carefully evaluating memory performance in disparate groups of trauma survivors, using the same test that allows a thorough decomposition of the multiple components of the memory system within specific populations, would ultimately help us in understanding differences in memory performance related to PTSD and/or aging.

The investigation of aging combat veterans revealed some patterns similar to what was observed in younger combat veterans and some patterns similar to what was observed in Holocaust survivors. Table 9.1 provides a comprehensive summary of the cognitive alterations that were found in each of the two studies as well as a summary of the alterations present when the two cohorts are combined. The comparisons show the findings distinguishing between trauma-exposed subjects with PTSD (PTSD+), trauma-exposed subjects without PTSD (PTSD−) and appropriately matched nonexposed controls.

As can be clearly seen in the first two panels in Table 9.1, the most consistent alterations pertained to the comparison between trauma-exposed subjects with PTSD and nonexposed controls. However, the two studies appeared to demonstrate different patterns with respect to PTSD-related alterations as demonstrated by the results of post hoc testing comparing

TABLE 9.1. CVLT Memory Measures: A Comparison of Significant Findings across the Holocaust Study, Combat Study, and the Two Cohorts Combined

	Combat			Holocaust			Combined		
	A[a]–B[b]	A–C[c]	B–C	A–B	A–C	B–C	A–B	A–C	B–C
Free recall									
Trial 1 (initial learning/ attention)					*			*	
Trials 1–5 (total learning)		*		*	*		*	*	*
List B[d]		*	*		*	*		*	*
Short delay		*		*		*	*	*	
Long delay		*	*		*		*	*	
Cued recall									
Short delay	*	*			*		*	*	
Long delay	*	*			*		*	*	
Contrast measures									
Proactive interference[d]		*	*			*			*
Retroactive interference[d]									
Retention (LDFR–SDFR) [d]									
Recognition hits		*			*			*	
Response bias[e]									

[a]PTSD+.
[b]PTSD−.
[c]Nonexposed.
[d]Measures not looked at in the 2004 Holocaust CVLT paper. These results were obtained at a later date for the purpose of this comparison. One subject was used in both groups since he is both a combat veteran and a child Holocaust survivor.
[e]Response bias score, sample sizes within Holocaust PTSD+, PTSD−, and Nonexposed groups are 33, 23, and 35, respectively. No missing data from the Combat sample.

trauma-exposed subjects with and without PTSD. The finding that different patterns emerged with respect to differences between trauma-exposed subjects without PTSD and nonexposed subjects, suggests that cohort differences between Holocaust survivors and combat-exposed veterans might be due to potential differences in the trauma-exposed controls across the two studies.

In this chapter, we take a closer look at the results of the two studies we performed in Holocaust survivors and aging combat veterans by combining the two data sets. This allows us to perform a direct comparison of the two cohorts and to systematically evaluate the potential contribution of individual differences to any observed group differences. As will be evident, this analysis revealed Holocaust survivors and aging combat veterans with

PTSD are far more similar to each other, in terms of learning and memory, than would be obvious when simply comparing the results of statistical analyses of the two studies. By systematically examining demographic and other potential differences between the two cohorts, it also became clear that differences in the findings of the two studies may hinge on differences in the makeup of the trauma-exposed group without PTSD. Following a presentation of the methods and statistical analyses, we discuss in detail the cognitive alterations that may be associated with PTSD and aging as well as the factors that appear to contribute variance in analyses which purport to test relationships between trauma-exposed subjects with PTSD and other groups.

METHODS

The sample from the "Holocaust cohort" consisted of 62 Holocaust survivors (20 males, 42 females) and 40 Jewish comparison subjects (18 males, 22 females) previously reported in Golier et al. (2002). The "Combat veteran cohort" consisted of 65 male veterans, 50 of whom served in combat in one or more war zones including World War II (n = 30), the Korean War (n = 6), and the Vietnam War (n = 30), and 15 veterans who did not engage in combat (Yehuda, Golier, Tischler, Stavitsky, & Harvey, in press). The ages of the combat veterans ranged from 50 to 83 years; the ages of the Holocaust survivors and the nonexposed subjects ranged from 57 to 85 years. The Vietnam veterans included in the present study do not include subjects from our previous study, who were on average 44.7 years at the time of study (Yehuda, Keefe, et al., 1995).

In both samples, the same exclusion criteria were applied: history of psychosis, bipolar disorder, organic mental disorder, amnestic disorder, or dementia. Subjects who met criteria for substance dependence within the past 2 years were excluded, but those with substance abuse were not. Subjects with an active medical or neurological illness (e.g., seizure disorder, transient ischemic attack, stroke), a history of bypass surgery, or significant head trauma were also excluded, as these conditions have been known to affect cognitive performance. Subjects with other illnesses common in this age group (e.g., hypertension, hyperlipidemia, arthritis) were studied if they were medically stabilized. Participants were not withdrawn from any medications to participate in this protocol. Commonly used medications included antihypertensives, lipid-lowering medication, gastrointestinal medications, and nonsteroidal anti-inflammatory medications. A small proportion of both cohorts were also taking psychotropic medications, on which they had been stabilized for at least several months.

Diagnoses were made according to the fourth edition of the *Diagnostic and Statistical Manual of Mental Disorders* (DSM-IV; American Psychiatric

Association, 1994) criteria using the Structured Clinical Interview for DSM-IV (SCID; Spitzer, Williams, & Gibbon, 1995) and the Clinician Administered PTSD Scale (CAPS; Blake et al., 1995). This scale has recently been validated for use in elderly trauma survivors (Hyer, Summers, Boyd, Litaker, & Boudewyns, 1996). The Combat Exposure Scale (Keane et al., 1989) and Trauma History Questionnaire (Green, unpublished scale) were used to identify traumatic events that would qualify as DSM-IV Criterion A stressors.

Neuropsychological Testing

The Wechsler Adult Intelligence Scale—Revised (WAIS-R; Wechsler, 1981) Vocabulary and Block Design subtests were administered to assess current verbal and nonverbal intelligence, and the CVLT was used to assess learning and memory. In the CVLT, a list of sixteen words (List A) is presented five times in succession, and subjects are instructed to recall as many of the words as possible after each presentation of the word list. After the five test trials of List A, a new list of words (List B) is read to the subjects, who are instructed to recall as many words as possible from List B. Subjects are then asked to recall List A again (short-delay free recall; SDFR) and, after a 20-minute interval, are asked to recall List A (long-delay free recall; LDFR). A test of cued recall is also included after the short- and long-delay free recall conditions and recognition memory is examined after the long-delay cued recall.

The dependent variables were number of words recalled following Trial 1 (initial learning), performance on learning Trials 1 through 5 (total learning), after a short delay (SDFR) and after a longer delay (LDFR), as well as short-delay and long-delay cued recall (SDCR and LDCR), and a recognition test, which yields the number of "hits" (i.e., correctly identified target words). In addition, subjects were evaluated for differences in proactive interference (List B minus List A, Trial 1; difficulty in subsequent learning as a result of initial learning), retroactive interference (SDFR—List A, Trial 5; difficulty recalling previously learned information as a result of newly learned information), retention (LDFR–SDFR; short-term retention compared to long-term retention) and response bias (based on the recognition hits). The data were examined for consistency and for outliers. One subject's score on the recognition hits was well below chance (this was a World War II subject with PTSD), thus this subject was removed from the sample, making the final sample size 65. (The pattern and significance of results was the same with or without this subject.)

Statistical Methods

The main analyses of memory performance by group (PTSD+, PTSD–, nonexposed) and cohort (Holocaust vs. Combat) were carried out in several stages. First, multivariate analysis of variance (MANOVA) was used to evaluate main effects and interactions in overall CVLT performance. These analyses were followed by two-way analyses of variance (ANOVA) to examine differences in individual items and contrast measures of the CVLT. Pair-wise post hoc comparisons were carried out using Bonferroni adjustment to the statistical significance level. In a second set of analyses, we repeated what we had done but omitted the women from the sample, since women were only present in the Holocaust cohort. In addition, we decided to examine the impact of current and past substance use and/or dependence by performing the identical sets of analyses on a more limited data set including only combat-exposed subjects with no current or lifetime substance abuse-related diagnoses. This was also done to make the groups more comparable in terms of potential covariates. For both analyses, potential confounds were defined through a combination of a theoretical selection of variables (e.g., presence or absence of a depressive disorder) and also through screening the data for variables that either differentiated the groups or were correlated with scores on the CVLT outcome measures (e.g., education, age). The use of analysis of covariance is somewhat controversial and because the covariates related to IQ may also reflect risk factors for PTSD, we analyzed the data with and without covariates.

RESULTS

Evaluation of Potential Confounds

Demographic and clinical information is provided in Table 9.2. The Holocaust and Combat cohorts differed in age ($F = 3.88$, $df = 1,159$, $p = .051$), with the Holocaust cohort being slightly older; WAIS-R Vocabulary age-corrected scaled scores ($F = 4.33$, $df = 1,150$, $p = .039$) and WAIS-R Block design age-corrected scaled scores ($F = 8.08$, $df = 1,152$, $p = .005$), differed, with the Holocaust cohort scoring higher; and age of the focal trauma ($F = 43.68$, $df = 1,108$, $p < .0005$) differed, with Holocaust survivors having been younger when traumatized than combat veterans. There were no significant differences with respect to the three trauma exposure groups (i.e., PTSD+, PTSD−, and nonexposed), nor were there group-by-cohort interactions in age or WAIS-R Block Design scores, but trauma-exposed groups had lower WAIS-R Vocabulary scores ($F = 10.38$, $df = 2,150$, $p < .0005$) and attained fewer years of formal education ($F = 12.91$, $df = 2,158$, $p < .0005$) than did the nonexposed group.

With respect to severity of PTSD and diagnostic comorbidities, neither Mississippi PTSD nor CAPS scores differed significantly by cohort but, as would be expected, differences were apparent across the trauma exposure groups. Importantly, no significant interactions between cohort and trauma

TABLE 9.2. Demographic and Clinical Characteristics in the Total Sample

	PTSD+		PTSD–		Nonexposed	
	Combat (n = 29)	Holocaust (n = 37)	Combat (n = 20)	Holocaust (n = 26)	Combat (n = 15)	Holocaust (n = 38)
	Means (standard deviations) within each group					
Age	65.8(9.8)	67.9(5.7)	67.6(12.1)	68.4(6.4)	65.1(9.6)	70.2(6.9)
Education (years)[a]	12.9(3.4)	12.0(4.3)	14.5(3.0)	15.8(3.7)	15.1(3.3)	16.1(2.9)
Vocabulary score[b]	10.3(3.5)	11.1(2.8)	11.7(4.0)	13.7(2.5)	13.2(4.6)	14.1(3.2)
Block design score[c]	9.0(3.2)	9.8(3.1)	8.9(3.0)	11.3(2.3)	10.2(3.9)	11.3(2.7)
Age focal trauma[d]	20.8(3.7)	14.8(5.9)	20.4(5.7)	11.9(7.0)	N/A	N/A
Mississippi PTSD scores[e]	113.6(20.3)	94.8(54.6)	76.7(16.9)	70.8(41.7)	65.1(11.3)	64.0(30.5)
Severity of PTSD (CAPS scores)[f]						
Reexperiencing	18.7(9.2)	21.4(7.7)	2.9(3.9)	6.3(4.2)	N/A	N/A
Avoidance	26.1(8.2)	25.3(9.6)	7.3(8.1)	7.4(5.0)	N/A	N/A
Hyperarousal	23.8(5.8)	22.8(7.1)	8.6(7.5)	8.3(5.8)	N/A	N/A
Diagnoses other than PTSD[g]	Number (percent) within each group					
Current MDD	12(42.9%)	12(32.4%)	1(5.0%)	4(15.4%)	0	0
Past MDD	16(57.1%)	19(51.4%)	4(20.0%)	8(30.8%)	3(20.0%)	0
Current substance abuse	1(3.4%)	0	1(5.0%)	0	0	0
Past substance abuse	11(37.9%)	0	7(35.0%)	0	8(53.3%)	0

Note. Results are reported as means (standard deviations in parentheses).

[a]One subject in the PTSD+ (Combat) group does not have education years data.

[b]WAIS-R age-scaled vocabulary score, sample sizes for PTSD+ (Combat), PTSD+ (Holocaust), PTSD– (Combat), PTSD– (Holocaust), and Nonexposed (Combat), and (Holocaust) groups are 29, 32, 19, 24, 15, and 37, respectively.

[c]WAIS-R age-scaled block design score, sample sizes for PTSD+ (Combat), PTSD+ (Holocaust), PTSD– (Combat), PTSD– (Holocaust), and Nonexposed (Combat) and (Holocaust) groups are 27, 36, 20, 23, 15, and 37, respectively.

[d]Age focal trauma, sample sizes for PTSD+ (Combat), PTSD+ (Holocaust), PTSD– (Combat), and PTSD– (Holocaust) groups are 29, 36, 19, and 25. Nonexposed sample has no focal trauma.

[e]Mississippi 35 score, sample sizes for PTSD+ (Combat), PTSD+ (Holocaust), PTSD– (Combat), PTSD– (Holocaust), Nonexposed (Combat), and (Holocaust) groups are 27, 33, 18, 20, 13, and 35, respectively.

[f]CAPS scores, sample sizes for PTSD+ (Combat), PTSD+ (Holocaust), PTSD– (Combat), PTSD– (Holocaust) are 27, 36, 19, and 26, respectively.

[g]MDD status and history missing for 1 PTSD+ (Combat).

exposure group were present when each of these variables was considered separately. However, it is interesting to note that the magnitude of difference in the PTSD+ group between combat veterans and Holocaust survivors was far greater on the patient-rated Mississippi than on the clinician-rated CAPS. Specifically, combat veterans with PTSD rated themselves to be 20% more symptomatic than Holocaust survivors with PTSD rated themselves, whereas there was only a 1% difference in CAPS scores between Combat veterans and Holocaust survivors with PTSD. This suggests either a tendency to overendorse symptoms in combat veterans, or underreport them in Holocaust survivors. With respect to depression comorbidity, no cohort differences were present. However, with respect to substance abuse, 4.6% of the combat sample met criteria for current substance abuse and 40% met criteria for past substance abuse/dependence; no current or past substance abuse/dependence was present in the Holocaust sample. There were significant trauma exposure group differences in both current (χ^2 = 29.38, df = 2, p < .0005) and past (χ^2 = 32.57, df = 2, p < .0005) depressive disorder owing to the high rate of comorbidity in the PTSD group. Based on these analyses, the WAIS-R Block Design and Vocabulary scores were used as covariates in a second set of analyses, as they had been in the individual papers reporting on each cohort respectively.

Differences in Attention, Learning, Retention and Recall

Table 9.1 summarizes findings observed in all analyses with the combined cohorts and contrasts these with the findings observed separately. Table 9.3 shows the means for all CVLT measures combining the two cohorts. In an initial analysis that did not consider the contribution of covariates, a significant cohort effect (Pillai's F = 2.51, df = 7,153, p = .018) on overall CVLT performance was observed using MANOVA. There were also significant trauma exposure group differences (Pillai's F = 4.47, df = 14,308, p < .0005) and interestingly, also a significant interaction effect (Pillai's F = 1.86, df = 14,308, p = .03) on overall CVLT performance. Univariate tests for each of the individual CVLT measures (listed in Table 9.3) were then performed. Significant cohort differences were observed in total learning (F = 8.91, df = 1,159, p = .005), initial learning (F = 11.21, df = 1,159, p = .001), SDFR (F = 7.69, df = 1,163, p = .006) and SDCR (F = 4.36, df = 1,163, p = .038), each characterized by a more proficient performance in the Holocaust cohort. Significant trauma exposure group differences, indicating performance decrements in trauma survivors relative to the non-exposed group, were observed in all of the individual CVLT components, as previously reported. However, no significant interactions were observed.

By post hoc testing with Bonferroni adjustment to the confidence inter-

TABLE 9.3. Comparison of CVLT Memory Measures

	PTSD+		PTSD−		Nonexposed	
	Combat (n = 29)	Holocaust (n = 37)	Combat (n = 20)	Holocaust (n = 26)	Combat (n = 15)	Holocaust (n = 38)
Free recall						
Trial 1 (initial learning/ attention)	5.2(1.7)	5.4(2.4)	5.5(1.8)	6.6(2.3)	5.2(1.3)	7.3(2.2)
Trials 1–5 (total learning)	36.6(10.6)	39.7(13.4)	41.9(9.4)	47.2(10.7)	47.1(7.6)	53.9(10.1)
List B	4.5(1.9)	5.1(2.4)	4.7(1.9)	5.1(2.2)	6.5(2.2)	7.2(2.3)
Short delay (SDFR)	6.4(2.5)	7.9(3.2)	8.2(3.1)	9.2(3.1)	9.9(2.4)	10.4(3.0)
Long delay (LDFR)	7.2(3.1)	8.1(3.6)	8.7(2.7)	9.8(3.7)	11.0(2.0)	10.5(3.1)
Cued recall						
Short delay	8.3(2.7)	9.3(3.0)	10.2(2.6)	10.4(3.3)	10.6(2.8)	11.5(2.6)
Long delay	8.3(3.1)	9.1(3.4)	10.6(2.5)	10.5(3.4)	11.3(2.3)	11.6(2.6)
Contrast measures						
Proactive interference	−.79(1.8)	−.32(2.2)	−.80(2.1)	−1.46(2.0)	1.3(2.1)	−.10(2.2)
Retroactive interference	−2.1(1.7)	−1.6(1.6)	−2.3(2.0)	−1.8(2.2)	−2.4(1.6)	−2.2(2.0)
Retention (LDFR–SDFR)	.79(1.8)	.24(1.6)	.55(2.4)	.70(1.7)	1.1(2.4)	.03(1.7)
Recognition hits	13.1(2.8)	12.9(2.9)	13.8(1.8)	14.0(1.8)	15.1(.92)	14.2(1.8)
Response bias[a]	−.05(.48)	−3.1(17.2)	−.07(.41)	−.02(.32)	−.002(.32)	−.03(.40)

Note. Results are reported as means (standard deviation in parentheses).
[a]Response bias score, sample sizes within Holocaust PTSD+, PTSD−, and Nonexposed groups are 33, 23, and 35, respectively. No missing data from the Combat sample.

val, the PTSD+ group performed more poorly than the nonexposed group for all measures for which there were overall trauma exposure group differences (total learning p < .0005, initial learning p = .002, SDFR p < .0005, SDCR p = .03, LDFR p < .0005, LDCR p < .0005, and List B recall p < .0005). The PTSD+ group performed more poorly than the PTSD− group in total learning (p = .007), SDFR (p = .034), SDCR (p = .025), LDFR (p = .030) and LDCR (p = .005). When comparing the PTSD− and nonexposed groups, the PTSD− group performed less proficiently on total learning (p = .005), List B recall (p < .0005) and SDFR (p = .029).

Because total learning is dependent on initial attention, the analyses were repeated using Trial 1 performance as a covariate. All group differences persisted, but no cohort differences persisted in any of the variables that had previously demonstrated a cohort difference. Interestingly, cohort by group interactions, emerged in SDFR (F = 3.23, df = 2,158, p = .042),

LDFR (F = 5.12, df = 2,158, p = .007) and LDCR (F = 3.11, df = 2,158, p = .047) driven by the finding that there were group differences in the initial attention within the Holocaust cohort but not within the combat cohort. The above analyses were all repeated using WAIS-R Vocabulary and Block Design scores as covariates. For the few cases in which there were missing WAIS scores (eight subjects from the Holocaust group and one subject from the combat group were missing the Vocabulary score and five subjects from the Holocaust group and two from the combat group were missing Block Design scores), the mean values of these measures were substituted for the missing values. By MANCOVA there remained a significant cohort (Pillai's F = 2.67, df = 7,151, p = .012) and group (Pillai's F = 3.38, df = 14,304, p < .0005) effect on overall CVLT performance. Using the WAIS scores as covariates an interaction of cohort and group became apparent (Pillai's F = 1.99, df = 14,304, p = .018) which was again driven by the significantly better performance of the nonexposed group versus the PTSD group within the Holocaust cohort. Significant cohort differences remained for total learning and initial learning, but were no longer present for short-delay free or cued recall. Significant group differences remained for all CVLT components other than initial learning.

Contrast Measures

No cohort differences were observed in any of the contrast measures, which included proactive interference (List B minus List A, Trial 1), retroactive interference (SDFR—List A, Trial 5), recognition hits, retention (LDFR–SDFR), and response bias. There were, however, differences between the groups in recognition hits (F = 7.15, df = 2,159, p = .001) and proactive interference (F = 7.74, df = 2,159, p = .001). No cohort-by-group interaction was observed. Post hoc tests demonstrate that the group differences were between the PTSD+ and nonexposed groups for recognition hits (p = .002) and between the PTSD– and nonexposed group for proactive interference (p = .002) (Table 9.1). Thus, the nonexposed group had better ability for recognition hits than the PTSD+ group, but the PTSD– group had better performance with respect to proactive interference than the nonexposed group.

Evaluation of the Effects of Gender

One of the main differences in the sample was that the Holocaust cohort included women, whereas the combat group did not. When women were eliminated from the analyses, it became clear how much their presence likely contributed to cohort or group differences in participant characteristics. Table 9.4 provides the demographic and clinical information of the samples when men only are considered, and underscores the fact that after removing the women, only the WAIS-R Block Design scores ($F = 13.02$, $df = 1,95$, $p < .0005$) and age of focal trauma ($F = 24.59$, $df = 1,66$, $p < .0005$) remained significantly different between the two cohorts, but note the substantial reduction in subject number.

Table 9.5 shows that the exclusion of women also abolished any effect of cohort on overall CVLT performance as well as cohort differences in all individual measures that had been apparent when both men and women were an-

TABLE 9.4. Demographic and Clinical Characteristics in the Male-Only Sample

	PTSD+		PTSD–		Nonexposed	
	Combat ($n = 29$)	Holocaust ($n = 12$)	Combat ($n = 20$)	Holocaust ($n = 9$)	Combat ($n = 15$)	Holocaust ($n = 16$)
	Means (standard deviations) within each group					
Age	65.8(9.8)	68.7(6.5)	67.6(12.1)	68.2(5.9)	65.1(9.6)	71.3(7.5)
Education (years)[a]	12.9(3.4)	13.1(3.9)	14.5(3.0)	15.3(3.7)	15.1(3.3)	17.1(2.5)
Vocabulary score[b]	10.3(3.5)	10.5(2.8)	11.7(4.0)	13.4(2.9)	13.2(4.6)	15.2(2.9)
Block design score[c]	9.0(3.2)	10.4(2.4)	8.9(3.0)	12.2(2.4)	10.2(3.9)	12.2(1.9)
Age focal trauma[d]	20.8(3.7)	13.9(6.0)	20.4(5.7)	13.6(7.4)	N/A	N/A
Mississippi PTSD scores[e]	113.6(20.3)	114.1(18.9)	76.7(16.9)	80.6(15.6)	65.1(11.3)	70.4(14.0)
Severity of PTSD (CAPS scores)[f]						
Reexperiencing	18.7(9.2)	21.7(8.0)	2.9(3.9)	6.8(5.2)	N/A	N/A
Avoidance	26.1(8.2)	25.0(5.3)	7.3(8.1)	7.1(5.5)	N/A	N/A
Hyperarousal	23.8(5.8)	22.8(7.0)	8.6(7.5)	9.6(7.1)	N/A	N/A
Diagnoses other than PTSD[g]	Number (percent) within each group					
Current MDD	12(42.9%)	3(25.0%)	1(5.0%)	1(11.1%)	0	0
Past MDD	16(57.1%)	7(58.3%)	4(20.0%)	3(33.3%)	3(20.0%)	0
Current substance abuse	1(3.4%)	0	1(5.0%)	0		
Past substance abuse	11(37.9%)	0	7(35.0%)	0	8(53.3%)	0

Note. Results are reported as means (standard deviations in parentheses).

[a]One subject in the PTSD+ (Combat) group does not have education years data.

[b]WAIS-R age-scaled vocabulary score, sample sizes for PTSD+ (Combat), PTSD+ (Holocaust), PTSD– (Combat), PTSD– (Holocaust), Nonexposed (Combat), and (Holocaust) groups are 29, 11, 19, 9, 15, and 16, respectively.

[c]WAIS-R age-scaled block design score, sample sizes for PTSD+ (Combat), PTSD+ (Holocaust), PTSD– (Combat), PTSD– (Holocaust), Nonexposed (Combat), and (Holocaust) groups are 27, 12, 20, 9, 15, and 15, respectively.

[d]One subject in the PTSD– (Combat) group does not have age focal trauma data. Nonexposed sample has no focal trauma.

[e]Mississippi 35 score, sample sizes for PTSD+ (Combat), PTSD+ (Holocaust), PTSD– (Combat), PTSD– (Holocaust), Nonexposed (Combat), and (Holocaust) groups are 27, 10, 18, 8, 13, and 14, respectively.

[f]CAPS scores, sample sizes for PTSD+ (Combat), PTSD+ (Holocaust), PTSD– (Combat), PTSD– (Holocaust) are 27, 11, 19, and 9, respectively.

[g]MDD status and history missing for 1 PTSD+ (Combat).

alyzed. There were still significant group effects on overall CVLT performance (Pillai's $F = 3.54$, $df = 18,176$, $p < .0005$) and in all of the individual CVLT components that had previously been significant with the exception of initial learning, which was no longer significant. Parallel to the total sample, significant differences were also seen in recognition hits ($F = 10.14$, $df = 2,95$, $p < .0005$) and proactive interference ($F = 6.73$, $df = 2,95$, $p = .002$). That removing women from the analyses erased cohort effects suggests that some of the differences between the two samples must have been related to gender, rather than other individual differences between the cohorts.

Effect of Substance Abuse

The two samples also differed in that the combat cohort contained subjects who met criteria for current and/or past substance abuse. To evaluate the impact of substance abuse on our results, we ran additional analyses excluding current and past substance abusers. With this smaller sample (combat $N = 38$; holocaust $N = 101$), there were still significant group effects on overall CVLT performance (Pillai's $F = 1.96$, $df = 9,125$, $p = 0.05$). On individual CVLT components, the cohort differences for SDFR and SDCR were no longer present while the differences in initial attention ($F = 7.63$, $df = 1,133$, $p = .007$) and total learning remained ($F = 3.95$, $df = 1,133$, $p = .049$).

Effect of Age at Trauma Exposure

As can be seen in Figures 9.1–9.4, the age of focal trauma was negatively correlated with all individual CVLT measures that were initially found to be significantly different between the two cohorts; specifically total learning ($r = -.426$, p .0005), initial learning ($r = -.417$, $p < .0005$), SDFR ($r = -.387$, $p < .0005$) and SDCR ($r = -.331$, $p < .0005$).

Due to these correlations and the significant difference between the two cohorts in age of focal trauma, we evaluated the effect of age of focal trauma on CVLT measures. This necessitated performing an analysis of only trauma survivors and omitting the nonexposed subjects. This variable was significantly associated with overall CVLT performance (Pillai's $F = 2.80$, $df = 9,99$, $p < .006$), and when used as a covariate to assess its effect on the individual CVLT measures, completely eliminated any effects of cohort on CVLT performance.

DISCUSSION

The opportunity to combine Holocaust and aging combat samples for the purpose of specifically identifying cohort effects and determining whether

TABLE 9.5. Comparison of CVLT Memory Measures in Combat Veterans and Male Holocaust Survivors

	PTSD+		PTSD−			Nonexposed	
	Combat (n = 29)	Combat (n = 30)	Holocaust (n = 12)	Combat (n = 20)	Holocaust (n = 9)	Combat (n = 15)	Holocaust (n = 16)
Free recall							
Trial 1 (initial learning/attention)	5.2(1.7)	5.1(1.7)	4.9(2.6)	5.5(1.8)	6.0(2.2)	5.2(1.3)	6.8(2.2)
Trials 1–5 (total learning)	36.6(10.6)	36.2(10.6)	32.7(10.6)	41.9(9.4)	43.3(11.2)	47.1(7.6)	51.9(9.3)
List B	4.5(1.9)	4.4(2.0)	4.2(1.9)	4.7(1.9)	4.4(1.7)	6.5(2.2)	6.9(2.3)
Short delay (SDFR)	6.4(2.5)	6.3(2.5)	6.1(1.5)	8.2(3.1)	7.9(3.6)	9.9(2.4)	9.9(2.9)
Long delay (LDFR)	7.2(3.1)	7.1(3.2)	6.3(2.5)	8.7(2.7)	8.3(4.4)	11.0(2.0)	10.2(2.9)
Cued recall							
Short delay	8.3(2.7)	8.2(2.7)	7.8(2.4)	10.2(2.6)	9.0(3.9)	10.6(2.8)	10.9(2.3)
Long delay	8.3(3.1)	8.2(3.1)	7.8(2.9)	10.6(2.5)	8.7(4.1)	11.3(2.3)	10.8(2.4)
Contrast measures							
Proactive interference	−.79(1.8)	−.73(1.7)	−.75(2.3)	−.80(2.1)	−1.6(1.7)	1.3(2.1)	.06(2.1)
Retroactive interference	−2.1(1.7)	−2.1(1.7)	−1.5(1.0)	−2.3(2.0)	−.1(1.9)	−2.4(1.6)	−2.7(2.4)
Retention (LDFR–SDFR)	.79(1.8)	.73(1.8)	.25(1.8)	.55(2.4)	.44(2.0)	1.1(2.4)	.31(2.2)
Recognition hits	13.1(2.8)	12.6(3.7)	11.5(3.0)	13.8(1.8)	13.4(2.1)	15.1(.92)	14.4(1.3)
Response bias[a]	−.05(.48)	−.08(.50)	−.31(.50)	−.07(.41)	−.26(.27)	−.002(.32)	−.02(.42)

Note. Results are reported as means (standard deviations in parentheses).
[a]Response bias score, sample sizes within Holocaust PTSD+, PTSD−, and Nonexposed groups are 10, 7, and 15, respectively. No missing data from the Combat sample.

and to what extent conclusions made in these groups separately would persist in the larger more heterogeneous sample provided us with a different set of conclusions than we have previously made about the impact of aging and PTSD in considering the two reports separately. In addition, we were able to look at contributions of factors that differed in the two cohorts, such as gender and age of focal trauma, and assess their impact on memory performance on the CVLT.

All told, there were four essential differences between the two cohorts, three of which were not obvious to us until we did this analysis, and would not have been observable by simply comparing our two papers side by side. The first distinguishing characteristic was the importance of the initial learning variable, which we interpret to reflect initial attention to the stimuli. In the two studies a different pattern of finding was reported. Specifically, this variable was not different across groups in the combat study, but was significantly different in Holocaust survivors with PTSD compared to nonexposed controls. The current analyses demonstrate that the impact of initial attention on CVLT data was so strong that, when this variable was used as a covariate, all other cohort differences disappeared.

The second important observation was the impact of gender. When women were removed from the sample, differences that seemed to be present between the two cohorts were drastically minimized. Interestingly, one of these differences was in initial attention. Thus, it appears that cohort and group differences in initial attention (demonstrating higher attention in the Holocaust cohort and in nonexposed subjects) were primarily due to the women having higher initial attention scores in general compared to men.

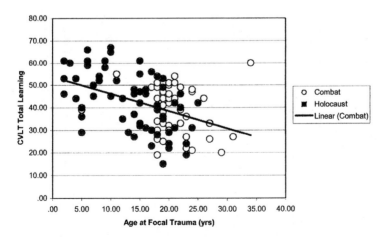

FIGURE 9.1. Relationship between total learning on the CVLT and age at the focal trauma.

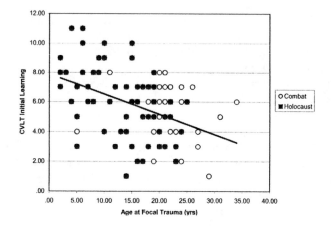

FIGURE 9.2. Relationship between initial learning and age at the focal trauma.

Therefore, in a male-only cohort such as combat veterans, this effect was not present. The presence of women in the Holocaust cohort also accounted for the higher WAIS-R Vocabulary scores in this cohort. Interestingly, however, gender differences were far more present in the non-PTSD groups than the PTSD groups. Thus, the impact of PTSD outweighs gender effects on cognitive measures. Nevertheless, because there is a gender effect, this is an important variable in considering the overall landscape of group differences.

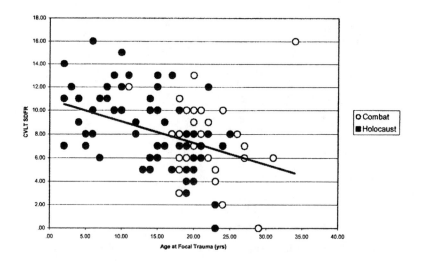

FIGURE 9.3. Relationship between short-delay recall and age at the focal trauma.

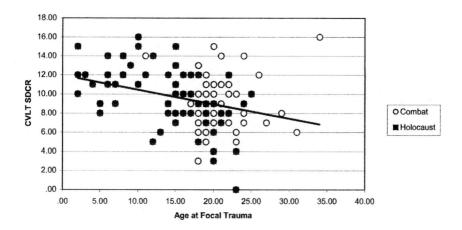

FIGURE 9.4. Relationship between short-delay cued recall and age at the focal trauma.

The third difference between the two cohorts is the impact of substance abuse on the findings. It has been suggested that controlling for substance abuse in Vietnam veteran samples reduces the memory interference phenomenon (Barrett et al., 1996) but does not increase the relative differences in other aspects of learning and recall measured by the CVLT. In the current study, removing persons with any substance abuse history eliminated the short-delay recall measures (cued and free recall), while maintaining cohort differences for both initial attention and total learning, suggesting that individuals with a history of substance abuse experience greater difficulty retaining information over time but that this difficulty may not be a sign of PTSD per se. The differential treatment of substance use might be partially responsible for the inconsistent findings in retention measures across studies using younger cohorts of veterans (see Vasterling & Brailey, Chapter 8, this volume).

The fourth observation that was made here, and not discussed in prior reports, was the relationship of cognitive performance to age at trauma exposure. Holocaust survivors in our sample were younger than combat veterans at the time of their focal trauma, with a larger age range within which the trauma occurred. However, there are no significant differences for the age at focal trauma between the PTSD+ and PTSD− groups within the Holocaust cohort. The relationship between age at trauma exposure and cognitive performance was striking, not only because of how clear the association was, but also because of its direction. Persons who were younger at the age of focal trauma showed better performance on all measures. There can be many reasons for this finding. For example, years of education and age at focal trauma are highly correlated, indicating that with respect to very young Holocaust survivors, it may have been easier for them to make up for educational losses if they were younger at the end of the war. However, controlling for years of education did not significantly change the relationship between the learning measures and age at focal trauma, nor was this relationship obliterated when controlling for current age.

The effect of age at trauma exposure obscured our ability to identify the impact of age on cognitive performance when the two samples were combined, even though this relationship was present in the two cohorts separately, particularly in the Holocaust cohort, which was older. Thus, combining cohorts may help bring some important facets contributing to memory alterations to light, while obscuring others.

Nonetheless, by combining two samples that are qualitatively different in ways that may impact cognitive performance, but similar with respect to having experienced an event of sufficient magnitude to produce lifelong, chronic PTSD, we learned that subjects with PTSD can in fact be distinguished on the basis of cognitive performance. On the other hand, because of differences in the populations from which these two PTSD groups were drawn, the overall landscape of group differences may be specific to a particular study. For example, there is no question that impairments in total learning are present in relation to aging and PTSD, but whether this may manifest itself as a specific group difference within a specific study will very much depend on which comparison groups are studied and how similar those comparison groups are to the PTSD group.

Indeed, one of the more subtle discoveries in our analysis was that the biggest differences were observed not between the two PTSD+ groups, who were surprisingly similar with respect to both cognitive performance and demographic and clinical features, but rather, between the two non-PTSD groups. Thus, decisions about not only the inclusion/exclusion criteria of a study, but the nature and number of the comparison groups are critical in examining issues of generalizeablity. The PTSD– group, in particular, can be a challenging group to include because they are not asymptomatic, and their symptoms may be quite variable within the group. There are also differences in the nonexposed group (i.e. initial attention and total learning).

Because in different studies even by the same investigators the non-PTSD groups can vary substantially, the current practice of literature review in which we take the bottom line conclusions as reflected by group comparisons within a specific study, may not be the best strategy in achieving the goal of understanding the generalizability of findings across different studies. Indeed, it was more useful to look at a comparison of means side by side in Tables 9.3 and 9.5, than the summary of findings in Table 9.1. Ultimately, by encouraging investigators to use clear guidelines in describing both PTSD and non-PTSD subjects, as well as using standardized measures, it will be possible to make comparisons across cohorts to differentiate true PTSD alterations from those associated with other individual differences.

ACKNOWLEDGMENTS

This work was supported by Grant Nos. NIMH R01-2- 49555 and NIMH R01-0-64675 and by VA MERIT review funding (to Rachel Yehuda).

REFERENCES

American Psychiatric Association (1994). *Diagnostic and statistical manual of mental disorders* (4th ed.). Washington, DC: Author.

Barrett, D. H., Green, M. L., Morris, R., Giles, W. H., & Croft, J. B. (1996). Cognitive functioning and posttraumatic stress disorder. *American Journal of Psychiatry, 153*, 1492–1494.

Blake, D. D., Weathers, F. W., Nagy, L. M., Kaloupek, D. G., Gusman, F. D., Charney, D. S., et al. (1995). The development of a clinician-administered PTSD scale. *Journal of Traumatic Stress, 8*, 75–90.

Boscarino, J. A. (1996). PTSD, exposure to combat, and lower plasma cortisol among Vietnam Veterans: Findings and clinical implications. *Journal of Consulting and Clinical Psychology, 64*, 191–201.

Bremner, J. D., Randall, P., Scott, T. M., Bronen, R. A., Seibyl, J. P., Southwick, S., et al. (1995). MRI-Based measurement of hippocampal volumes in patients with combat-related posttraumatic stress disorder. *American Journal of Psychiatry, 152*, 973–981.

Bremner, J. D., Randall, P., Vermetten, E., Staib, L., Bronen, R. A., Mazure, C., et al. (1997). Magnetic resonance imaging-based measurement of hippocampal volume in posttraumatic stress disorder related to childhood physical and sexual abuse: A preliminary report. *Biological Psychiatry, 41*, 23–32.

de Leon, M. J., Convit, A., George, A. E., Golumb, J., deSanti, S., Tarshish, C., et al. (1996). In vivo structural studies of the hippocampus in normal aging and in incipient Alzheimer's disease. *Annals of the New York Academy of Sciences, 777*, 1–13.

de Leon, M. J., George, A. E., Golomb, J., Tarshish, C., Convit, A., Kluger, A., et al. (1997). Frequency of hippocampal formation atrophy in normal aging and Alzheimer's disease. *Neurobiology of Aging, 18*, 1–11.

de Leon, M. J., Golumb, J., George, A. E., Convit, A., Tarshis, C. Y., McRae, T., et al. (1993). The radiologic prediction of Alzheimer Disease: The atrophic hippocampal formation. *American Journal of Radiology, 14*, 897–906.

de Leon, M. J., McRae, T., Rusinek, H., DeSanti, S., Taeshish, C., Golumb, J., et al. (1997). Cortisol reduces hippocampal glucose metabolism in normal elderly, but not in Alzheimer's disease. *Journal of Clinical Endocrinology and Metabolism, 82*, 3251–3259.

de Leon, M. J., McRae, T., Tsai, J. R., George, A. E., Marcus, D. L., Freedman, M., et al. (1998). Abnormal cortisol responses in Alzheimer's disease linked to hippocampal atrophy. *Lancet, 8607,* 391–392.

Delis, D. C., Kramer, J., Kaplan, E., & Ober, B. A. (1987). *California Verbal Learning Test (CVLT) Research Edition–Adult Version* . New York: Psychological Corporation.

Deuschle, M., Gotthardt, U., Schweiger, U., Weber, B., Korner, A., Schmider, J., et al. (1997). With aging in humans the activity of the hypothalamus–pituitary–adrenal system increases and its diurnal amplitude flattens. *Life Science, 61,* 2239–2246.

Dori, D., Casale, G., Solerte, S. B., Fioravanti, M., Migliorati, G., Cuzzoni, G., et al. (1994). Chrononeuroendocrinological aspects of physiological aging and senile dementia. *Chronobiologia, 21,* 121–126.

Golier, J. A., Yehuda, R., Lupien, S. J., Harvey, P. D., Grossman, R., & Elkin, A. (2002). Memory performance in Holocaust survivors with posttraumatic stress disorder. *American Journal of Psychiatry, 159,* 1682–1688.

Golomb, J., de Leon, M. J., Kluger, A., George, A. E., Tarshish, C., & Ferris, S. H. (1993). Hippocampal atrophy in normal aging. An association with recent memory impairment. *Archives of Neurology, 50,* 967–973.

Golomb, J., Kluger, A., de Leon, M. J., Ferris, S., Convit, A., Mittelman, M. S., et al. (1994). Hippocampal formation size in normal human aging: A correlate of delayed secondary memory performance. *Learning and Memory, 1,* 45–54.

Golomb, J., Kluger, A., de Leon, M. J., Ferris, S. H., Mittelman, M., Cohen, J., et al. (1996). Hippocampal formation size predicts declining memory performance in normal aging. *Neurology, 47,* 810–813.

Gurvits, T. V., Shenton, M. E., Hokama, H., Ohta, H., Lasko, N. B., Gilbertson, M. W., et al. (1996). Magnetic resonance imaging study of hippocampal volume in chronic, combat-related posttraumatic stress disorder. *Biological Psychiatry, 40,* 1091–1099.

Hyer, L., Summers, M. N., Boyd, S., Litaker, M., & Boudewyns, P. (1996). Assessment of older combat veterans with the clinician-administered PTSD scale. *Journal of Traumatic Stress, 3,* 587–593.

Keane, T., Fairbank, J., Caddell, J., Zimering, R., Taylor, K., & Mora, C. (1989). Clinical evaluation of a measure to assess combat exposure. *Psychological Assessment, 1,* 53–55.

Klonoff, H., McDougall, G., Clark, C., Kramer, P., & Horgan, J. (1976). The neuropsychological, psychiatric, and physical effects of prolonged and severe stress: 30 years later. *Canadian Psychiatric Association Journal, 12,* 175–181.

Mason, J. W., Giller, E. L., Kosten, T. R., Ostroff, R., & Podd, L. (1986). Urinary-free cortisol levels in posttraumatic stress disorder patients. *Journal of Nervous and Mental Diseases, 174,* 145–159.

Sandyk, R., Anninos, P. A., & Tsagas, N. (1991). Age-related disruption of circadian rhythms: Possible relationship to memory and implications for therapy with magnetic fields. *International Journal of Neuroscience, 59,* 259–262.

Sapolsky, R. (1997). Why stress is bad for your brain. *Science, 273,* 749–750.

Sherman, B., Wysham, C., & Pfohl, B. (1985). Age-related changes in the circadian rhythm of plasma cortisol in man. *Journal of Clinical Endocrinology and Metabolism, 61,* 439–443.

Spitzer, R. L., Williams, J. B. W., & Gibbon, M. (1995). *Structured Clinical Interview for DSM-IV (SCID)*. New York: New York State Psychiatric Institute, Biometrics Research.

Stein, M. B., Koverola, C., Hanna, C., Torchia, M. C., & McClarty, B. (1997). Hippocampal volume in women victimized by childhood sexual abuse. *Psychological Medicine, 27*, 951–959.

Sutker, P. B., Allain, A. N., & Johnson, J. L. (1993). Clinical assessment of long-term cognitive and emotional sequelae to World War II prisoner-of-war confinement: Comparison of pilot twins. *Psychological Assessment, 5*, 3–10.

Sutker, P. B., Allain, A. N., Jr., Johnson, J. L., & Butters, N. M. (1992). Memory and learning performances in POW survivors with history of malnutrition and combat veteran controls. *Archives of Clinical Neuropsychology, 7*, 431–444.

Sutker, P. B., Galina, Z. H., West, J. A., & Allain, A. N. (1990). Trauma-induced weight loss and cognitive deficits among former prisoners of war. *Journal of Consulting and Clinical Psychology, 58*, 323–328.

Sutker, P. B., Vasterling, J. J., Brailey, K., & Allain, A. N. (1995). Memory, attention, and executive deficits in POW survivors: Contributing biological and psychological factors. *Neuropsychology, 9*, 118–125.

Sutker, P. B., Winstead, D. K., Galina, Z. H., & Allain, A. N. (1991). Cognitive deficits and psychopathology among former prisoners of war and combat veterans of the Korean conflict. *American Journal of Psychiatry, 148*, 67–72.

Yehuda, R., Boisoneau, D., Lowy, M. T., & Giller, E. L. (1995). Dose response changes in plasma cortisol and lymphocyte glucocorticoid receptors following dexamethasone administration in combat veterans with and without posttraumatic stress disorder. *Archives of General Psychiatry, 52*, 583–593.

Yehuda, R., Boisoneau, D., Mason, J. W., & Giller, E. L. (1993). Relationship between lymphocyte glucocorticoid receptor number and urinary-free cortisol excretion in mood, anxiety, and psychotic disorder. *Biological Psychiatry, 34*, 18–25.

Yehuda, R., Golier, J., & Kaufman, S. (in press). Circadian rhythm of salivary cortisol in Holocaust Survivors with and without PTSD. *American Journal of Psychiatry.*

Yehuda, R., Golier, J. A., Tischler, L., Stavitsky, K., & Harvey, P. D. (in press). Learning and memory in aging combat veterans with PTSD. *Journal of Clinical and Experimental Neuropsychology.*

Yehuda, R., Keefe, R. S. E., Harvey, P. D., Levengood, R. A., Gerber, D. K., Geni, J., et al. (1995). Learning and memory in combat veterans with posttraumatic stress disorder. *American Journal of Psychiatry, 152*, 137–139.

Yehuda, R., Southwick, S. M., Nussbaum, G., Wahby, V., Mason, J. W., & Giller, E. L. (1990). Low urinary cortisol excretion in patients with PTSD. *Journal of Nervous and Mental Disease, 178*, 366–309.

Yehuda, R., Teicher, M. H., Trestman, R. L., Levengood, R. A., & Siever, L. J. (1996). Cortisol regulation in posttraumatic stress disorder and major depression: A chronobiological analysis. *Biological Psychiatry, 40*, 79–88.

Wechsler, D. (1981): *Wechsler Adult Intelligence Scale-Revised* . New York: Psychological Corporation.

CHAPTER 10

PTSD and Traumatic
Brain Injury

ALLISON G. HARVEY, MICHAEL D. KOPELMAN,
and CHRIS R. BREWIN

A traumatic brain injury (TBI) can be *open*, resulting from the skull and dura being penetrated by a sharp object (such as a missile wound), or *closed*, resulting from a blow to the head, rapid acceleration–deceleration, or severe rotational forces (as when a car turns over). An ongoing topic of debate is whether an individual who has sustained a TBI during a trauma can subsequently develop acute stress disorder (ASD) or posttraumatic stress disorder (PTSD) (e.g., Bryant, 2001; Harvey, Brewin, Jones, & Kopelman, 2003; McMillan, 1997). This chapter begins with a brief overview of the empirical literature that addresses the debate. We then discuss three theoretical arguments against the proposal that PTSD/ASD and TBI can coexist and we present possible resolutions of these arguments. Finally, we outline the priorities for future research and comment on the methodology of research conducted on this topic and the confusion and overlap in defining key terms.

Most of the studies we review in this chapter have based the diagnosis of TBI on an estimate of the length of posttraumatic amnesia (PTA). PTA is the length of time after the trauma during which the patient is (almost) completely unable to store current events in memory. It is clinically defined as the period between the onset of the injury and the return of continuous personal memories (Russell & Smith, 1961). It involves disorientation, confusion, and an inability to "store and retrieve new information" (Schacter & Crovitz, 1977, p. 151). During PTA "islands of memory," or brief periods of apparently normal encoding and retrieval, are evident in approximately one third of mild and moderate TBIs (Forrester, Encel, & Geffen, 1994). The resolution of PTA has been defined as the point from which the patient can give an accurate and continuing account of happenings in his or her surrounding environment (Symonds & Russell, 1943). Duration of PTA is most reliably assessed prospectively over at least 3 days, using measures typically comprising orientation and memory components (e.g., Westmead PTA Scale, Shores, Marosszeky, Sandanam, & Batchelor, 1986; Galveston Orientation and Amnesia Test, Sohlberg & Mateer, 1989). However, when such assessment is not possible, the less reliable retrospective procedure of repeatedly asking patients about their trauma with the persistent question "And then what happened . . . ?", until their account is continuous (Gronwall & Wrightson, 1980) must suffice. It should be noted that it is not clear whether the prospective and the retrospective method assesses exactly the same construct. PTA has been used to categorize the severity of the TBI with 0–60 minutes of PTA indicating a mild TBI, 1–24 hours of PTA indicating a moderate TBI, and more than 24 hours of PTA indicating a severe TBI (Russell & Smith, 1961).

Retrograde amnesia (RA) refers to the period prior to the trauma that, in some TBI cases, is not remembered (Russell, 1971). RA is usually (but not always) briefer than PTA, and recovery is characterized by the emergence of islands of memory, which gradually converge, with the more distant memories recovering first (Russell & Nathan, 1946; Zangwill, 1966). Schacter and Crovitz (1977) distinguished between two types of RA (cf. Squire, Cohen, & Nadel, 1984; Symonds, 1966): (1) a temporary retrograde amnesia which initially extends for days, weeks or months but gradually shrinks with time posttrauma, and (2) a permanent but very short retrograde amnesia (often just a few seconds). Some have included retrograde amnesia as part of PTA (Sisler & Penner, 1975)—this is perhaps better described as the "amnesic gap." In this chapter we adopt the more standard definition of PTA that excludes retrograde amnesia (Schachter & Crovitz, 1977).

DO PTSD/ASD AND TBI COEXIST?

It has been repeatedly argued that, if patients are amnesic for the trauma, they will not display several of the key symptoms of ASD and PTSD: Specifically, they will be unable to have experienced intense affect during the trauma, and they will not reexperience memories of the trauma or avoid these memories. Consistent with this position, several studies of the coexistence of PTSD and TBI have indicated a lack of association between PTSD and TBI with Mayou, Bryant, and Duthie (1993), Sbordone and Liter

(1995) and Warden et al. (1997) reporting a 0% rate of PTSD following TBI. However, other investigators have reported case studies documenting that PTSD and TBI can coexist (e.g., Bryant, 1996; King, 1997; McMillan, 1991), and the majority of studies based on reasonably large samples of consecutively admitted patients report rates of PTSD in head-injured victims ranging from 20% to 40% (e.g., Bryant & Harvey, 1995; Hickling, Gillen, Blanchard, Buckley, & Taylor, 1998; Ohry, Rattock, & Solomon, 1996; Rattock & Ross, 1993). These rates are consistent with the rates of PTSD in non-TBI samples (e.g., Blanchard et al., 1996; McFarlane, 1988; Riggs, Rothbaum, & Foa, 1995).

The coexistence of ASD and TBI has received much less attention but those studies that have been conducted indicate that in trauma survivors who experienced a period of PTA ranging from 5 minutes to 24 hours (i.e., mild or moderate PTA) ASD was diagnosed in 14% of the sample (Harvey & Bryant, 1998a). This rate is comparable to that found in non-TBI samples (19%: Brewin, Andrews, Rose, & Kirk, 1999a; 13%: Harvey & Bryant, 1998b).

We note that Bryant, Marosszeky, Crooks, and Gurka (2000) identified cases of PTSD occurring among 27% of moderate and severe TBIs. These interesting findings contradict the picture that emerged from earlier studies which suggested that TBI and PTSD coexist relatively rarely (Joseph & Masterson, 1999; McMillan, 1996), and that PTSD is more likely in the context of mild rather than severe TBI (Joseph & Masterson, 1999).

In summary, the majority of the evidence that has accrued indicates that PTSD/ASD can coexist with TBI (see Harvey et al., 2003 for a detailed critique of the literature in this area). We now address how this coexistence might be accounted for theoretically.

HOW DO PTSD/ASD AND TBI COEXIST?

Given the argument that if patients are amnesic for the trauma they will not display key symptoms of ASD and PTSD, discussion of how PTSD/ASD might come to coexist is warranted.

Lack of Affect Problem

The DSM-IV definition of PTSD/ASD requires that a person "has been exposed to a traumatic event in which both of the following were present: (1) the person experienced, witnessed or was confronted with an event or events that involved actual or threatened death or serious injury, or a threat to the physical integrity of self or others and (2) the person's response involved intense fear, helplessness or horror" (p. 427). With regard to the first requirement, whether or not a person with a TBI fully "experienced" or "witnessed" an event can be debated and will depend on the level of TBI sustained and whether 'islands of memory' (Forrester et al., 1994) were experienced, but patients who sustained a TBI can certainly be said to have been "confronted" by it. What is perhaps more debatable is the second requirement. That is, can a person who suffers PTA and disturbed consciousness experience the intense emotion required for the diagnosis? At least two resolutions of this paradox are plausible. *Resolution 1* states that patients with TBI do not experience intense affect but this is not a barrier to them developing PTSD or ASD. *Resolution 2* states that patients with TBI do experience intense affect after all.

Resolution 1

In considering this resolution, it is important to recall that the requirement to experience intense affect was not present in previous formulations of the DSM and is not part of the criteria for PTSD laid down in the ICD (World Health Organization, 1993). Evidence on the ubiquity of intense emotions in individuals who later develop PTSD is lacking at this time. In the DSM-IV Field Trials, Kilpatrick et al. (1998) reported that some individuals with PTSD did not have this symptom. Similarly, Brewin, Andrews, and Rose (1999b) found that although intense emotions were very much the norm, a small proportion of violent crime victims did not report intense fear, helplessness, or horror at the time of the trauma but subsequently developed PTSD. Thus, the evidence that the experiencing of intense emotion is essential for the development of PTSD or ASD is not yet compelling. It is possible that data from victims of sudden violent assaults and motor vehicle accidents may yield a different picture from studies of combat veterans and rape victims where the trauma is typically more prolonged and there may be more opportunity to experience overwhelming emotions.

Resolution 2

Consistent with this resolution, Bryant and Harvey (1999b) found that some TBI patients reported fear and helplessness (41%), although not as frequently as non-TBI patients (68%). There are at least three pathways by which TBI patients might experience intense affect. First, as mentioned previously, during PTA there may be "islands of memory" that are sufficient for intense affect to be experienced. One study suggested that these occur in approximately one-third of all mild and moderate TBI cases (Forrester et al., 1994). Of those reporting "islands," 44% reported them as occurring for a specific event within 5 minutes of the injury and 71% as occurring within 15 minutes of the injury (Gronwall & Wrightson, 1980). It has been proposed that islands of memory during PTA may be the precipitant of PTSD as they would allow encoding of at least some aspects of the trauma. Indeed, King (1997) and McMillan (1996) both presented case studies where islands of memory appear to be the precipitant of intrusive symptoms.

Second, intense affect may be associated with periods immediately prior to or subsequent to the period of amnesia surrounding a traumatic impact. McMillan (1996) reported that emotionally distressing thoughts and dreams reported by patients with a TBI covered various time points including just before impact and after the resolution of PTA (e.g., on the way to the hospital). Kopelman's (2000) description of Patient C reported a similar phenomenon in a policeman who was beaten over the head with his own truncheon and sustained severe head injuries. This patient had PTSD for events immediately preceding loss of consciousness. Further, Di Gallo, Barton, and Parry-Jones (1997) assessed a sample of child motor vehicle accident survivors at 2 weeks and 3–4 months posttrauma. Ten of the fifty-seven patients assessed reported intrusive thoughts of their last preaccident memories and of their first recollections in hospital. This evidence suggests that intact memories before and after event-related amnesia may permit the experiencing of intense levels of affect.

A third possibility is that information encountered after the trauma may lead to intense affect being generated by events that at the time elicited low or moderate levels of affect. This process is well known in the literature on human conditioning and is known as "stimulus revaluation" (e.g., Davey, 1989). For example, a physical assault may have minimal psychological consequences until the victim later learns that their attacker has previously or subsequently killed someone. This new information alters the representation of the traumatic event, dramatically increasing fear and the perception of threat. As a result, attentional and memory biases may be exacerbated. Equally, information that decreases the perception of threat may result in a reduction in affect and in selective cognitive biases.

Lack of Reexperiencing Problem

A period of disturbed consciousness occurs in most head injuries involving brain injury. It has been suggested that the complete absence of recall of the trauma will preclude PTSD (Boake, 1996; Bontke, 1996; Price, 1994; Sbordone, 1991), or at least reduce the risk of PTSD developing (Taylor & Koch, 1995). It is argued that when there is no memory for the trauma there can be no intrusive reexperiencing of the trauma that is necessary for a diagnosis of PTSD. At least two resolutions of this paradox are plausible. As in the case of the "Lack of affect" argument, *Resolution 1* states that patients with TBI do not reexperience the trauma but this is not a barrier to them developing PTSD. *Resolution 2* states that patients with TBI do reexperience the traumatic incident after all.

Resolution 1

In evaluating this resolution, it is important to recall that the diagnostic criteria for PTSD require only one "reexperiencing" symptom. These symptoms include intrusive thoughts, dreams, and distress or physiological arousal on exposure to trauma-related cues. None of these symptoms are dependent on having a conscious memory of the traumatic incident itself (although such intrusive memories are a very common form of "reexperiencing"). Thus, it is possible that the use of more inclusive structured diagnostic interviews has enabled additional individuals to qualify for a PTSD diagnosis on the basis of intrusive thoughts or conditioned emotional responses and despite an absence of any explicit memory for the traumatic incident. For example, in the Warden et al. (1997) study, no cases of PTSD were reported although six patients (13%) met criteria for all other symptoms except reexperiencing. However, the method employed to assess reexperiencing symptoms in this study was limited as it comprised two questions; one from the Present State Examination and one composed by the authors.

Perhaps, therefore, the reexperiencing symptoms reported by individuals who sustained a TBI are qualitatively different to those reported by PTSD patients who did not sustain a TBI. McMillan's (1996) observation that relatively few of the 10 cases reported in his paper experienced "vivid flashbacks" provides some evidence for this position. On the other hand, Bryant and Harvey (1995) examined a sample of six TBI patients selected for reporting intrusive imagery of events during the period of loss of consciousness. The intrusions described by this group were indistinguishable from those of non-TBI patients in terms of vividness, involuntariness, control, belief associated with the image, affect, sensory detail, whether the image involved movement, which perspective it was from, and the management of the image. Data on larger samples are urgently needed to characterize the exact nature of the reexperiencing symptoms reported by TBI patients.

Resolution 2

Resolution 1 implies that overall fewer TBI patients than non-TBI patients will report reexperiencing symptoms as enumerated in the DSM-IV Criterion B. Within the first month posttrauma, reexperiencing was reported by 19% of mild-TBI and 40% of non-TBI patients (Bryant & Harvey, 1999b). However, at 6-month follow-up this difference had disappeared, 24% of mild-TBI and 21% of non-TBI patients reported these symptoms. Perhaps, therefore, some TBI patients do have intrusive memories of the traumatic event. At least four possible explanations can be outlined in support of Resolution 2. Two of these have already been described in connection with the "Lack of affect" argument, and involve the possibility of preserved "islands of memory" and of memory for events immediately preceding and/or following the period of PTA or loss of consciousness (LOC). The other explanations consider processes of confabulation and the laying down of different kinds of representations in memory.

In principle, theoretical conceptualizations of memory fall into two camps (Zola, 1998). One postulates that memories for an event can be fixed and that all aspects of the memory can be accurately retrieved regardless of the conditions of encoding or retrieval. An alternative view highlights the possibility that memories for an event may be altered, distorted, and reconstructed. Well known are memory distortions caused by source amnesia, unintentional integration of information not part of the original memory, and false memory construction (Burgess & Shallice, 1996; Hyman & Loftus, 1998; Johnson, 1988; Kopelman, 1999; Kopelman, Ng, & Van den Brouke, 1997; McNally, 2003; Moscovitch & Melo, 1997).

A number of studies testify to the malleability of intrusive memories. Reynolds and Brewin (1998) examined the most prominent intrusive cognitions in patients with PTSD and depression and nonclinical controls. A small number of patients reported what Reynolds and Brewin termed "elaborative cognitions," cognitions that had some basis in actual experience but had then been elaborated into a scenario that had not actually occurred. Similarly, Merckelbach, Muris, Horselenberg, and Rassin (1998) reported that in normal subjects intrusive recollections of a traumatic event were not necessarily veridical. Rather, in about 20% of cases, they were exaggerations of the event or "worst-case scenarios."

In this context it is interesting that out of 50 survivors who were assessed within 1 month as having no memory for their trauma, 40% reported full recall of the traumatic event when reassessed after 2 years (Harvey & Bryant, 1999). There are several processes that may have contributed to the reconstruction of these memories. Involvement in compensation or treatment following a trauma is common. Given that "probably any activity that encourages people to think about, imagine, and talk about events will lead to the construction of an image and narrative" (Hyman & Loftus, 1998, p. 939) and that a person's belief in a memory increases with rehearsal (Johnson, 1988), the processes of treatment and seeking compensation are likely to be precipitants for the reconstruction of memory. Both require the trauma survivor to report the details of the trauma repeatedly and, in the case of the legal process, there may be pressure to recall the traumatic event in order that it be used as evidence. Previous research has shown that repeated instructions to recall nonevents can lead to false memories (Roediger, McDermott, & Goff, 1997). However, data collected by Harvey and Bryant (1999) indicated that being involved in treatment or compensation was not associated with the subsequent recall of previously inaccessible memories.

It is also possible that memories of the event can be cued and reconstructed through the use of photographs, discussion with witnesses, and fantasy (Harvey & Bryant, 1999). Alternatively, islands of memory may be fertile ground for the reconstruction of memories (Harvey & Bryant, 1999; Hyman & Loftus, 1998). Finally, it is possible that such reconstruction processes may be fuelled by a need to process or make sense of the traumatic event (Christianson & Engelberg, 1997). This proposal is consistent with the predictions of cognitive models of PTSD that emphasize that trauma resolution is propelled by a desire to make sense of the trauma and integrate the trauma memories with existing networks (Foa, Steketee, & Rothbaum, 1989) or assumptions about the world (Janoff-Bulman, 1992).

The fourth explanation to be considered under Resolution 2 involves the encoding of events at more than one level in memory, a subject of renewed investigation since the early 1980s (e.g., Schacter, 1987; Squire, 1992; Tulving & Schacter, 1990). One influential distinction that has been drawn is between explicit or declarative memory and implicit or nondeclarative memory. The former includes conscious recollection of episodes and autobiographical events, whereas the latter includes procedural memory, conditioning, and indirect demonstrations that (perceptual or semantic) information has been encoded without conscious recollection of the learning episode (e.g., through tests involving "subliminal priming") (Schacter, 1987; Tulving & Schacter, 1990). Layton and Wardi-Zonna (1995) proposed that PTSD can occur in the absence of explicit memory through implicit learning.

PTSD patients do often report vivid and fragmented reexperiencing of the sensory aspects of their traumas, particularly in the form of visual images but also sometimes in the modality of sound, smell, and touch. Unlike participants in implicit memory experiments, however, who are obliged to rely on some kind of indirect judgment or guess, they are usually aware that these experiences originate from the traumatic event. Consequently, this type of remembering does not correspond to the term implicit memory as it is usually employed. For this reason, a dual-representation theory of PTSD was proposed that made a distinction between "verbally accessible" and "situationally accessible" memories (Brewin, 2001, 2003; Brewin, Dalgleish, & Joseph, 1996). Information that receives sufficient conscious attention is encoded in a way that permits interaction with the rest of the autobiographical memory system, and facilitates later memory search and deliberate retrieval ("verbally accessible knowledge"). In contrast, information that receives minimal processing (e.g., stimuli in peripheral vision that are not attended to) is encoded using a lower-level, largely perceptual system that does not interact with the rest of the autobiographical knowledge base. This information cannot be accessed using ordinary retrieval strategies but can be retrieved automatically in the presence of the appropriate cues, and mediates the vivid reexperiencing phenomena that are a unique feature of PTSD.

Dual-Representation theory implies, therefore, that some degree of consciousness is essential for the creation of any kind of trauma memory. However, temporary impairments in consciousness such as coma or PTA might interfere with the creation of verbally accessible memories while still permitting some information to be retained within situationally accessible memory. (This could occur in the *absence* of preserved islands of memory in which encoding is normal). These periods of impaired consciousness could later form the basis of the reexperiencing of fragmentary sensations encoded during the trauma, even in the absence of a conscious memory for what had transpired. Of course, these sensations could also be involved in a more general process of memory reconstruction.

Joseph and Masterson (1999) recently elaborated the idea that dual-representation theory may account for the coexistence of PTSD and TBI. These authors further proposed that the absence of a conscious memory for the trauma might impede the normal processes of adjustment to the event and put the individual at greater risk of chronic or delayed PTSD.

Lack of Avoidance Problem

In patients diagnosed with PTSD, refusal to talk about the trauma, blockage of thoughts relating to the trauma, or the avoidance of places or people associated with the trauma (Criterion C) are commonly reported. O'Brien and Nutt (1998) argued that if a trauma survivor is completely amnesic for the event, they will have no negative association with trauma-related thoughts or stimuli and thus no desire to avoid these. As in the case of the previous two arguments, *Resolution 1* states that patients with TBI do not avoid reminders of the trauma but this is not a barrier to them developing PTSD. *Resolution 2* states that patients with TBI do avoid reminders of the traumatic incident after all.

Resolution 1

Although avoidance of reminders of the trauma, whether internal reminders such as thoughts and memories, or external reminders such as situations and television programs, is very common in PTSD, the diagnostic criteria do not actually require it. The necessary three symptoms from the Criterion

C cluster could consist of restricted affect, detachment from other people, and hopelessness about the future. Theoretically, therefore, under this resolution TBI patients could receive a PTSD diagnosis because of emotional numbing and despite showing little evidence of cognitive or behavioral avoidance.

Resolution 2

The presence of avoidance symptoms has been reported following mild (Harvey & Bryant, 1998b), moderate (Warden et al., 1997), and severe (Bryant et al., 2000) TBI. Warden et al. (1997) argued that the development of avoidance symptoms is independent of memory for the event and that there may occur the "uncoupling between conscious memories of the event and fear-conditioned behaviour, such as avoidance and arousal symptoms" (p. 21). In essence, this is a similar proposal for dual representations of the traumatic experience in memory that has already been made in relation to reexperiencing.

Summary

We have argued that each of the points of debate concerning the coexistence of TBI with ASD and PTSD are potentially resolvable. One resolution involves accepting that TBI patients do not experience a particular set of symptoms that are common among non-TBI patients with PTSD, but that this is nevertheless no barrier to them receiving a PTSD diagnosis. Essentially, this resolution focuses attention on the set of diagnostic criteria for PTSD that have been proposed in the DSM-IV, and to the many different combinations of symptoms that will result in a PTSD diagnosis. The second resolution involves accepting that TBI patients do experience the same symptoms as other PTSD patients, but that there may be crucial differences in symptom content (e.g., the time period of intrusive memories) or in the relative importance of specific underlying cognitive processes (e.g., memory reconstruction, situationally accessible memory). At present the kind of detailed information about symptoms that would enable us to choose between these various possibilities has not been collected.

FUTURE RESEARCH

Methodology

When reviewing the empirical literature that addresses the coexistence of PTSD/ASD and TBI it became apparent that the methodology of these studies could be improved in various ways. First, several studies diagnosed

PTSD/ASD on the basis of an informal clinical interview. The diagnosis of PTSD was based on a clinician-administered structured clinical interview in only a small proportion of the studies. In future research, a structured interview with established psychometric properties should be employed. Second, von Wowern (1966) reported on the inaccuracy of self-report among TBI patients. Hence, it is of concern that the method of determining TBI is often not described fully or based on self-report. Third, although an increasing number of studies recruit consecutively admitted patients, several are based on convenience samples. In these studies the representativeness of the sample is difficult to evaluate. Differences in the quality of methodology may well account for the variation in the findings we reviewed earlier in this chapter. It is hoped that with improved methods more consistency in results will emerge. Further, it will be possible to evaluate the evidence for the various "resolutions" that we have proposed above.

Overlapping Terminology

There are a number of terms used in the PTSD and TBI literatures that require clarification in future research. First, TBI is often said to be compounded by the presence of postconcussion symptoms (Binder, 1986). Common symptoms include headaches, sensitivity to light and sound, concentration problems, memory deficits, fatigue, dizziness, and irritability (Bohnen & Jolles, 1992). Postconcussive symptoms are typically reported by mild-TBI (as opposed to moderate and severe) patients and often occur in the absence of objective neurological or radiological findings (Bazarian et al., 1999). There has been considerable debate over the etiology of the postconcussional syndrome. The two etiological camps are those who attribute the symptoms to neurological damage (Levin et al., 1987) and those who argue that the symptoms may be initiated by a transient physiological disturbance but are maintained by psychological distress (Lishman, 1988; Rutherford, 1989). Rimel, Giordani, Barth, Boll, and Jane (1981) postulated three explanations for the postconcussional syndrome as follows: (1) chronic or residual central nervous system damage, (2) secondary gain, and (3) emotional response or PTSD. An issue to be resolved in future research is that the literature to date has failed to clearly distinguish between postconcussional syndrome and PTSD/ASD. This terminological confusion is compounded by the overlap between the symptoms of postconcussional syndrome and PTSD/ASD. Symptoms common in both conditions include poor concentration, depression, anxiety, sleep disturbance and irritability (Davidoff, Laibstain, Kessler, & Mark, 1988). In an examination of the interplay between TBI and PTA, Bryant and Harvey (1999a) concluded that the heightened anxiety and frequent memory intrusions experienced by PTSD patients may result in greater demands on cognitive resources, and that this may contribute to the occurrence of postconcussional symptoms.

Second, whiplash injuries are caused by the sudden acceleration and/or deceleration of the head and neck when the former is free to move, although very many differing clinical definitions of the syndrome have been given. Some studies have shown that postconcussional syndrome can develop from whiplash injury (Evans, 1992) and others that the two syndromes are highly comorbid (Miller, 1998). The major distinguishing feature is that whiplash typically involves bruising to ligaments and soft tissues of the head and neck. The symptoms accompanying the physical injury include complaints of concentration and memory problems, headache, irritability, loss of libido, anxiety, and depression. Clearly, there is considerable overlap between whiplash, postconcussional syndrome, and PTSD. Future research is required to develop methods to establish the extent to which these are distinct or overlapping entities.

Subsyndromal Symptoms

Many patients exhibit features of PTSD, but fall just short of a strict formal diagnosis in some way. Consequently, it is sensible to recognize that PTSD is essentially a syndrome or cluster of symptoms whose number and severity vary along a continuum, and that strict hard-and-fast categories (PTSD/ no PTSD) may miss important pathology and may be the source of apparent conflicts in the literature. Hence, symptom severity may be just as important, if not more so, than a categorical diagnosis. However, decisions about what are significant clinical thresholds may have to be changed to reflect the presence of comorbid TBI.

Clinical Implications

New treatments specifically designed for the treatment of TBI patients with ASD and PTSD need to be developed and tested. Several case studies (Horton, 1993; McGrath, 1997) and one small randomized controlled trial (Bryant, Moulds, Guthrie, & Nixon, 2003) have reported on the effectiveness of cognitive behavioral approaches. However, given that individuals who have sustained a TBI may be more likely to report recurring thoughts rather than vivid images of the trauma (McMillan, 1996), it is possible that cognitive approaches should be emphasized, rather than exposure-based approaches. The development of treatments specifically designed to inhibit the activation of situationally accessible memories (Brewin, 2001, 2003) may be particularly relevant to TBI patients.

CONCLUSION

It has frequently been argued that PTSD cannot be diagnosed in individuals who have experienced a severe TBI. Specifically, the amnesia accompanying a moderate or severe TBI was thought to preclude qualification for three PTSD diagnostic criteria: the experience of intense affect, reexperiencing symptoms, and avoidance symptoms. When studies using established, previously validated measures of PTSD are considered, the evidence clearly favors the coexistence of PTSD and TBI, even when the TBI is moderate or severe. We have proposed that there are two resolutions to these apparent contradictions: (1) accepting that these symptoms are absent but recognizing the ways in which it is nonetheless possible to meet diagnostic criteria for PTSD, or (2) accepting that these symptoms can occur following TBI, albeit taking a different form compared to their presentation in non-TBI patients. None of the available evidence provides a basis for choosing between these two possible resolutions. In addition to identifying an important issue for future research, our review argues for mandatory assessment of ASD and PTSD among those who sustain a TBI during a traumatic event and for more systematic consideration of possible brain injury in patients presenting with ASD and PTSD.

REFERENCES

Bazarian, J. J., Wong, T., Harris, M., Leahey, N., Mookerjee, S., & Dombovy, M. (1999). Epidemiology and predictors of post-concussive syndrome after minor head injury in an emergency population. *Brain Injury, 13*, 173–89.

Binder, L. M. (1986). Persisting symptoms after mild head injury: A review of the postconcussive syndrome. *Journal of Clinical and Experimental Neuropsychology, 8*, 323–346.

Blanchard, E. B., Hickling, E. J., Barton, K. A., Taylor, A. E., Loos, W. R., & Jones-Alexander, J. (1996). One-year prospective follow-up of motor vehicle accident victims. *Behaviour Research and Therapy, 34*, 775–786.

Boake, C. (1996). Do patients with mild brain injuries have posttraumatic stress disorder too? *Journal of Head Trauma Rehabilitation, 11*, 95–102.

Bohnen, N., & Jolles, J. (1992). Neurobehavioral aspects of postconcussive symptoms after mild head injury. *Journal of Nervous and Mental Disease, 180*, 183–192.

Bontke, C. F. (1996). Do patients with mild brain injuries have posttraumatic stress disorder too? *Journal of Head Trauma Rehabilitation, 11*, 95–102.

Brewin, C. R. (2001). A cognitive neuroscience account of posttraumatic stress disorder and its treatment. *Behaviour Research and Therapy, 39*, 373–393.

Brewin, C. R. (2003). *Posttraumatic stress disorder: Malady or myth?* New Haven: Yale University Press.

Brewin, C. R., Andrews, B., Rose, S., & Kirk, M. (1999a). Acute stress disorder and posttraumatic stress disorder in victims of violent crime. *American Journal of Psychiatry, 156*, 360–366.

Brewin, C. R., Andrews, B., & Rose, S. (1999b). Fear, helplessness, and horror in posttraumatic stress disorder: Investigating DSM-IV criterion A2 in victims of violent crime. *Journal of Traumatic Stress, 13*, 499–509.

Brewin, C. R., Dalgleish, T., & Joseph, S. (1996). A dual representation theory of posttraumatic stress disorder. *Psychological Review, 103*, 670–686.

Bryant, R. A. (1996). Posttraumatic stress disorder, flashbacks, and pseudomemories in closed head injury. *Journal of Traumatic Stress, 9*, 621–629.

Bryant, R. A. (2001). Posttraumatic stress disorder and traumatic brain injury: Can they co-exist? *Clinical Psychology Review, 21*, 931–945.

Bryant, R. A., & Harvey, A. G. (1995). Acute stress response: A comparison of head injured and non-head injured patients. *Psychological Medicine, 25*, 869–874.

Bryant, R. A., & Harvey, A. G. (1999a). Postconcussive symptoms and posttraumatic stress disorder after mild traumatic brain injury. *Journal of Nervous and Mental Disease, 187*, 302–305.

Bryant, R. A., & Harvey, A. G. (1999b). The influence of traumatic brain injury on acute stress disorder and post-traumatic stress disorder following motor vehicle accidents. *Brain Injury, 13*, 15–22.

Bryant, R. A., Marosszeky, J. E., Crooks, J., & Gurka, J. A. (2000). Posttraumatic stress disorder following severe traumatic brain injury. *American Journal of Psychiatry, 157*, 629–631.

Bryant, R. A., Moulds, M., Guthrie, R., & Nixon, R. D. V. (2003). Treating acute stress disorder following mild traumatic brain injury. *American Journal of Psychiatry, 160*, 585–587.

Burgess, P. W., & Shallice, T. (1996). Confabulation and the control of recollection. *Memory, 4*, 359–411.

Christianson, S. A., & Engelberg, E. (1997). Remembering and forgetting traumatic experiences: A matter of survival. In M. A. Conway (Ed.), *Recovered memories and false memories* (pp. 230–250). Oxford, UK: Oxford University Press.

Davey, G. C. L. (1989). UCS revaluation and conditioning models of acquired fear. *Behaviour Research and Therapy, 27*, 521–528.

Davidoff, D. A., Laibstain, D. F., Kessler, H. R., & Mark, V. H. (1988). Neurobehavioural sequelae of minor head injury: A consideration of post-concussive syndrome versus post-traumatic stress disorder. *Cognitive Rehabilitation, March/April*, 8–13.

Di Gallo, A., Barton, J., & Parry-Jones, W. (1997). Road traffic accidents: Early psychological consequences in children and adolescents. *British Journal of Psychiatry, 170*, 358–362.

Evans, R. W. (1992). Some observations on whiplash injuries. *Neurology Clinics, 10*, 975–997.

Foa, E. B., Steketee, G., & Rothbaum, B. O. (1989). Behavioral/cognitive conceptualizations of post-traumatic stress disorder. *Behavior Therapy, 20*, 155–176.

Forrester, G., Encel, J., & Geffen, G. (1994). Measuring post-traumatic amnesia (PTA): An historical review. *Brain Injury, 8*, 175–184.

Gronwall, D., & Wrightson, P. (1980). Duration of post-traumatic amnesia after mild head injury. *Journal of Clinical Neuropsychology, 2,* 51–60.

Harvey, A. G., Brewin, C. R., Jones, C., & Kopelman, M. (2003). Coexistence of traumatic brain injury and posttraumatic stress disorder: Resolving the paradox. *Journal of the International Neuropsychological Society, 9,* 663–676.

Harvey, A. G., & Bryant, R. A. (1998a). Acute stress disorder following mild traumatic brain injury. *Journal of Nervous and Mental Disease, 186,* 333–337.

Harvey, A. G., & Bryant, R. A. (1998b). The relationship between acute stress disorder and posttraumatic stress disorder: A prospective evaluation of motor vehicle accident survivors. *Journal of Consulting and Clinical Psychology, 66,* 507–512.

Harvey, A. G., & Bryant, R. A. (1999). Reconstructing Trauma Memories: A Prospective Study of "Amnesic" Trauma Survivors. *Manuscript submitted for publication.*

Hickling, E. J., Gillen, R., Blanchard, E. B., Buckley, T., & Taylor, A. (1998). Traumatic brain injury and posttraumatic stress disorder: A preliminary investigation of neuropsychological test results in PTSD secondary to motor vehicle accidents. *Brain Injury, 12,* 265–274.

Horton, A. H. (1993). Posttraumatic stress disorder and mild head trauma: Follow up of a case study. *Perceptual and Motor Skills, 76,* 243–246.

Hyman, I. E., & Loftus, E. F. (1998). Errors in autobiographical memory. *Clinical Psychology, 18,* 933–947.

Janoff-Bulman, R. (1992). *Shattered assumptions: Towards a new psychology of trauma.* New York: The Free Press.

Johnson, M. K. (1988). Discriminating the origin of information. In T. F. Oltmanns & B. A. Maher (Eds.), *Delusional beliefs* (pp. 34–65). New York: Wiley.

Joseph, S., & Masterson, J. (1999). Posttraumatic stress disorder and traumatic brain injury: Are they mutually exclusive? *Journal of Traumatic Stress, 12,* 437–453.

Kilpatrick, D. G., Resnick, H. S., Freedy, J. R., Pelcovitz, D., Resick, P., Roth, S., & van der Kolk, B. (1998). Posttraumatic stress disorder field trial: Evaluation of the PTSD construct—Criteria A through E. In T. Widiger, A. Frances, H. Pincus, R. Ross, M. First, W. Davis, & M. Kline (Eds.), *DSM-IV sourcebook* (Vol. 4, pp. 803–844). Washington, DC: American Psychiatric Press.

King, N. S. (1997). Post-traumatic stress disorder and head injury as a dual diagnosis: "Islands of memory" as a mechanism. *Journal of Neurology, Neurosurgery, and Psychiatry, 62,* 82–84.

Kopelman, M. D. (1999). Varieties of false memory. *Cognitive Neuropsychology, 16,* 197–214.

Kopelman, M. D. (2000). Focal retrograde amnesia and the attribution of causality— An exceptionally critical review. *Cognitive Neuropsychology, 17,* 585–621.

Kopelman, M. D., Ng, N., & Van den Brouke, O. (1997). Confabulation extending across episodic memory, personal and general semantic memory. *Cognitive Neuropsychology, 14,* 683–712.

Layton, B. S., & Wardi-Zonna, K. (1995). Posttraumatic stress disorder with neurogenic amnesia for the traumatic event. *The Clinical Neuropsychologist, 9,* 2–10.

Levin, H. S., Amparo, E., Eisenberg, H. M., Williams, P. H., High, W. M., McArdle, C. B., & Weiner, R. L. (1987). Magnetic reasonance imaging and computerised tomography in relation to the neurobehavioural sequelae of mild and moderate head injuries. *Journal of Neurosurgery, 66,* 706–713.

Lishman, W. A. (1988). Physiogenesis and psychogenesis in the "post-concussional syndrome." *British Journal of Psychiatry, 153,* 460–469.

Mayou, R., Bryant, B., & Duthie, R. (1993). Psychiatric consequences of road accidents. *British Medical Journal, 307,* 647–651.

McFarlane, A. C. (1988). The phenomenology of posttraumatic stress disorder following a natural disaster. *The Journal of Nervous and Mental Disease, 176,* 22–29.

McGrath, J. (1997). Cognitive impairment associated with post-traumatic stress disorder and minor head injury: A case report. *Neuropsychological Rehabilitation, 7,* 231–239.

McMillan, T. M. (1991). Posttraumatic stress disorder and severe head injury. *British Journal of Psychiatry, 159,* 431–433.

McMillan, T. M. (1996). Post-traumatic stress disorder following minor and severe closed head injury: 10 single cases. *Brain-Injury, 10,* 749–758.

McMillan, T. M. (1997). Minor head injury. *Current Opinion in Neurology, 10,* 479–483.

McNally, R. J. (2003). *Remembering trauma.* Cambridge, MA: Harvard University Press.

Merckelbach, H., Muris, P., Horselenberg, R., & Rassin, E. (1998). Traumatic intrusions as "worst case scenarios." *Behaviour Research and Therapy, 36,* 1075–1079.

Miller, L. (1998). Motor vehicle accidents: Clinical, neuropsychological and forensic considerations. *Journal of Cognitive Rehabilitation, 16,* 10–12.

Moscovitch, M., & Melo, B. (1997). Strategic retrieval and the frontal lobes: Evidence from confabulation and amnesia. *Neuropsychologia, 35,* 1017–1034.

O'Brien, M., & Nutt, D. (1998). Loss of consciousness and post-traumatic stress disorder. *British Journal of Psychiatry, 173,* 102–104.

Ohry, A., Rattock, J., & Solomon, Z. (1996). Post-traumatic stress disorder in brain injury patients. *Brain Injury, 10,* 687–695.

Price, K. P. (1994). Posttraumatic stress disorder and concussion: Are they incompatible? *Defense Law Journal, 43,* 113–120.

Rattock, J., & Ross, B. (1993). Post traumatic stress disorder in the traumatically head injured. *Journal of Clinical and Experimental Neuropsychology (Abstract), 6,* 243.

Reynolds, M., & Brewin, C. R. (1998). Intrusive cognition, coping strategies and emotional responses in depression, post-traumatic stress disorder and a nonclinical population. *Behaviour Research and Therapy, 36,* 135–148.

Riggs, D. S., Rothbaum, B. O., & Foa, E. B. (1995). A prospective examination of symptoms of posttraumatic stress disorder in victims of non-sexual assault. *Journal of Interpersonal Violence, 10,* 201–214.

Rimel, R. W., Giordani, B., Barth, J. T., Boll, T. J., & Jane, J. A. (1981). Disability caused by minor head injury. *Neurosurgery, 9,* 221–228.

Roediger, H. L., McDermott, K. B., & Goff, L. M. (1997). Recovery of true and false: Paradoxical effects of repeated testing. In M. A. Conway (Ed.), *Recovered memories and false memories* (pp. 118–149). Oxford, UK: Oxford University Press.

Russell, W. R. (1971). *The traumatic amnesias.* London: Oxford University Press.

Russell, W. R., & Nathan, P. W. (1946). Traumatic amnesia. *Brain, 69,* 280–300.

Russell, W. R., & Smith, A. (1961). Post-traumatic amnesia in closed head injury. *Archives of Neurology, 5,* 4–17.

Rutherford, W. H. (1989). Postconcussion symptoms: Relationship to acute neurological indices, individual differences and circumstances of injury. In H. S. Levin, H. M. Eisenberg, & A. L. Benton (Eds.), *Mild head injury* (pp. 217–228). New York: Oxford University Press.

Sbordone, R. J. (1991). *Neuropsychology for the attorney*. Orlando: Deutsch Press.

Sbordone, R. J., & Liter, J. C. (1995). Mild traumatic brain injury does not produce post-traumatic stress disorder. *Brain Injury, 9*, 405–412.

Schacter, D. L. (1987). Implicit memory: History and current status. *Journal of Experimental Psychology: Learning, Memory and Cognition, 13*, 501–518.

Schacter, D. L., & Crovitz, H. F. (1977). Memory function after closed head injury: A review of the quantitative research. *Cortex, 13*, 150–176.

Shores, A., Marosszeky, J. E., Sandanam, J., & Batchelor, J. (1986). Preliminary validation of a clinical scale for measuring the duration of post-traumatic amnesia. *Medical Journal of Australia, 144*, 569–572.

Sisler, G., & Penner, H. (1975). Amnesia following severe head injury. *Canadian Psychiatric Association Journal, 20*, 333–336.

Sohlberg, M. M., & Mateer, C. A. (1989). *Introduction to cognitive rehabilitation: Theory and practice*. New York: Guilford Press.

Squire, L. R. (1992). Declarative and nondeclarative memory: Multiple brain systems supporting learning and memory. *Journal of Cognitive Neuroscience, 4*, 232–243.

Squire, L. R., Cohen, N. J., & Nadel, L. (1984). The medial temporal region and memory consolidation: A new hypothesis. In H. Weingartner & E. Parker (Eds.), *Memory consolidation* (pp. 185–210). Hillsdale, NJ: Erlbaum.

Symonds, C. (1966). Disorders of memory. *Brain, 89*, 625–644.

Symonds, C. P., & Russell, W. R. (1943). Accidental head injuries: Prognosis in service patients. *Lancet, 1*, 7–10.

Taylor, S., & Koch, W. J. (1995). Anxiety disorders due to motor vehicle accidents: Nature and treatment. *Clinical Psychology Review, 15*, 721–738.

Tulving, E., & Schacter, D. L. (1990). Priming and human memory systems. *Science, 247*, 301–306.

von Wowern, F. (1966). Post-traumatic amnesia and confusion as an index of severity in head injury. *Acta Neurologica Scandinavia, 42*, 373–378.

Warden, D. L., Labbate, L. A., Salazar, A. M., Nelson, R., Sheley, E., Staudenmeier, J., & Martin, E. (1997). Posttraumatic stress disorder in patients with traumatic brain injury and amnesia for the event? *Journal of Neuropsychiatry and Clinical Neurosciences, 9*, 18–22.

World Health Organization. (1993). *The ICD-10 classification of mental and behavioural disorders*. Geneva: WHO.

Zangwill, O. L. (1966). The amnesic syndrome. In C. W. M. Whitty & O. L. Zangwill (Eds.), *Amnesia* (pp. 61–82). London: Butterworth.

Zola, S. M. (1998). Memory, amnesia, and the issue of recovered memory: Neurobiological aspects. *Clinical Psychology Review, 18*, 915–932.

PART V

Clinical Applications

CHAPTER 11

Clinical Neuropsychological Evaluation

JENNIFER J. VASTERLING
and JENNIFER SUE KLEINER

The subjective impression of cognitive impairment is sufficiently common in posttraumatic stress disorder (PTSD) that attentional and memory deficits are incorporated as part of the diagnostic criteria. With increasing awareness of the objective neuropsychological performance deficits experienced among at least subsets of individuals suffering PTSD (see Vasterling & Brailey, Chapter 8, this volume), referrals for neuropsychological evaluation of PTSD patients are becoming more commonplace. Moreover, neuropsychological evaluation is conducted routinely in certain populations (e.g., motor vehicle accidents survivors) in which the stressor also involves potential brain injury. Thus, the influence of PTSD on neuropsychological functioning is frequently relevant in both psychiatric and nonpsychiatric (e.g., primary care) settings.

Many questions remain regarding the neuropsychological profile of PTSD and the potential influence of individual difference variables, trauma characteristics, and treatments on cognitive performance in PTSD. As such, caution limits the degree to which empirically based knowledge can be translated to the clinical context. Nonetheless, the growing neuropsychological and neurobiological literatures summarized in previous chapters of this text provide a basis from which to develop neuropsychological assessment strategies when PTSD is a potential clinical feature.

In this chapter, we integrate current knowledge of the neuropsychological correlates of PTSD with epidemiological factors in an attempt to outline the fundamental considerations that a clinician faces when conducting a clinical neuropsychological evaluation on a patient potentially suffering from PTSD. In the first section, we discuss clinical assessment procedures relevant to establishing a PTSD diagnosis, evaluating concurrent psychopathology, and conducting the core neuropsychological assessment. The second section addresses interpretive issues, including differential diagnosis and assessment of motivation.

CLINICAL ASSESSMENT PROCEDURES

Establishing a Diagnosis of PTSD

Prior to determining the degree to which possible neuropsychological impairment is related to PTSD, a diagnosis of PTSD should first be established. Because of the symptom overlap with other emotional disorders (e.g., depression, non-PTSD anxiety disorders), two of the most important steps in evaluating PTSD are (1) establishing that a traumatic event occurred and (2) conducting a thorough assessment of symptom criteria that can be linked to the traumatic event(s). A full discussion of the methodological and conceptual issues related to PTSD assessment is beyond the scope of this chapter; however, a number of informative reviews are available (e.g., Everly & Lating, 2004; Flack, Litz, Weathers, & Beaudreau, 2002; Keane, Buckley, & Miller, 2003; Keane, Weathers, & Foa, 2000; Sutker, Uddo-Crane, & Allain, 1991; Uddo, Allain, & Sutker, 1996; Weathers & Keane, 1999). In addition, a summary of current assessment tools may be found on the website for the National Center for PTSD. The following sections provide a brief summary of issues relevant to establishing the occurrence of a trauma event and assessing symptom criteria.

Elicitation of the Trauma History

A core element of PTSD diagnosis is the experience of a traumatic event. The fourth edition of the *Diagnostic and Statistical Manual of Mental Disorders* (DSM-IV; American Psychiatric Association, 1994) specifies that "the person experienced, witnessed, or was confronted with an event or events that involved actual or threatened death or serious injury, or a threat to the physical integrity of self or other" (Criterion A1) and that the "person's response involved intense fear, helplessness, or horror" (Criterion A2). Although the optimal range of accepted traumatic stressors remains somewhat controversial (see Breslau, 2001; McNally, 2003), trauma events are typically conceptualized as differing in severity and response from more typical life stressors (e.g., divorce, loss of employment).

There are several relevant factors to consider in eliciting description of the trauma event. First, knowledge of the chronology of the trauma event relative to symptom development aids in linking both psychological and neuropsychological symptoms to the stressor. Secondly, information relative to trauma intensity, duration, and frequency bears on understanding symptom presentation (Uddo et al., 1996). For example, if there is a history of multiple traumatic events, attributing symptoms to the trauma and establishing the course of the disorder can be difficult (Keane et al., 2000; Weathers & Keane, 1999).

Neuropsychological factors also potentially influence evaluation of Criterion A. Specifically, a neurological event may coincide with psychological trauma, as is the case with some motor vehicle accidents, falls, assaults, and combat blast injuries. When consciousness is altered at the time of traumatization, poor initial encoding potentially degrades explicit memory processes and subsequent recall of the trauma (Klein, Caspi, & Gil, 2003; McMillan, Williams, & Bryant, 2003). In the most extreme scenario, the individual may have experienced neural insult sufficiently severe to preclude any conscious recollection of the event. Whether PTSD can develop in this circumstance has been a source of much debate (see Harvey, Kopelman, & Brewin, Chapter 10, this volume). However, even without frank neurological insult at the time of traumatization, recall of the trauma may be subject to certain types of memory distortion (e.g., Loftus & Burns, 1982; Smith, Ellsworth, & Kassin, 1989) and may not remain consistent over time (Schwarz, Kowalski, & McNally, 1993; Southwick, Morgan, Nicolaou, & Charney, 1997). As described by Brewin (Chapter 6, this volume), increased arousal and narrowing of attention may serve to highlight some features of the event while diminishing others. Thus, it may be necessary to seek methods of verifying the trauma beyond the self-report of the person assessed, given the potential for both emotional and externally induced, neurogenic contamination.

Despite the potential usefulness of assessment tools specific to Criterion A traumatic events, there are far fewer of such instruments as compared to those assessing PTSD symptoms (Weathers & Keane, 1999). However, multiple trauma assessment methods do exist, including interview formats, cued recall, checklists, and records review, each characterized by strengths and weaknesses regarding the balance between time efficiency and comprehensiveness. The reader is referred to Everly and Lating (2004), Norris and Riad (1997), and Weathers and Keane (1999) for more extensive discussion of trauma assessment methods.

Assessment of PTSD Symptom Criteria

PTSD symptoms are grouped in the DSM-IV into three criterion clusters: reexperiencing of the trauma; avoidance and emotional numbing; and heightened arousal. Additional criteria require that symptoms have endured for more than 1 month and cause clinically significant distress or functional impairment. We have noted that overattention to reexperiencing symptoms with disregard for other symptom criteria ranks among the most common mistakes in diagnosing PTSD in neuropsychological and non-mental health contexts. Although subthreshold presentations may reflect partial remissions of PTSD that nonetheless impact neuropsychological functioning, basing a diagnosis on one or two reexperiencing symptoms (e.g., nightmares or intrusive thoughts) may result in misdiagnosis (e.g., misattributing depressive ruminations to PTSD).

Similar to assessment of the trauma event, PTSD symptom criteria may be assessed using several methods including face-valid, DSM-based paper-and-pencil inventories, paper-and-pencil measures that do not correspond directly to DSM symptom criteria but instead rely on cut-off scores, and structured, semistructured, and unstructured clinical interviews. Whereas comprehensive interview formats permit integration of behavioral observations and greater depth in probing for symptoms (with semistructured and structured interviews also facilitating reliability within the diagnostic process), interviews are often more time consuming than other methods of assessment and may be subject to perceived response demands. DSM-based paper-and-pencil inventories are typically briefer while maintaining direct correspondence to disorder criteria; however, like structured and semi-structured interviews, the face-validity of DSM-based checklists renders them particularly susceptible to response bias (i.e., shaping responses in a desired direction) (Meier, 1994; Weathers, Keane, King, & King, 1997). Conversely, whereas non-DSM-based measures are less face valid, the spec ificity of such instruments to PTSD diagnosis has been questioned (Weathers et al., 1997). The current gold standard is multimethod assessment, which provides converging evidence through capitalization of the strengths of each methodology (Weathers & Keane, 1999).

A limitation of all of the most commonly used assessment methods listed above is that they are reliant on self-report and each, to varying degrees, may be subject to distortion. There are several partial solutions to this problem. One is consideration of collateral sources of information, such as medical record review, family observations, and clinician-based observations. Although not currently normed for diagnostic purposes, ancillary methods such as psychophysiological (Blanchard & Buckley, 1999; Keane et al., 1998; Orr & Roth, 2000) and electrophysiological (see Metzger, Gilbertson, & Orr, Chapter 4, this volume) assessment and experimental cognitive paradigms (e.g., emotional Stroop paradigm; see Constans, Chapter 5, this volume) that are less susceptible to intentional distortion also hold promise to provide confirmatory evidence for a diagnosis.

Assessment of Behavioral and Other Contributory Factors

Comprehensive neuropsychological evaluation includes assessment of presenting symptoms, behavioral observations, and individual historical fac-

tors that potentially contribute to objective neuropsychological performances, diagnosis, and treatment recommendations. We focus on those
historical and clinical features that warrant special emphasis when PTSD is
germane to the evaluation. For examples and discussions of general
neuropsychological interviews and checklists, please refer to Freed (2003),
Sbordone (2000), and White (1992).

Comorbid Psychopathology

As described in Duke and Vasterling (Chapter 1, this volume), the prevalence of some comorbid mental disorders (e.g., depression, substance use
disorder, anxiety disorders) in PTSD is high (see also Brady, Killeen,
Brewerton, & Lucierni, 2000; Uddo, et al., 1996; Weathers & Keane,
1999). The National Comorbidity Study, for example, revealed that more
than half of PTSD cases were accompanied by a comorbid depressive disorder (Kessler, Sonnega, Bromet, Hughes, & Nelson, 1995). Such comorbidities may complicate neuropsychological evaluation in several respects.
First, there is overlap in symptom criteria (e.g., anhedonia, concentration
difficulties) between PTSD and other psychiatric disorders, such as depression, potentially leading to diagnostic ambiguities in psychopathology diagnosis. Second, the combination of PTSD and depression may put individuals at increased risk for suicidal behaviors (Oquendo et al., 2003), some of
which (e.g., gunshots wounds to the head, drug overdoses resulting in
coma) may result in lasting neuropsychological impairment. Finally, certain
comorbidities (e.g., alcohol use disorders, depression) may influence neuropsychological performance directly.
    Thus, neuropsychological evaluation should include assessment of
potential psychiatric comorbidities, as well as behaviors (e.g., suicide attempts, excessive alcohol consumption) that potentially influence neuropsychological performance and clinical outcome. A review of psychopathology assessment methods is beyond the scope of the chapter; however,
similar to PTSD assessment, a number of interview-based (e.g., Structured
Clinical Interview for Axis I DSM-IV Diagnoses; First, Spitzer, Gibbon, &
Williams, 1994), observer-rated (e.g., Hamilton Anxiety Rating Scale;
Hamilton, 1959) and paper-and-pencil self-report (Beck Depression Inventory—II; Beck, Steer, & Brown, 1996; Beck Anxiety Inventory; Beck, Epstein, Brown, & Steer, 1988; Alcohol Timeline Followback; Sobell &
Sobell, 1996; Self-Administered Short Michigan Alcoholism Screening Test;
Selzer, Vinokur, & van Rooijen, 1975) assessment tools are available. At a
minimum, consideration of potential comorbid disorders should be integrated into medical record review, the clinical interview, and behavioral observations of displayed affect during the evaluation (Brady et al., 2000).
    The chronology of non-PTSD mental disorders also bears on the clini-

cal neuropsychological evaluation of PTSD cases. For example, knowing the chronology of substance use in relation to the onset of cognitive impairment and PTSD symptoms is useful to interpretation of neuropsychological test data. Preliminary evidence that neurodevelopmental disorders such as attention-deficit/hyperactivity disorder (ADHD) may be associated with increased risk of PTSD (Gilbertson, Gurvits, Lasko, Orr, & Pitman, 2001; Gurvits et al., 2000; Gurvits et al., 1993) highlights the need to assess mental disorders that predate PTSD onset. Likewise, neurobehavioral disorders (e.g., dementia) with onset postdating trauma exposure may be associated with recurrence or exacerbation of PTSD symptoms (van Achterberg, Rohrbaugh, & Southwick, 2001). Such neurobehavioral disorders, while possibly related to PTSD as risk factors, also potentially affect neuropsychological performance independently of PTSD.

Associated Medical and Somatic Disorders

As summarized in Schnurr and Green (2004), stress exposure can lead to significant health consequences, some of which (e.g., cardiovascular disease, immune disorders, cerebrovascular disease, pain disorders) may put individuals at increased risk for neuropsychological dysfunction either directly via disease-related neural dysfunction (Hart, Martelli, & Zasler, 2000; Shucard et al., 2004; Waldstein, Snow, Muldoon, & Katzel, 2001) or indirectly via iatrogenic (e.g., chemotherapy, radiation, neurosurgery) side effects (e.g., Forsyth & Cascino, 1995; Jennings, 1995; Keime-Guibert, Napolitano, & Delattre, 1998; Walch, Ahles, & Saykin, 1998). As discussed earlier, brain injury at the time of trauma may also be present and potentially impact neuropsychological performance (Gioia & Isquith, 2004; Goldstein & Levin, 2001; Levin & Kraus, 1994; McDonald, Flashman, & Saykin, 2002).

Other Associated Clinical Features

Disruption of sleep is a core of feature of PTSD that may lead to impaired neuropsychological performance. PTSD is associated with abnormalities in sleep arousal, rapid eye movement sleep, and disruptive movements during sleep (e.g., Breslau et al., 2004; Harvey, Jones, & Schmidt, 2003; Krakow et al., 2001; Mellman, Kulick-Bell, Ashlock, & Nolan, 1995; Ohayon & Shapiro, 2000; Singareddy & Balon, 2002). Although little is known about the direct effects of PTSD sleep disturbance on neuropsychological functioning, sleep deprivation in non-PTSD populations is associated with neuropsychological compromise (e.g., Falleti, Maruff, Collie, Darby, & McStephen, 2003; Hood & Bruck, 2002; Kelly & Coppel, 2001; Lee, Kim,

& Suh, 2003; McCann et al., 1992; Szelenberger & Niemcewicz, 2000). Thus, information about both the immediate context of the prior night's sleep and the more general pattern of sleep is relevant to interpretation of neuropsychological test data.

The arousal disturbances associated with PTSD may also affect test performances. Both hyper- and hypoarousal have been shown to influence neuropsychological test performances (Robbins, 1998). As described in previous chapters (see Southwick, Rasmusson, Barron, & Arnsten, Chapter 2, this volume; Metzger, Gilbertson, & Orr, Chapter 4, this volume), it is becoming increasingly apparent that centrally mediated disturbances in arousal may accompany PTSD, and the pattern of neuropsychological impairment documented in some PTSD studies (e.g., Vasterling, Brailey, Constans, & Sutker, 1998) is consistent with induced hyperarousal states in animal studies (e.g., Robbins, 1998). In addition to querying for behavioral symptoms (e.g., sleep disturbance, hypervigilance) associated with arousal alteration, level of arousal may also be observed behaviorally during the evaluation.

Finally, dissociative features may accompany PTSD (Bremner et al., 1992; Koopman et al., 2001) particularly following physical abuse, sexual abuse, and rape (Spiegel & Cardena, 1991). These symptoms have been defined as a three-fold construct: difficulty recalling critical aspects of the trauma as a result of alterations in memory processes; alteration in one's sense of engagement with the environment; and alterations in consciousness (Feeny, Zoellner, Fitzgibbons, & Foa, 2000). Little is known about the impact of acute dissociative symptoms on neuropsychological performance, although dissociative disorders have been linked to amnesia for personal information (Spiegel & Cardena, 1991). However, because symptoms of dissociation are often described subjectively as episodes of forgetting or limited encoding that may be confused with a less transient cognitive impairment, such symptoms typically require further elaboration for appropriate diagnostic consideration.

Medications

Like many other psychiatric disorders, PTSD is commonly treated with psychotropic medications, ranging in potential impact on cognitive functioning from negative to positive. Similarly, as described above, because chronic PTSD confers additional risk of somatic illness, it is not uncommon for PTSD-diagnosed individuals to also take medications for somatic conditions. Thus, as with any thorough neuropsychological interview, it is helpful to assess the onset (or remission) of cognitive complaints in relation to changes in medications, particularly those with central nervous system properties.

NEUROPSYCHOLOGICAL TESTING ISSUES

Selection of Neurobehavioral Instruments

In this section, we emphasize review of general considerations in test selection for neuropsychological evaluation of PTSD, giving only representative examples of commonly used instruments (especially those found to be sensitive to PTSD) rather than a prescribed "how to" approach. Our overarching approach is based on conceptual domains rather than the specific instruments to assess those domains. As there are often multiple test instrument alternatives and the development and refinement of neuropsychological assessment methods continually evolves, we reason that a conceptual approach will ultimately be more informative than a rigid prescription of specific tests. There are several compendiums that describe the existing pool of neuropsychological assessment instruments (e.g., Lezak, 1995; Spreen & Strauss, 1998).

As with any comprehensive neuropsychological examination, a broad assessment across multiple functional domains is necessary for clinical hypothesis testing. That is, an evaluation should be structured to provide *both* confirmatory and disconfirmatory evidence. Otherwise, evaluation results are vulnerable to subjective clinical biases. What this means concretely is that the evaluation should assess functional domains that have high probability of impairment if PTSD is the suspected etiology of cognitive dysfunction, as well as those that have low probability of impairment if PTSD is the primary etiological factor. Assessment of functional domains not typically impaired in PTSD may also help develop alternative etiological hypotheses (i.e., that a condition other than PTSD is contributing to cognitive dysfunction).

A second consideration in selecting neuropsychological tests is level of difficulty. As reviewed in Vasterling and Brailey (Chapter 8, this volume), the mean neuropsychological test scores of PTSD-diagnosed individuals reported in the empirical literature suggest that the level of cognitive impairment associated with PTSD is typically relatively mild. Although mean performance scores distinguish PTSD-diagnosed individual from those without PTSD diagnosis, the scores nonetheless often fall within normal limits. The relatively subtle impairment associated with PTSD has two implications for evaluation: (1) tasks must be sufficiently challenging to be sensitive, and (2) as in any neuropsychological evaluation, the overall pattern of relative strengths and weaknesses is often more important to interpretation than normative scores considered in isolation.

Finally, the tradition of clinical neuropsychological evaluation emphasizes use of performance-based assessment methodologies. As with other mental disorders such as depression (Kalska, Punamaeki, Maekinen-Pelli, & Saarinen, 1999) and Alzheimer's disease (Duke, Seltzer, Seltzer, &

Vasterling, 2002; Kaszniak & Zak, 1996), self-report of cognitive symptoms and objective performances have been found to diverge in PTSD (Roca & Freeman, 2001). Thus, application of objective, performance-based assessment instruments is critical to adequate neuropsychological assessment of PTSD.

Which Domains Are Most Likely to Be Sensitive to PTSD?

Overall, as reviewed in Vasterling and Brailey (Chapter 8, this volume), although there continues to be controversy regarding the profile of neuropsychological impairment associated with PTSD, the domains for which the most evidence of PTSD-related impairment exists are attention and memory.

Attention is a multifaceted construct, for which multiple conceptual models exist. For example, Mirsky, Anthony, Duncan, Ahearn, and Kellam (1991) proposed a model that breaks attention into four constructs: focus–execute, sustain, shift, and encode. As an additional example, Posner, Walker, Friedrich, and Rafal (1984) posited that attention involves a three-stage process involving disengagement from the current stimuli, movement (or shift) of attention to a new stimulus, and engagement with the new stimulus. Regardless of the model adopted, the empirical literature suggests that PTSD is not associated with global impairment of attention but instead may be associated with impairment of only certain aspects (i.e., working memory, vigilance) of attention. Thus, based on the current literature, measures of attention that might be expected to be relatively more sensitive to PTSD include those assessing working memory, such as Digit Span backward and Arithmetic from the Wechsler Adult Intelligence Scale, Third Edition (WAIS-III, Wechsler, 1997a) or those measuring sustained attention or vigilance such as continuous performance test paradigms. Conversely, tasks that measure simple attention (e.g., digit repetition) or basic attentional scanning (e.g., cancellation tasks) would not be expected to be particularly sensitive to PTSD.

Memory can be conceptualized as a series of processes that involve the registration, encoding, and reconstruction of an event (Lezak, 1995). Various models of memory, while often overlapping conceptually, categorize component processes differently with such distinctions as anterograde versus retrograde, short- versus long-term, declarative versus nondeclarative, implicit versus explicit, and semantic versus episodic memory (Bauer, Grande, & Valenstein, 2003). Much of the clinical neuropsychological PTSD literature focuses on examination of explicit (memory with conscious awareness), anterograde (formation of new memories), episodic (personally dated or contextually encoded information) processes. Standard clinically administered memory instruments such the Rey Auditory Verbal Learning

Test (AVLT; Rey, 1964), California Verbal Learning Test (CVLT; Delis, Kramer, Kaplan, & Ober, 1987) or its more recent revision (CVLT-II), Continuous Visual Memory Test (Trahan & Larrabee, 1988), verbal and nonverbal subtests of the Wechsler Memory Scale, Third Edition (Wechsler, 1997b), and Recognition Memory Test (Warrington, 1984) are examples of widely used standardized memory tests characterized as reflecting explicit, episodic, anterograde processes.

The empirical literature points in particular to memory impairment at the levels of initial registration and learning (see Vasterling & Brailey, Chapter 8, this volume), corresponding to test of memory immediately after presentation of study materials and during the initial trials of a multiple exposure memory task (e.g., AVLT, CVLT). Findings are less robust regarding test of memory following a delayed interval, especially if the proficiency of immediate recall is taken into account (e.g., as computed by savings ratios or difference scores). There also appears to be a dissociation between spontaneous recall and recognition memory, with recall typically less proficient than recognition memory. Thus, memory tests that differentiate between initial learning and retention over time and include recall and recognition test formats currently hold the greatest potential to inform clinical evaluation.

Which Domains Are Likely to Be Least Sensitive to PTSD?

As summarized in Chapter 8, there is scant evidence that PTSD is associated with impairment of basic language functions (e.g., language comprehension, repetition, spontaneous speech), motor speed (e.g., finger tapping), or visuospatial skills (e.g., visual construction, visual object recognition, left–right orientation). However, there is some evidence that when executive control or strategic planning is required on motor (e.g., Gurvits et al., 1993; Gurvits et al., 2000) and visual–organizational tasks (Gurvits et al., 2002), PTSD may be associated with performance deficits. Likewise, there is limited evidence that word-list generation, a task sensitive to prefrontal integrity, may be impaired in PTSD (Gil, Calev, Greenberg, Kugelmass, & Lerer, 1990; Bustamante, Mellman, David, & Fins, 2001; Koenen et al., 2001; Uddo, Vasterling, Brailey, & Sutker, 1993).

Prefrontal Cognitive Functions

Executive control and other functions that are often associated with the functional integrity of the prefrontal cortex require special mention. Although there is not strong evidence that PTSD is associated with deficits on more commonly used clinical tasks of executive functioning (see Vasterling & Brailey, Chapter 8, this volume) such as the Wisconsin Card Sorting Test

(WCST; Berg, 1948; Heaton, Chelune, Talley, Kay, & Curtiss, 1993), aspects of "prefrontal" functioning not assessed by these tasks may nonetheless be impaired in PTSD. Studies that have included error analysis (e.g., Vasterling et al., 1998) have provided evidence that PTSD is associated with impaired inhibitory functions on memory and attentional tasks. Likewise, as described above, deficits on motor, visual–organizational, and word-list generation tasks with strong executive demands have also been noted in PTSD-diagnosed individuals. Finally, Koenen and her colleagues (2001) documented PTSD-related deficits on comparative neuropsychology tasks (e.g., object alternation) linked in both the animal and human literatures to prefrontal cortical dysfunction. Thus, it may be necessary for the clinician to extend beyond the most widely used clinical executive tasks to multifaceted instruments (e.g., Behavioral Assessment of the Dysexecutive System [Wilson, Alderman, Burgess, Emslie, & Evans, 1996] and Delis–Kaplan Executive Function System [Delis, Kaplan & Kramer, 2003]) and paradigms derived from the animal (cf. Koenen et al., 2001) and human (e.g., Bechara, Damasio, Tranel, & Anderson, 1994) experimental literatures to examine aspects of executive and prefrontal functioning not tapped by more traditional tasks.

Intellectual and Achievement Testing

As reviewed in Chapter 8, there is evidence that PTSD is associated with less proficient performance on intellectual tasks, especially those that assess verbal intelligence (e.g., Gil et al., 1990; Vasterling, Brailey, Constans, Borges, & Sutker, 1997). Whereas screening tasks such as the Shipley Institute of Living Scale—Revised (Zachary, 1986) or the Vocabulary subtest of the Wechsler intelligence scales (WAIS-R; Wechsler, 1981; WAIS-III; Wechsler, 1997a) that estimate intellectual functioning have been found to be sensitive to PTSD (Brandes et al., 2002; Gil et al., 1990; Gurvits et al., 1993; Gurvits et al., 2000; Macklin et al., 1998; Vasterling et al., 1997; Vasterling et al., 2002), more comprehensive tests such as the full Wechsler intelligence scales provide information about multiple dimensions of intellectual functioning. Although little is known about performance on achievement tasks by individuals diagnosed with PTSD, findings that neurodevelopmental disorders (Gilbertson et al., 2001; Gurvits et al., 2000; Gurvits et al., 1993), lower proficiency on military entrance tests (Centers for Disease Control Vietnam Experiences Study, 1988; Macklin et al., 1998; Pitman, Orr, Lowenhagen, Macklin, & Altman, 1991), and lower educational attainment (Green, Grace, Lindy, Gleser, & Leonard, 1990; Kulka et al., 1990) are among the risk factors for PTSD that suggest that achievement testing may provide useful clinical information in neuropsychological evaluations of PTSD.

DIFFERENTIAL DIAGNOSIS OF NEUROPSYCHOLOGICAL DEFICITS

Common Differentials

As described above, individuals with PTSD may also suffer from medical or mental disorders that lead to neuropsychological deficits independent of those associated with PTSD. When such conditions are known and are already being managed appropriately, the etiological differentiation of known neuropsychological deficits may have only minimal impact on clinical care. That is, in the context of multiple neuropsychological risk factors, an understanding of neuropsychological strengths and weaknesses is typically more important to treatment planning than is an estimation of the relative contribution of each condition to the neuropsychological impairment. However, when concurrent disorders associated with potential neuropsychological compromise exist but are not yet identified, the detection of cognitive compromise not attributable to PTSD may have significant clinical impact, particularly when undetected disorders are potentially treatable or amenable to intervention. Similarly, misdiagnosis of another disorder as PTSD has significant clinical implications.

While not a comprehensive listing of differential diagnoses, the more common conditions that may both accompany PTSD and confer additional risk for neuropsychological compromise include traumatic brain injury, alcohol and other substance use disorders, and depression. Likewise, among individuals with chronic PTSD, both age and the experience of chronic stress may result in health problems such as vascular disease (e.g., hypertension and cerebrovascular disease) that potentially lead to neuropsychological compromise. In children, potential concomitant disorders associated with cognitive compromise may include development disorders such as ADHD. Mental disorders that may be misdiagnosed as PTSD because of symptom overlap or misclassification of similar symptoms include adjustment disorder, other anxiety disorders, psychotic disorders, and mood disorders.

Considerations in Differentiating Diagnostic Etiologies

Among the potential factors to consider in differentiating neuropsychological symptoms attributable to PTSD from those attributable to other disorders or conditions are the onset and course of the emotional and neuropsychological symptoms, the pattern of neuropsychological deficits, and the severity of neuropsychological impairment. As described earlier in this chapter, linkage of psychological symptoms to the trauma event is helpful in establishing a PTSD diagnosis. However, linking onset of neuropsychological symptoms to trauma exposure and PTSD onset may in some cases be less relevant to differential diagnosis. Specifically, because the direction of causality between PTSD and neuropsychological performance remains ambiguous (see Vasterling & Brailey, Chapter 8, this volume), whether cognitive impairment precedes or follows PTSD onset is not necessarily informative. Nonetheless, a dramatic decline in neuropsychological functioning in a person who has suffered PTSD for a prolonged period without prior significant neuropsychological dysfunction may indicate the development of a non-PTSD disorder.

Both the pattern and the severity of neuropsychological deficits also potentially inform differential diagnosis. For example, primary language dysfunction or aphasia (e.g., impairment of auditory comprehension or speech output), visuoperceptual impairment (e.g., visual agnosia), or significant fine motor impairment would strongly suggest the possibility of a non-PTSD etiology for observed neuropsychological impairment. Similarly, PTSD would not be expected to be associated with pronounced unilateral deficits or sensorimotor impairment, despite preliminary findings of more subtle interhemispheric differences on information-processing tasks (e.g., Metzger et al., 2004; Vasterling, Duke, Tomlin, Lowery, & Kaplan, 2004). Finally, the neuropsychological deficits associated with PTSD would not be expected to be severe. In fact, some have argued that PTSD is not associated with cognitive deficits but instead, that enhanced cognitive processing serves as a protective factor for PTSD development or mitigates PTSD symptom severity following trauma exposure (Gilbertson et al., 2001). Thus, severe neuropsychological deficits would likely indicate an alternative etiology.

Malingering and Motivational Disorders

There is no evidence that the intentional feigning of symptoms is the norm among individuals presenting with PTSD; however, because PTSD may be associated with trauma events that are compensable or involve litigation (e.g., motor vehicle accidents, occupational injuries or events), there is the possibility in select contexts that secondary gain may factor into symptom presentation in subsets of individuals (e.g., DeViva & Bloem, 2003; Gold & Frueh, 1999; Larrabee, 1998). Further, as in other psychiatric disorders, symptom distortion may occur among treatment-seeking individuals as a means to convey the need for help (e.g., Hyer et al., 1988). Although there is a growing literature examining methods of detecting PTSD symptom exaggeration (e.g., Bury & Bagby, 2002; Elhai, Gold, Frueh, & Gold, 2000; Elhai et al., 2004; Franklin, Repasky, Thompson, Shelton, & Uddo, 2003; Franklin, Repasky, Thompson, Shelton, & Uddo, 2002), few PTSD studies have included motivational assessment of neuropsychological deficits (cf. Sullivan et al., 2003). However, a number of measures of motivation are available that are geared specifically to assessment of effort on cognitive tasks such as the Test of Memory Malingering (Tombaugh, 1996), Rey Fifteen Item Memory Test (Rey, 1964), and Victoria Symptom Validity Test (Hiscock & Hiscock, 1989), a more comprehensive listing of which may be found in Bianchini, Mathias, and Greve (2001).

CONCLUSIONS AND FUTURE DIRECTIONS

Neuropsychological evaluation of PTSD may be applied to the clinical context in several ways. First, neuropsychological evaluation can rule out or identify other, non-PTSD etiologies of neural dysfunction that may require a different treatment protocol than that associated with PTSD. Second, as discussed in more detail in the following two chapters on pharmacological and behavioral interventions, the neuropsychological profile of PTSD can inform treatment strategies. Third, understanding the neuropsychological strengths and weaknesses of an individual can aid in vocational planning and modification of existing treatment plans (e.g., use of written versus oral instructions, note-taking during psychoeducational interventions).

In some respects, the clinical demands for conducting neuropsychological evaluation of PTSD have outpaced the knowledge provided by the empirical literature addressing neuropsychological functioning in PTSD. As such, translation of findings from the empirical literature should be implemented with the appropriate caution inherent to a developing knowledge base. Nonetheless, integration of findings from the neurobiological, electrophysiological, neuroimaging, and cognitive and clinical neuropsychology PTSD literatures provides a basis from which to apply general principles of clinical neuropsychological evaluation in the PTSD context.

Basic principles that can be applied to the clinical evaluation include thorough assessment of the trauma event, PTSD symptom profile, and comorbid disorders; broad survey of neuropsychological functional domains with objective, performance-based instruments to ascertain individual strengths and weaknesses and provide confirmatory and disconfirmatory evidence relative to the general pattern of dysfunction that would be expected to accompany PTSD; consideration of the severity of cognitive deficits; and, documentation of the onset and course of emotional and neuropsychological symptoms. The current body of empirical evidence suggests that when neuropsychological deficits accompany PTSD, they are most likely characterized by mild attentional and memory impairment and do not reflect basic language, visual recognition, or fine motor dysfunction.

Potentially fruitful future directions include the clinical application of comparative neuropsychological tasks, cognitive paradigms from the human experimental literature, and multifaceted test instruments to the assessment of executive functioning in PTSD. In addition, concurrent use of neuroimaging and electrophysiological methods with clinical neuropsychological evaluation procedures will potentially provide converging or discordant evidence of neural dysfunction. Finally, electrophysiological and cognitive information-processing paradigms that are difficult to distort volitionally may serve as useful ancillary methods of establishing PTSD diagnosis.

REFERENCES

American Psychiatric Association. (1994). *Diagnostic and statistical manual of mental disorders* (4th ed.). Washington, DC: Author.

Bauer, R. M., Grande, L., & Valenstein, E. (2003). Amnestic disorders. In K. M. Heilman & E. Valenstein (Eds.), *Clinical neuropsychology* (pp. 495–573). New York: Oxford University Press.

Bechara, A., Damasio, H., Tranel, D., & Anderson, S. (1994). Insensitivity to future consequences following damage to human prefrontal cortex. *Cognition, 50,* 7–15.

Beck, A. T., Epstein, N., Brown, G., & Steer, R. A. (1988). An inventory for measuring clinical anxiety: Psychometric properties. *Journal of Consulting and Clinical Psychology, 56,* 893–897.

Beck, A. T., Steer, R. A., & Brown, G. K. (1996). *Manual for the Beck Depression Inventory–II* . San Antonio, TX: Psychological Corporation.

Berg, E. A. (1948). A simple objective treatment for measuring flexibility in thinking. *Journal of General Psychology, 39,* 15–22.

Bianchini, K. J., Mathias, C. W., & Greve, K. W. (2001). Symptom validity testing: A critical review. *Clinical Neuropsychologist, 15,* 19–45.

Blanchard, E. B., & Buckley, T. C. (1999). Psychophysiological assessment of posttraumatic stress disorder. In P. A. Saigh & J. D. Bremner (Eds.), *Posttraumatic stress disorder: A comprehensive text* (pp. 248–266). Needham Heights, MA: Allyn & Bacon.

Brady, K. T., Killeen, T. K., Brewerton, T., & Lucerini, S. (2000). Comorbidity of psychiatric disorders and posttraumatic stress disorder. *Journal of Clinical Psychiatry, 61*(Suppl. 7), 22–32.

Brandes, D., Ben-Schachar, G., Gilboa, A., Bonne, O., Freedman, S., & Shalev, A. Y. (2002). PTSD symptoms and cognitive performance in recent trauma survivors. *Psychiatry Research, 110,* 231–238.

Bremner, J. D., Southwick, S., Brett, E., Fontana, A., Rosenheck, R., & Charney, D. S. (1992). Dissociation and posttraumatic stress disorder in Vietnam combat veterans. *American Journal of Psychiatry, 149,* 328–332.

Breslau, N. (2001). The epidemiology of posttraumatic stress disorder: What is the extent of the problem? *Journal of Clinical Psychiatry, 62*(Suppl. 17), 16–22.

Breslau, N., Roth, T., Burduvali, E., Kapke, A., Schultz, L., & Roehrs, T. (2004). Sleep in lifetime posttraumatic stress disorder: A community-based polysomnographic study. *Archives of General Psychiatry, 61,* 508–516.

Bury, A. S., & Bagby, R. M. (2002). The detection of feigned uncoached and coached posttraumatic stress disorder with the MMPI-2 in a sample of workplace accident victims. *Psychological Assessment, 14*, 472–484.

Bustamante, V., Mellman, T. A., David, D., & Fins, A. I. (2001). Cognitive functioning and the early development of PTSD. *Journal of Traumatic Stress, 14*, 791–797.

Centers for Disease Control Vietnam Experiences Study. (1988). Health status of Vietnam veterans I: Psychosocial characteristics. *Journal of the American Medical Association, 259*, 2701–2707.

Delis, D. C., Kaplan, E., & Kramer, J. H. (2003) *Delis-Kaplan Executive Function Scale.* San Antonio, TX: Psychological Corporation.

Delis, D. C., Kramer, J., Kaplan, E., & Ober, B. A. (1987). *The California Verbal Learning Test manual.* New York: Psychological Corporation.

DeViva, J. C., & Bloem, W. D. (2003). Symptom exaggeration and compensation seeking among combat veterans with posttraumatic stress disorder. *Journal of Traumatic Stress, 16*, 503–507.

Duke, L. M., Seltzer, B., Seltzer, J. E., & Vasterling, J. J. (2002). Cognitive components of deficit awareness in Alzheimer's disease. *Neuropsychology, 16*, 359–369.

Elhai, J. D., Gold, P. B., Frueh, B. C., & Gold, S. N. (2000). Cross-validation of the MMPI-2 in detecting malingered posttraumatic stress disorder. *Journal of Personality Assessment, 75*, 449–463.

Elhai, J. D., Naifeh, J. A., Zucker, I. S., Gold, S. N., Deitsch, S. E., & Frueh, B. C. (2004). Discriminating malingered from genuine civilian posttraumatic stress disorder: A validation of three MMPI-2 infrequency scales (F, Fp, and Fptsd). *Assessment, 11*, 139–144.

Everly, G. S., Jr., & Lating, J. M. (2004). Psychological and psychophysiological assessment of posttraumatic stress. In G. S. Everly, Jr. & J. M. Lating (Eds.), *Personality-guided therapy for posttraumatic stress disorder* (pp. 73–88). Washington, DC: American Psychological Association.

Falleti, M. G., Maruff, P., Collie, A., Darby, D. G., & McStephen, M. (2003). Qualitative similarities in cognitive impairment associated with 24 hours of sustained wakefulness and a blood alcohol concentration of 0.05%. *Journal of Sleep Research, 12*, 265–274.

Feeny, N. C., Zoellner, L. A., Fitzgibbons, L. A., & Foa, E. B. (2000). Exploring the roles of emotional numbing, depression, and dissociation in PTSD. *Journal of Traumatic Stress, 13*, 489–499.

First, M. B., Spitzer, R. L., Gibbon, M., & Williams, J. B. W. (1994). *Structured Clinical Interview for Axis I DSM-IV.* New York: New York State Psychiatric Institute.

Flack, W. F., Litz, B. T., Weathers, F. W., & Beaudreau, S. A. (2002). Assessment and diagnosis of PTSD in adults: A comprehensive psychological approach. In M. B. Williams & J. F. Sommer, Jr. (Eds.), *Simple and complex post-traumatic stress disorder: Strategies for comprehensive treatment in clinical practice* (pp. 9–22). Binghamton, NY: Haworth Maltreatment and Trauma Press/Haworth Press.

Forsyth, P. A., & Cascino, T. L. (1995). Neurological complications of chemotherapy. In R. G. Wiley (Ed.), *Neurological complications of cancer* (pp. 241–266). New York: Marcel Dekker.

Franklin, C. L., Repasky, S. A., Thompson, K. E., Shelton, S. A., & Uddo, M. (2003).

Assessment of response style in combat veterans seeking compensation for posttraumatic stress disorder. *Journal of Traumatic Stress, 16*, 251–255.

Franklin, C. L., Repasky, S. A., Thompson, K. E., Shelton, S. A., & Uddo, M. (2002). Differentiating overreporting and extreme distress: MMPI-2 use with compensation-seeking veterans with PTSD. *Journal of Personality Assessment, 79*, 274–285.

Freed, D. M. (2003). Considerations of neuropsychological factors in interviewing. In. M. Hersen (Ed.), *Diagnostic interviewing* (3rd ed., pp. 67–82). New York: Kluwer Academic/Plenum Publishers.

Gil, T., Calev, A., Greenberg, D., Kugelmass, S., & Lerer, B. (1990). Cognitive functioning in post-traumatic stress disorder. *Journal of Traumatic Stress, 3*, 29–45.

Gilbertson, M. W., Gurvits, T. V., Lasko, N. B., Orr, S. P., & Pitman, R. K. (2001). Multivariate assessment of explicit memory function in combat veterans with posttraumatic stress disorder. *Journal of Traumatic Stress, 14*, 413–432.

Gioia, G. A., & Isquith, P. K. (2004). Ecological assessment of executive function in traumatic brain injury. *Developmental Neuropsychology, 25*, 135–158.

Gold, P. B., & Frueh, B. C. (1999). Compensation-seeking and extreme exaggeration of psychopathology among combat veterans evaluated for posttraumatic stress disorder. *Journal of Nervous and Mental Disease, 187*, 680–684.

Goldstein, F. C., & Levin, H. S. (2001). Cognitive outcome after mild and moderate traumatic brain injury in older adults. *Journal of Clinical and Experimental Neuropsychology, 23*, 739–753.

Green, B. L., Grace, M. C., Lindy, J. D., Gleser, G. C., & Leonard, A. (1990). Risk factors for PTSD and other diagnoses in a general sample of Vietnam veterans. *American Journal of Psychiatry, 147*, 729–733.

Gurvits, T. V., Carson, M. A., Metzger, L., Croteau, H. B., Lasko, N. B., Orr, S. P., & Pitman, R. K. (2002). Absence of selected neurological soft signs in Vietnam nurse veterans with post-traumatic stress disorder. *Psychiatry Research, 110*, 81–85.

Gurvits, T. V., Gilbertson, M. W., Lasko, N. B., Tarhan, A. S., Simeon, D., Macklin, M. L., Orr, S. P., & Pitman, R. K. (2000). Neurologic soft signs in chronic posttraumatic stress disorder. *Archives of General Psychiatry, 57*, 181–186.

Gurvits, T. V., Lasko, N. B., Schacter, S. C., Kuhne, A. A., Orr, S. P., & Pitman, R. K. (1993). Neurological status of Vietnam veterans with chronic posttraumatic stress disorder. *Journal of Neuropsychiatry and Clinical Neurosciences, 5*, 183–188.

Hamilton, M. (1959). The assessment of anxiety states by rating. *British Journal of Medical Psychology, 32*, 50–55

Hart, R. P., Martelli, M. F., & Zasler, N. D. (2000). Chronic pain and neuropsychological functioning. *Neuropsychology Review, 10*, 131–149.

Harvey, A. G., Jones, C., & Schmidt, D. A. (2003). Sleep and posttraumatic stress disorder: A review. *Clinical Psychology Review, 23*, 377–407.

Heaton, K., Chelune, G. J., Talley, J. L., Kay, G. G., & Curtiss, G. (1993). *Wisconsin Card Sorting Test Manual-Revised and expanded* . Odessa, FL: Psychological Assessment Resources.

Hiscock, M., & Hiscock, C. K. (1989). Refining the forced choice method for the detection of malingering. *Journal of Consulting and Experimental Neuropsychology, 11*, 967–974.

Hood, B., & Bruck, D. (2002). A comparison of sleep deprivation and narcolepsy in terms of complex cognitive performance and subjective sleepiness. *Sleep Medicine, 3,* 259–266.

Hyer, L., Boudewyns, P., Harrison, W. R., O'Leary, W. C., Bruno, R. D., Saucer, R. T., & Blount, J. B. (1988). Vietnam veterans: Overreporting versus acceptable reporting of symptoms. *Journal of Personality Assessment, 52,* 475–486.

Jennings, M. T. (1995). Neurological complications of radiotherapy. In R. G. Wiley (Ed.), *Neurological complications of cancer* (pp. 219–240). New York: Marcel Dekker.

Kalska, H., Punamaeki, R. L., Maekinen-Pelli, T., & Saarinen, M. (1999). Memory and metamemory functioning among depressed patients. *Applied Neuropsychology, 6,* 96–107.

Kaszniak, A. W., & Zak, M. G. (1996). On the neuropsychology of metamemory: Contributions from the study of amnesia and dementia. *Learning and Individual Differences, 8,* 355–381.

Keane, T. M., Buckley, T. C., & Miller, M. W. (2003). Forensic psychological assessment in PTSD. In R. I. Simon (Ed.), *Posttraumatic stress disorder in litigation: Guidelines for forensic assessment* (2nd ed., pp. 119–140). Washington, DC: American Psychiatric Publishing.

Keane, T. M., Kaloupek, D. G., Blanchard, E. B., Hsieh, F. Y., Kolb, L. C., Orr, S. P., Thomas, R. G., & Lavori, P. W. (1998). Utility of psychophysiological measurement in the diagnosis of posttraumatic stress disorder: Results from a Department of Veterans Affairs Cooperative Study. *Journal of Consulting and Clinical Psychology, 66,* 914–923.

Keane, T. M., Weathers, F. W., & Foa, E. B. (2000). Diagnosis and assessment. In E. B. Foa, T. M. Keane, & M. J. Friedman (Eds.), *Effective treatments for PTSD: Practice guidelines from the International Society for Traumatic Stress Studies* (pp. 18–36). New York: Guilford Press.

Keime-Guibert, F., Napolitano, M., & Delattre, J. Y. (1998). Neurological complications of radiotherapy and chemotherapy. *Journal of Neurology, 245,* 695–708.

Kelly, D. A., & Coppel, D. B. (2001). Sleep disorders. In R. Tarter & M. Butters (Eds.), *Medical neuropsychology* (pp. 267–284). New York: Kluwer Academic.

Kessler, R. C., Sonnega, A., Bromet, E., Hughes, M., & Nelson, C. B. (1995). Posttraumatic stress disorder in the national comorbidity survey. *Archives of General Psychiatry, 52,* 1048–1060.

Klein, E., Caspi, Y., & Gil, S. (2003). The relation between memory of the traumatic event and PTSD: Evidence from studies of traumatic brain injury. *Canadian Journal of Psychiatry, 48,* 28–33.

Koenen, K. C., Driver, K. L., Oscar-Berman, M., Wolfe, J., Folsom, S., Huang, M. T., & Schlesinger, L. (2001). Measures of prefrontal system dysfunction in posttraumatic stress disorder. *Brain and Cognition, 45,* 64–78.

Koopman, C., Drescher, K., Bowles, S., Gusman, F., Blake, D., Dondershine, H., Chang, V., Butler, L., & Spiegel, D. (2001). Acute dissociative reactions in veterans with PTSD. *Journal of Trauma and Dissociation, 2,* 91–111.

Krakow, B., Germain, A., Warner, T. D., Schrader, R., Koss, M., Hollifield, M., Tandberg, D., Melendrez, D., & Johnston, L. (2001). The relationship of sleep quality and posttraumatic stress to potential sleep disorders in sexual assault survivors with nightmares, insomnia, and PTSD. *Journal of Traumatic Stress, 14,* 647–665.

Kulka, R. A., Schlenger, W. E., Fairbank, J. A., Hough, R. L., Jordan, B. K., Marmar, C. R., & Weiss, D. S. (1990). *Trauma and the Vietnam war generation: Report of findings from the National Vietnam Veterans Readjustment Study.* New York: Brunner/Mazel.

Larrabee, G. J. (1998). Somatic malingering on the MMPI and MMPI-2 in personal injury litigants. *The Clinical Neuropsychologist, 12,* 179–188.

Lee, H. J., Kim, L., & Suh, K. Y. (2003). Cognitive deterioration and changes of P300 during total sleep deprivation. *Psychiatry and Clinical Neurosciences, 57,* 490–496.

Levin, H., & Kraus, M. F. (1994). The frontal lobes and traumatic brain injury. *Journal of Neuropsychiatry and Clinical Neurosciences, 6,* 443–454.

Lezak, M. (1995). *Neuropsychological assessment* (3rd ed.). New York: Oxford University Press.

Loftus, E. F., & Burns, T. E. (1982). Mental shock can produce retrograde amnesia. *Memory and Cognition, 10,* 318–323.

Macklin, M. L., Metzger, L. J., Litz, B. T., McNally, R. J., Lasko, N. B., Orr, S. P., & Pitman, R. K. (1998). Lower precombat intelligence is a risk factor for posttraumatic stress disorder. *Journal of Consulting and Clinical Psychology, 66,* 323–326.

McCann, U. D., Penetar, D. M., Shaham, Y., Thorne, D. R., Gillin, J. C., Sing, H. C., Thomas, M. A., & Belenky, G. (1992). Sleep deprivation and impaired cognition: Possible role of brain catecholamines. *Biological Psychiatry, 31,* 1082–1097.

McDonald, B. C., Flashman, L. A., & Saykin, A. J. (2002). Executive dysfunction following traumatic brain injury. *Neurorehabilitation, 17,* 333–344.

McMillan, T. M., Williams, W. H., & Bryant, R. (2003). Posttraumatic stress disorder and traumatic brain injury: A review of causal mechanisms, assessment, and treatment. *Neuropsychological Rehabilitation, 13,* 149–164.

McNally, R. J. (2003). Progress and controversy in the study of posttraumatic stress disorder. *Annual Review of Psychology, 54,* 229–252.

Meier, S. (1994). *The chronic crisis in psychological measurement and assessment.* New York: Academic Press.

Mellman, T. A., Kulick-Bell, R., Ashlock, L. E., & Nolan, B. (1995). Sleep events among veterans with combat-related posttraumatic stress disorder. *American Journal of Psychiatry, 152,* 110–115.

Metzger, L. J., Paige, S. R., Carson, M. A., Lasko, N. B., Paulus, L. A., Pitman, R. K., & Orr, S. P. (2004). PTSD arousal and depression symptoms associated with increased right-sided parietal EEG asymmetry. *Journal of Abnormal Psychology, 113,* 324–329.

Mirsky, A. F., Anthony, B. J., Duncan, C. C., Ahearn, M. B., & Kellam, S. G. (1991). Analysis of the elements of attention: A neuropsychological approach. *Neuropsychology Review, 2,* 109–145.

Norris, F. H., & Riad, J. K. (1997). Standardized self-report measures of civilian trauma and posttraumatic stress disorder. In J. P. Wilson & T. M. Keane (Eds.), *Assessing psychological trauma and PTSD* (pp. 69–97). New York: Guilford Press.

Ohayon, N. M., & Shapiro, C. M. (2000). Sleep disturbance and psychiatric disorders associated with posttraumatic stress disorder in the general population. *Comprehensive Psychiatry, 41*, 469–478.

Oquendo, M. A., Friend, J. M., Halberstam, B., Brodsky, B. S., Burke, A. K., Grunebaum, M. F., Malone, K. M., & Mann, J. J. (2003). Association of comorbid posttraumatic stress disorder and major depression with greater risk for suicidal behavior. *American Journal of Psychiatry, 160*, 580–582.

Orr, S. P., & Roth, W. T. (2000). Psychophysiological assessment: Clinical applications for PTSD. *Journal of Affective Disorders, 61*, 225–240.

Pitman, R. K., Orr, S. P., Lowenhagen, M. J., Macklin, J. L., & Altman, B. (1991). Pre-Vietnam contents of posttraumatic disorder veterans' service medical and personnel records. *Comprehensive Psychiatry, 32*, 416–422.

Posner, M. I., Walker, J., Friedrich, F. J., & Rafal, R. D. (1984). Effects of parietal lobe injury on covert orienting of visual attention. *Journal of Neuroscience, 4*, 163–187.

Rey, A. (1964). *L'examen clinique en psychologie* [The clinical examination in psychology]. Paris: Presses Universitaires France.

Robbins, T. W. (1998). Arousal and attention: Psychopharmacological and neuropsychological studies in experimental animals. In R. Parasuraman (Ed.), *The attentive brain* (pp. 189–220). Cambridge, MA: MIT Press.

Roca, V., & Freeman, T. W. (2001). Complaints of impaired memory in veterans with PTSD. *American Journal of Psychiatry, 158*, 1738–1739.

Sbordone, R. J. (2000). The assessment interview in clinical neuropsychology. In. G. Groth-Marnat (Ed.), *Neuropsychological assessment in clinical practice: A guide to test interpretation and integration* (pp. 94–126). New York: Wiley.

Schnurr, P. P., & Green, B. L. (2004). *Trauma and health: Physical health consequences of exposure to extreme stress*. Washington, DC: American Psychological Association.

Schwarz, E. D., Kowalski, J. M., & McNally, R. J. (1993). Malignant memories: Posttraumatic changes in memory in adults after a school shooting. *Journal of Traumatic Stress, 6*, 545–553.

Selzer, M. L., Vinokur, A., & van Rooijen, L. A. (1975). A self-administered Short Michigan Alcoholism Screening Test (SMAST). *Journal of Studies on Alcohol Abuse, 36*, 117–126.

Shucard, J. L., Parrish, J., Shucard, D. W., McCabe, D. C., Benedict, R. H., & Ambrus, J. (2004). Working memory and processing speed deficits in systemic lupus erythematosus as measured by the paced auditory serial addition test. *Journal of the International Neuropsychological Society, 10*, 35–45.

Singareddy, R. K., & Balon, R. (2002). Sleep in posttraumatic stress disorder. *Annals of Clinical Psychiatry, 14*, 183–190.

Smith, V. L., Ellsworth, P. C., & Kassin, S. M. (1989). Eyewitness accuracy and confidence: Within- versus between-subjects correlations. *Journal of Applied Psychology, 74*, 356–359.

Sobell, L. C., & Sobell, M. B. (1996). *Alcohol Timeline Followback (TLFB) Users' Manual*. Toronto, Canada: Addiction Research Foundation.

Southwick, S. M., Morgan, A. C., Nicolaou, A. L., & Charney, D. S. (1997). Consistency of memory for combat-related traumatic events in veterans of Operation Desert Storm. *American Journal of Psychiatry, 154*, 173–177.

Spiegel, D., & Cardena, E. (1991). Disintegrated experience: The dissociative disorders revisited. *Abnormal Psychology, 100,* 366–378.

Spreen, O., & Strauss, E. (1998). *A compendium of neuropsychological tests: Administration, norms, and commentary* (2nd ed.). New York: Oxford University Press.

Sullivan, K., Krengel, M., Proctor, S. P., Devine, S., Heeren, T., & White, R. F. (2003). Cognitive functioning in treatment-seeking Gulf War veterans: Pyridostigmine bromide use and PTSD. *Journal of Psychopathology and Behavioral Assessment, 25,* 95–103.

Sutker, P. B., Uddo-Crane, M., & Allain, A. N. (1991). Clinical and research assessment of posttraumatic stress disorder: A conceptual overview. *Psychological Assessment, 3,* 520–530.

Szelenberger, W., & Niemcewicz, S. (2000). Severity of insomnia correlates with cognitive impairment. *Acta Neurobiologica, 60,* 373.

Tombaugh, T. N. (1996). *Test of Memory Malingering (TOMM).* New York: Multi-Health Systems.

Trahan, D. E., & Larrabee, G. J. (1988). *Continuous Visual Memory Test professional manual.* Odessa, FL: Psychological Assessment Resources.

Uddo, M., Allain, A. N., & Sutker, P. B. (1996). Assessment of posttraumatic stress disorder: A conceptual overview. In T. W. Miller (Ed.), *Theory and assessment of stressful life events* (pp. 181–207). Madison, CT: International University Press.

Uddo, M., Vasterling, J. J., Brailey, K., & Sutker, P. B. (1993). Memory and attention in combat-related post-traumatic stress disorder (PTSD). *Journal of Psychopathology and Behavioral Assessment, 15,* 43–52.

van Achterberg, M. E., Rohrbaugh, R. M., & Southwick, S. M. (2001). Emergence of PTSD in trauma survivors with dementia. *Journal of Clinical Psychiatry, 62,* 206–207.

Vasterling, J. J., Brailey, K., Constans, J. I., Borges, A., & Sutker, P. B. (1997). Assessment of intellectual resources in Gulf War veterans: Relationship to PTSD. *Assessment, 4,* 51–59.

Vasterling, J. J., Brailey, K., Constans, J. I., & Sutker, P. B. (1998). Attention and memory dysfunction in posttraumatic stress disorder. *Neuropsychology, 12,* 125–133.

Vasterling, J. J., Duke, L. M., Brailey, K., Constans, J. I., Allain, A. N., Jr., & Sutker, P. B. (2002). Attention, learning, and memory performances and intellectual resources in Vietnam veterans: PTSD and no disorder comparisons. *Neuropsychology, 16,* 5–14.

Vasterling, J. J., Duke, L. M., Tomlin, H., Lowery, N., & Kaplan, E. (2004). Global–local visual processing in posttraumatic stress disorder. *Journal of the International Neuropsychological Society, 10,* 709–718.

Walch, S. E., Ahles, T. A., & Saykin, A. J. (1998). Neuropsychological impact of cancer and cancer treatments. In J. C. Holland (Ed.), *Psycho-oncology* (pp. 500–508). New York: Oxford University Press.

Waldstein, S. R., Snow, J., Muldoon, M. F., & Katzel, L. I. (2001). Neuropsychological consequences of cardiovascular disease. In. R. E. Tarter & M. Butters (Eds.), *Medical neuropsychology* (2nd ed., pp. 51–83). New York: Kluwer Academic.

Warrington, E. K. (1984). *Recognition Memory Test*. Windsor, UK: NFER-Nelson.

Weathers, F. W., & Keane, T. M. (1999). Psychological assessment of traumatized adults. In P. A. Saigh & J. D. Bremner (Eds.), *Posttraumatic stress disorder: A comprehensive text* (pp. 219–247). Needham Heights, MA: Allyn & Bacon.

Weathers, F. W., Keane, T. M., King, L.A., & King, D.W. (1997). Psychometric theory in the development of posttraumatic stress disorder assessment tools. In J. P. Wilson & T. M. Keane (Eds.), *Assessing psychological trauma and PTSD* (pp. 98–135). New York: Guilford Press.

Wechsler, D. (1981). *Manual for the Wechsler Adult Intelligence Scale-Revised*. New York: Psychological Corporation.

Wechsler, D. (1997a). *Wechsler Adult Intelligence Scale-Third Edition*. San Antonio, TX: Psychological Corporation.

Wechsler, D. (1997b). *WAIS-III WMS-III technical manual*. San Antonio, TX: Psychological Corporation.

Wilson, B. A., Alderman, N., Burgess, P. W., Emslie, H., & Evans, J. J. (1996). *Behavioral assessment of the dysexecutive syndrome*. St. Edmunds, UK: Thames Valley Test Company.

White, R. F. (1992). Neuropsychological Interview. In R.F. White (Ed.), *Clinical syndromes in adult neuropsychology: The practitioner's handbook* (pp. 484–489). Amsterdam: Elsevier.

Zachary, R. A. (1986). *Shipley Institute of Living Scale: Revised manual*. Los Angeles: Western Psychological Services.

CHAPTER 12

Implications for Psychological Intervention

CHRIS R. BREWIN

PSYCHOLOGICAL TREATMENT OF PTSD

Posttraumatic stress disorder (PTSD) is a complex disorder involving a variety of quite distinct biological and psychological disturbances. Psychologically, changes can be observed in attention, memory, behavior, emotion, conscious appraisals, and sense of identity. It is important to note that it is not a disorder characterized exclusively, or even mainly, by fear. Although the emotions of fear, helplessness, and horror emphasized by DSM-IV are prominent, other emotions such as anger are extremely prevalent (Reynolds & Brewin, 1999). Guilt is frequently reported, and in some victim groups high levels of shame predict the course of the disorder (Andrews, Brewin, Rose, & Kirk, 2000). Critically, some of these emotions are not experienced during the trauma at all but only occur later. Thus, as many theorists have argued, there is a vital distinction between emotions that represent immediate wired-in responses to extreme threat and those that reflect a slower, higher-level cognitive appraisal of what is happening and why. These observations caution that models of PTSD based on the study of fear in animals, while of great interest, are unlikely on their own to provide a sufficiently comprehensive account of the disorder.

Similarly, two separate processes are involved in recovery from traumatic experiences (Brewin, 2003). One is bringing under control the vivid reexperiencing of the trauma through flashbacks and nightmares, a reaction that seems to be mainly reported in the context of extreme fear, helplessness, or horror. The second is the conscious reappraisal of the event and its impact. Corresponding to these two processes are contrasting types of therapy for PTSD. One type, which includes prolonged exposure, focuses primarily on the relief of flashbacks and nightmares whereas the other type, which includes cognitive therapy, places greater emphasis on issues of belief, interpretation, and identity. Both exposure and cognitive methods have been demonstrated to be clinically very effective although not all patients are able to tolerate them and not all patients become symptom-free as a result (Foa et al., 1999; Marks et al., 1998; Resick et al., 2002; Tarrier et al., 1999).

Why have two different kinds of treatment evolved? According to many theorists (e.g., Evans, 2003; Sloman, 1996) human reasoning is performed by two systems. One is associative and automatic, making use of basic principles such as the similarity between elements or the closeness of two elements in time. It searches for and bases conclusions on patterns and regularities between elements such as images and stereotypes. The second system is rule based and deliberate, and tries to describe the world in more conceptual terms by capturing a structure that is logical or causal. Exposure treatments, like extinction procedures in animal learning, appear to draw on associative reasoning in that they attempt to produce new patterns and regularities involving the same elements that were part of the traumatic experience. Although the steps demanded by the treatment are deliberate, the processes by which change occurs are automatic. This approach is particularly useful for altering reactions that arise from the original traumatic response. In contrast, cognitive methods involve the derivation of explicit rules that are then effortfully evaluated and modified verbally within therapy sessions. This approach is useful for altering reactions generated by higher-order cognitive appraisals.

During prolonged exposure (Foa & Rothbaum, 1998) patients typically close their eyes and are asked to relive the trauma as vividly as possible. This involves giving a very detailed narrative account of the trauma, reporting everything they recall seeing, hearing, touching, smelling, feeling, and thinking throughout the whole event. The reliving process often results in spontaneous flashbacks, providing additional detailed, image-based information to be incorporated into the narrative. The account may be tape recorded and the patient asked to listen to the tape every day until the next session. This provides an opportunity for further flashbacks and further elaborations of the narrative, as well as a gradual acclimatization to the most disturbing elements. The therapy requires that patients focus their attention on the traumatic material and do not distract themselves with other thoughts or activities or deliberately skip over uncomfortable moments.

Along with exposing themselves to the traumatic memory through thought, patients are encouraged to expose themselves to real-life situations linked to the trauma, such as the street in which they were attacked, the exact model and color of car that ran into them, or the hospital ward in which they nearly died. Again the aim is to provoke fear reactions and to extinguish them by staying in the same place, focusing on the trauma reminders, and waiting for the realization of safety to overcome the expectation of danger. This is a demanding therapy but if followed conscientiously usually leads to a rapid reduction in levels of fear and in the extent to which memories are relived in the present.

The primary focus of exposure therapy is the intense fear, helplessness, or horror experienced at the time of the trauma. In contrast, cognitive therapy addresses a variety of different emotions that may have been present during the trauma or may not have been experienced until later, when the person received additional information about what had happened and why. Whereas in prolonged exposure therapists have a clear-cut strategy but no direct control over associative changes within the memory system, the cognitive approach is in some ways more precisely targeted and involves a delicate dialogue between therapist and patient. The therapist's initial task is to find out as much as possible about how the trauma and the reactions that followed have been interpreted by the patient, and about the chains of reasoning that support these interpretations. In some cases this reasoning will be in the form of explicit rules or assumptions that the patient can articulate. For example, they may comment "It was my fault I was attacked because I knew this street was unsafe and I didn't look carefully enough before getting out of my car." At other times the reasoning may be associative, in the form of specific negative thoughts or images that come spontaneously to mind and influence the interpretive process. The basic premise of cognitive therapy is that emotions are more the product of beliefs and interpretations than of events themselves, and that changing beliefs is the most effective way to reduce unwanted emotion.

Cognitive therapy requires a high degree of respect for patients' beliefs and the ability to motivate them to explore the puzzling inconsistencies and the no-go areas of their inner world. As the founder of cognitive therapy for depression, Aaron Beck has insisted it is a collaborative enterprise designed to uncover mental patterns, assumptions, and secrets, not a tool for browbeating patients who appear to hold irrational beliefs. Even the most irrational thoughts generally have a logic that makes sense when it is related to a particular personal history. The skill of the therapist lies in uncovering the logic while simultaneously helping the patient to discover an alternative way of reasoning about the same events that makes equally good if not better sense.

In practice, cognitive therapy for PTSD usually contains some element of exposure (e.g., Ehlers et al., 2003; Resick & Schnicke, 1993). For example, Resick and Schnicke developed a version of cognitive therapy called cognitive processing therapy, specifically for rape victims. After an educational session, patients are asked to write about what it means to them that the event happened. This provides an early opportunity to identify negative beliefs and to explain the relationship between events, thoughts, and feelings. Patients then write a very detailed account of the event during which they are encouraged to relive their emotions in full, and reread it daily. They are then taught how to challenge their negative beliefs by asking themselves questions to do with how well their beliefs fit the facts and whether there are other beliefs that provide an equally good or better account of their reactions.

INSIGHTS FROM NEUROPSYCHOLOGY
AND COGNITIVE NEUROSCIENCE

Altering Old Memories or Creating New Memories?

The material reviewed in Chapters 3, 6, and 8 of this volume suggested that the extinction of fear memories, including those created by exposure to a trauma, does not come about through unlearning but through inhibition by new learning. This new learning consists of novel stimulus–stimulus and stimulus–response associations that link trauma reminders with alternative nonthreatening situations and nonfearful responses. Such associations may come about through repeatedly replaying the traumatic events or revisiting the trauma scene once the danger has passed, until negative responses are extinguished. They may develop because of the survivor's own spontaneous actions and mental processes or because of similar actions prompted by a therapist.

Specifically, it has been proposed that inhibitory projections from the prefrontal cortex to the amygdala enable these new associations to block inappropriate responses to no-longer-relevant trauma stimuli, while leaving the original learned associations intact (Brewin, 2001; Elzinga & Bremner, 2002; LeDoux, 1998; Rauch et al., 1998; see also Vasterling & Brailey, Chapter 8, this volume). This is an attractive approach because it is consistent with a great deal of evidence that fear responses can return even though they have been extinguished in the laboratory (Bouton & Swartzentruber, 1991; Jacobs & Nadel, 1985) or successfully treated with cognitive-behavioral therapy (Rachman, 1989). It is also supported by some evidence, reviewed in Shin, Rauch, and Pitman (Chapter 3, this volume), for reduced volume and hypoactivation of the prefrontal cortex in PTSD, and for an inverse relationship between levels of activation in the amygdala and prefrontal cortex.

Memory consolidation is dependent on a variety of mechanisms, including gene expression and protein synthesis, that operate during the hours and days following a learning episode. These mechanisms result in a labile memory sensitive to disruption being transformed into one that is robust and insensitive to disruption. Memory can be severely impaired by blocking protein synthesis during or immediately after learning. For example, consolidation of a learned tone–shock association can be blocked by infusing a protein synthesis inhibitor into the basolateral amygdala (Maren, Ferrario, Corcoran, Desmond, & Frey, 2003; Schafe & LeDoux, 2000). Whereas cortical structures do not appear essential for learning simple CS–UCS associations, the new learning required by extinction is believed to involve neuronal changes in the hippocampus and in the prefrontal cortex. Extinction is prevented from taking place by lesions to the prefrontal cortex (LeDoux, 1998), by blocking protein synthesis in the medial prefrontal cortex (Santini, Ge, Ren, de Ortiz, & Quirk, 2004) or hippocampus (Fischer, Sananbenesi, Schrick, Spiess, & Radulovic, 2004), or by blocking cytoskeletal rearrangement in the hippocampus (Fischer et al., 2004).

An alternative to the view that extinction involves new learning is provided by reconsolidation theory (e.g., Nader, 2003). According to this, memory consolidation is not permanent; rather, memories move in and out of active and inactive states. When a memory (for example of a tone–shock association) is retrieved, it becomes labile again and needs to be reconsolidated. Interfering with this process, it has been suggested, can produce the same dramatic memory impairment as blocking the original consolidation. Numerous studies have now demonstrated that if a previous memory of a tone–shock association is reactivated (by briefly representing the tone or the shock), and this is followed by giving a protein synthesis inhibitor, then the original memory no longer appears to exert any control over behavior (e.g., Debiec, LeDoux, & Nader, 2002). On the basis of such results it has been suggested that even well-consolidated memories are not permanent, that consolidation and reconsolidation are qualitatively similar processes that can be blocked at any stage, and that original memories of fearful experiences can be destabilized, altered, and even permanently erased.

Recent evidence has indicated that in fact the cellular basis of consolidation and reconsolidation is somewhat different (Lee, Everitt, & Thomas, 2004). Moreover, blocking reconsolidation with protein synthesis inhibitors does not invariably result in the abolition of the original learning. The more time that is allowed to elapse between the original training and memory reactivation, the less likely that blocking reconsolidation will have any effect (Milekic & Alberini, 2002). Initial impairments can also be reversed, either when the animal is prompted with a reminder (Fischer et al., 2004), or as a result of spontaneous recovery with time (Lattal & Abel, 2004). Thus reconsolidation appears to be a much more limited process than was first thought, and there are no grounds at present for thinking that original fear memories can be readily impaired or erased.

These studies of animal conditioning have important implications for psychotherapists. The most influential and widely accepted accounts of treatment for PTSD have proposed that therapy is concerned with "modifying" trauma memories. For example, as noted above, Foa and Rothbaum (1998) regard the memories of PTSD patients as containing faulty information. Like the reconsolidation theorists, they suggest that trauma memories should be reactivated and changed, not by blocking protein synthesis but by incorporating into them more accurate information. Ehlers and Clark (2000) and Conway and Pleydell-Pearce (2000) have suggested that trauma memories are vulnerable to being constantly triggered and brought into awareness because they are disorganized and fragmented. One of the functions of therapy, they propose, is to make them coherent and better structured, reducing the risk of unwanted intrusions.

All these approaches reflect the essentially rationalist assumptions of classical cognitive-behavioral therapy, in which patients are seen as possessing inaccurate or otherwise faulty memories or beliefs that have to be corrected. The basic concept of memory transformation is, however, shared by alternative therapeutic approaches that are more constructivist than rationalist. For example, it has often been suggested that the function of eliciting a detailed verbal or written account of a horrific experience is to assist the person in turning "traumatic memories" into "narrative memories." In this formulation, "traumatic memories" are seen as fixed and inflexible representations consisting largely of raw sensory data that need to be interpreted and anchored within a personal narrative framework that provides them with meaning. This approach is not rationalist in that the new narrative does not need to be more "correct" but simply to provide a coherent and acceptable account in the individual's own terms.

If original memories cannot be corrected, updated, or reorganized, however, therapists must be doing something different, such as the construction and consolidation of alternative memories. This possibility was considered by Brewin, Dalgleish, and Joseph (1996) and Foa and McNally (1996). More recently, Brewin (2003) elaborated the principles whereby newly constructed memories compete with the original memory for control of behavior, and these are discussed below.

Verbal and Nonverbal Processing in PTSD

Constans (Chapter 5, this volume) provided evidence that certain stimuli, such as threatening faces, are preferentially processed at a preattentive level by individuals with PTSD. In contrast, there was little indication that threatening words are preferentially processed at a preattentive level. If replicated, this suggests that the unconscious processes underlying heightened vigilance are primarily concerned with scanning and classifying perceptual features of the environment, and supports a functional separation between nonverbal and verbal processing in PTSD.

Further evidence for this functional separation was presented in Vasterling and Brailey (Chapter 8, this volume). Whereas there are few differences in visuospatial performance, some neuropsychological studies have found that PTSD patients are more likely to show deficits on verbal tasks than on visuospatial tasks. Interestingly, studies with normal participants also indicate that inducing withdrawal states by showing an aversive film improves spatial performance on a task thought to measure working memory while simultaneously impairing performance on a verbal version of the same task (Gray, 2001). Consistent with this, the few studies that have reported differences in lateralization of neural dysfunction in PTSD are suggestive of hypoactivation of the left hemisphere and corresponding advantages on right hemisphere tasks.

Similarly, Chemtob and Hamada (1984) proposed that individuals with a cerebral organization favoring right-hemisphere processing would be at greater risk for PTSD. This group was defined for research purposes as consisting of right-handers with evidence of reduced cerebral lateralization for language, as revealed by mixed lateral preference and familial left-handedness. Consistent with this hypothesis, there is evidence that right-handers who prefer to use their left hand, foot, or eye for some activities, or have a left-handed parent, are overrepresented among individuals with PTSD (Chemtob & Taylor, 2003; Spivak, Segal, Mester, & Weizman, 1998).

There are several reasons why verbal memory deficits are of particular interest in PTSD. As proposed by Vasterling and Brailey (Chapter 8, this volume), intact prefrontal skills such as the ability to hold and manipulate information in working memory are believed to be critical in inhibiting unwanted distraction from extraneous information. There is a clear parallel here with the studies of extinction in animals, and with neuropsychological theories of PTSD in which memory representations located in the prefrontal cortex inhibit lower-level representations created at the time of the trauma (Brewin, 2003). The implication is that verbal processing is one specific type of prefrontal activity that shares with others an inhibitory capability. Vasterling, Brailey, Constans, and Sutker (1998) found that the failure to inhibit irrelevant information on neutral tasks was related to the amount of reexperiencing of trauma-related symptoms, supporting the idea that both reflect a deficit in inhibition.

Wild, Baxendale, Scragg, and Gur (2002) investigated the relationship between verbal memory deficits and outcome in patients receiving treatment for PTSD. Various aspects of cognitive performance were measured at the beginning of therapy but it was verbal memory impairment, independent of overall intelligence, that was the only measure to predict a poorer outcome. Relatedly, two nonclinical studies have investigated the relationship between verbal working memory capacity and the ability to suppress unwanted thoughts. In both studies participants with lesser working memory capacity had more intrusions, whether of arbitrary thoughts of a white bear (Brewin & Beaton, 2002) or of personally relevant obsessional thoughts (Brewin & Smart, 2005).

Finally, verbal and nonverbal activity appear to be differentially related to the development of intrusive memories. Participants who watched a trauma film while carrying out a concurrent visuospatial task had a reduced number of intrusions, whereas a concurrent verbal task increased the probability of intrusions (Holmes, Brewin, & Hennessy, 2004). The authors interpreted this to mean that under normal circumstances intrusive visual memories are mediated by visuospatial processes, but that if a concurrent task competed for these resources at encoding, fewer intrusions would result. Similarly, they proposed that intrusions are normally suppressed by appropriately targeted verbal processing, but that if a concurrent task competed for these resources at encoding, more intrusions would result. Deficits in verbal abilities, whether inherited or a response to life stresses, might therefore be expected to increase the risk of PTSD in individuals exposed to trauma.

Thus, numerous findings using very different concepts and methods appear to converge on the conclusion that in PTSD there is likely to be a sensitization of and increased efficiency in the perceptual processing of trauma-related stimuli, coupled with a diminution of verbal memory-related abilities. It is too early to say whether this pattern is causally related to the likelihood of developing PTSD, but it does underscore the possible significance of an increased functional separation between verbal and nonverbal processing in this disorder. This separation may be reflected in the diverse nature of PTSD symptoms, some of which (flashbacks) are overwhelmingly perceptual in nature whereas others (negative beliefs and appraisals, concentration problems) are primarily verbal. But there are grounds for believing it may also be reflected much more widely in the risk of developing PTSD, in the way the disorder develops, and in the response to treatment.

Fast and Slow Learning Systems

Other research in cognitive neuroscience appears highly relevant to PTSD even in the absence of studies of traumatized populations. McClelland, McNaughton, and O'Reilly (1995) proposed that the hippocampus is a rapid learning system that can respond to momentarily changing circumstances, distinct from a neocortical memory system that provides for longer-term storage and that learns slowly about the underlying structure present in ensembles of similar experiences. The representation of an experience in the neocortical system depends on a widely distributed pattern of neural activity. The repeated reinstatement of hippocampally based memories— for example, through bringing them to mind and rehearsing them over and over again—permits the neocortex to learn by making a series of small adjustments to the connections between neurons.

In accounting for the existence of these different types of memory system, McClelland et al. (1995) pointed out that the neocortical system, although efficient at gradually extracting underlying rules and consistencies, is unable to respond rapidly to new information that contradicts what has already been learned. Such information tends to produce "catastrophic interference" (McCloskey & Cohen, 1989), with the network being unable to integrate the new data and responding by ignoring relevant past experiences. As an example of this problem, McClelland describes trying to teach a computer simulation of this neocortical memory system about the properties of birds. The network performs well when it is given lots of examples of birds, and is told that all of them can fly. However, when it is presented with a penguin, a bird that cannot fly, the network experiences catastrophic interference and responds either by classifying the penguin as a nonbird or by concluding that birds cannot fly after all.

The existence of a hippocampal system, however, may permit the rapid formation of representations of the new information (the penguin) in a way that avoids interference with the knowledge already available in the neocortical system (all birds can fly). McClelland et al. propose that the most efficient way of allowing the neocortical system to integrate the new information is via a process they call "interleaved learning," in which the system is gradually exposed to the new information interleaved with old examples from the same domain. In the case of the penguin, this would involve presenting the memory system with examples of birds that can fly interleaved with examples of birds that cannot fly (like the ostrich). This process enables the network to be slowly reorganized so that eventually it can successfully classify both eagles and ostriches as birds.

This description of "catastrophic interference" is clearly reminiscent of clinical accounts of how trauma overturns long-held assumptions and is hard to integrate with previous knowledge. In the process known as "overassimilation" (Resick & Schnicke, 1993) some traumatized people attempt to deny the reality of the event and turn it into a nontrauma, equivalent to trying to turn the penguin into a nonbird. In the process Resick and Schnicke term "overaccommodation," people let the fact of the trauma overturn everything they previously assumed to be true, equivalent to concluding that birds cannot fly. Equally strikingly, the procedures that therapists have traditionally used to help people adjust to trauma and other shocking experiences (sometimes called "working through" or "emotional processing") tend to involve the repeated appraisal and reappraisal of the event alongside preexisting expectations, plans, and goals.

"Interleaved learning" is an interesting way of conceptualizing the repeated verbal processing of the trauma and its implications. This process of repeated information review and comparison between pre- and posttrauma states may be impeded by negative emotions or "stuck points," resulting in avoidance or in the rehearsal of partial and/or distorted versions of the trauma. These overassimilated trauma memories require identification, challenge, and modification (Resick & Schnicke, 1993). Otherwise the person will have alternative, competing representations, some containing and some omitting important information about the event. As noted by McClelland et al. (1995), such knowledge systems are inherently unstable. Inputs such as unexpected trauma reminders may cause a switch in the version currently in consciousness, accompanied by strong emotional reactions.

IMPLICATIONS FOR UNDERSTANDING POSTTRAUMA REACTIONS

What are the implications of the insights provided by neuroscience for understanding the normal course of posttrauma reactions and the patterns that result in PTSD? As noted elsewhere in this volume, we are not currently able to draw conclusions about the causal role of the patterns of neuropsychological performance or brain responses associated with PTSD. These may represent preexisting risk factors for disorder, abnormal reactions to the traumatic event, or reactions to specific combinations of life circumstances and patterns of coping (such as avoidance of specific mental contents). It is important to note that many of the neural changes brought about by exposure to extreme stress need not be permanent. For example, many of the hippocampal changes such as reduced synaptic plasticity, retraction of dendritic processes, reduction in volume, and inhibition of neurogenesis, are potentially reversible (Alderson & Novack, 2002; Sapolsky, 2003).

Moreover, reductions in verbal memory or working memory capacity are not necessarily best explained by changes in neural functioning brought about specifically by trauma. Similar memory problems are associated with ordinary life stresses as well as traumatic events, and can be reversed by interventions such as expressive writing (Klein & Boals, 2001a, 2001b). It is quite possible that neuropsychological deficits are secondary to reductions in processing capacity brought about by effortful avoidance of specific thoughts and images. Nevertheless, neuropsychological deficits of whatever origin may affect the course of the disorder and response to treatment.

The evidence for a separation between verbal and nonverbal or image-based processing is consistent with the view that therapy for PTSD consists of two distinct aspects, one concerned with the reduction of flashbacks, nightmares, and conditioned responses, and one concerned with repair of the sense of self and associated negative beliefs (Brewin et al., 1996; Ehlers & Clark, 2000; van der Kolk, McFarlane, & van der Hart, 1996). The implications of having separate verbal and nonverbal processing and memory systems are central aspects of dual-representation theory (Brewin et al., 1996), according to which flashbacks and nightmares involve the activation of traces of the traumatic event recorded in the situationally accessible memory (SAM) system. This is a largely image-based system which encodes unattended sensory information but is unable to encode contextual detail including whether events belong to the present or the past. Immediately postincident, far more detail, particularly about sights, sounds, smells, movement, and so on, is encoded in the SAM system than in the verbally accessible memory (VAM) system which has recorded the corresponding conscious experience of the trauma. Information in the VAM system, unlike in the SAM system, can be retrieved at will, can be described in words, and is fully contextualized within the person's life history.

The most recent version of the theory (Brewin, 2001, 2003) proposes that when the trauma survivor deliberately maintains attention on the content of the flashbacks, and no longer tries to suppress them, information that was only present in the SAM system becomes reencoded into the VAM system, at which point the memories are assigned a spatial and temporal context. The process has to be repeated numerous times because there may be a lot of extra information in the SAM system that has to be transferred to the VAM system. Eventually, provided the person is now safe, detailed memories in the SAM system that signaled the continuing presence of danger are matched by detailed memories in the VAM system that locate the danger in the past. When the person encounters trauma reminders these VAM memories are accessed, inhibiting inappropriate amygdala activation and preventing the return of fear.

Unlike most other contemporary explanations of PTSD, dual-representation theory explicitly maintains that the original trauma memories are not altered in any way but remain intact and may be vividly reexperienced again in the future if the person unexpectedly comes across very detailed and specific reminders of the trauma. Rather, recovery is seen in terms of creating new trauma memories in the VAM system that are made more permanent and more easily accessible by repeatedly going over them. This process produces competing memories of the trauma, an original one associated with extreme fear, helplessness, or horror, and more recent ones in which the trauma is recalled in a place of safety as something that belongs to the past. So long as it is these new memories that are accessed when the person comes across reminders of the trauma, the victim will not feel in danger.

In addition to dealing with flashbacks, a separate task in the aftermath of trauma is to evaluate the implications of what has happened. The information provided by the trauma may initially produce catastrophic interference with existing knowledge about the self and its relation to the world. Integrating the new information will be slow and gradual in comparison to the rapid realization of the occurrence of the traumatic event. This "working through" or "emotional processing" will depend on the rehearsal of interleaved pre- and posttrauma memories, repeatedly comparing the beliefs, plans, and goals that used to exist with those that have now been forced upon the reluctant trauma victim. The repeated reinstatement of these contrasting hippocampally based memories will permit more complex neocortical knowledge structures to be gradually adjusted so that old and new data are combined together in a more coherent way. This is essentially a process of construction and the need felt by many survivors to talk over and over again about their trauma may reflect the ongoing work of putting together a version of events that is coherent and makes sense in all its details.

The proposed existence of fast and slow memory systems has the potential to explain several interesting aspects of the response to trauma. The rapid formation of limited memories in the hippocampal system allows some acknowledgment of the event, but an absence of integration with knowledge already available in the neocortical system may contribute to a sense of unreality surrounding the event. Here "unreality" reflects the comparative lack of neuronal connections between the initial hippocampal memory and other neocortical memory structures that are known to be closely related conceptually. Using the framework of fast and slow memory systems, "denial" may be construed as the refusal to consciously dwell on the traumatic experience and to initiate the process of interleaved learning. The existence of unchanged neocortical knowledge structures may be why certain people who have been traumatized describe being able to "live in the past" and to pretend to themselves that the event never really happened. Their unwillingness or inability to update their memory systems may reflect the feeling that it is simply too painful to acknowledge the reality of their loss.

How is it that certain people can block what Horowitz (1976) suggested was an innate impulse toward resolving this kind of discrepancy? Using Resick and Schnicke's (1993) concept of overassimilation, in which the reality of what happened is distorted, the discrepancy with previous beliefs and goals can be made to go away. I recently elaborated on this idea (Brewin, 2001) by proposing that what people have to do is to actively construct and rehearse a distorted version of the event from which awkward elements have been removed. Rehearsing this version often enough will lead to its becoming more accessible than the original memory which still contains the unwanted facts.

This strategy will only work if the person can limit or eradicate their exposure to trauma reminders that have more in common with the original memory and that will, if unexpectedly encountered, cause it to spontaneously come to mind. In practice someone can limit their exposure to trauma reminders in many ways, by avoiding anything to do with the incident, not talking about it, switching off certain television programs, moving to a new house, and changing their job or their friends. All these are things that trauma survivors frequently do. But if they are unexpectedly confronted with additional trauma reminders, the original trauma memory is likely to be automatically accessed in the form of flashbacks and the body will once again sense itself to be in immediate danger. In this form of interrupted recovery both the process of transferring information from an image-based to a verbally based memory, and the process of allowing hippocampal and neocortical representations to interact and gradually change, are prematurely blocked or inhibited.

Another form of interrupted recovery occurs when the survivor is unable to prevent trauma reminders from constantly activating negative images and thoughts and is engaged in an exhausting battle to stop them entering consciousness. This is the situation of most people presenting with active PTSD. The survivor is likely to label a wide variety of innocuous situations as potentially threatening, unpredictable, or unfair, to label themselves as weak, bad, or inadequate, or to label any positive goals as irrelevant or unattainable. This form of catastrophic interference has the effect of vastly increasing the number of cues that will potentially act as trauma reminders, thereby inducing a constant sense of current threat, inadequacy, or hopelessness.

IMPLICATIONS FOR PSYCHOLOGICAL TREATMENT

As we have noted, the ease with which fear responses can be reinstated following extinction in animals or following successful therapy in patients provides a strong hint that fear memories encoded in an image-based memory system remain intact and are not directly modified by psychological therapy. From the perspective of dual-representation theory, exposure treatment is a very good way of helping to construct detailed verbal memories which can then be used to exert inhibitory control over involuntary sensory and perceptual memories associated with amygdala activation. Brewin (2001) argued that what suppresses flashbacks is the reencoding of critical retrieval cues that were previously only encoded as images. These cues must be reencoded in a form that enables them to be deliberately recalled, and they must be associated with a past temporal context and a sense of current safety. That is, the cues must be identified as belonging to a specific past event which does not now constitute an ongoing threat. The value of adding real-life to imaginal exposure is that it provides an opportunity to reencode additional retrieval cues that might not spontaneously come to mind.

Consistent with therapists who emphasize a graduated approach to trauma recall, particularly when it has occurred early in life (e.g., Herman, 1992), dual-representation theory suggests that arousal levels must be carefully managed during this process. If arousal is too low, this may mean that traumatic images are not being accessed. If arousal becomes too high and the person starts to dissociate, becoming overabsorbed in the traumatic memory at the expense of contact with their immediate surroundings, frontal and hippocampal activity will again become impaired and the person will reexperience the trauma without transferring information from image-based to verbal memory. With complex or long-lasting traumas it is likely that repeated episodes of recall will be necessary, with the process being terminated each time the person dissociates to the extent that he or she is no longer able to reflect consciously on the material coming to mind.

In order to complete information transfer it may be necessary to divide the trauma episode or episodes into smaller units, and to construct a hierarchy from less distressing to more distressing moments. Other useful techniques may include having the person perform a visuospatial task such as knitting, model-building, or carrying out eye movements while recalling their trauma. These tasks should theoretically lessen absorption by competing for resources in the image-based memory system. There is also evidence that typing the trauma narrative on a typewriter or word processor may reduce levels of arousal compared to writing longhand (Brewin & Lennard, 1999), perhaps because typing is more effortful and once again limits absorption in the trauma memory. If information transfer is being implemented successfully, there should be a steady increase in the amount of the trauma narrative that the person is able to retrieve and reflect upon before beginning to dissociate.

Although effortful processing has the advantage of limiting absorption, the neuropsychological evidence of reduced verbal and working memory resources must also be borne in mind. The ability to hold traumatic images in mind and focus attention upon them is also effortful and is likely to be reduced in patients with PTSD. This is also consistent with the idea of a graduated approach to trauma recall if sufficiently detailed processing is to be successfully achieved. Limited working memory resources point furthermore to the need to provide patients with reminders of the material covered in therapy sessions and of the content of any homework. In prolonged exposure these reminders typically take the form of providing patients with an audiotape of the session to play at home.

Closer study of people reliving traumatic events has identified that most have a small number of "hotspots," often quite brief moments when emotions are exceptionally intense (Ehlers & Clark, 2000; Richards & Lovell, 1999), and it has been proposed that these hotspots correspond to the content of the flashbacks that people with PTSD experience (Grey, Young, & Holmes, 2002). Ehlers and Clark suggested that these moments might be associated with important meanings and that exposure treatment could be more efficient if it focused specifically on hotspots rather than the entire event. Although these moments usually involve intense fear, other emotions such as anger and shame do sometimes figure in them, particularly when the trauma has been prolonged (Grey, Holmes, & Brewin, 2001). From the perspective of dual-representation theory, hotspots may correspond to moments when there was maximal functional separation between visuospatial and verbal processing, leading to a large discrepancy between the contents of the respective memory systems. In other words, these are the moments when there are many potential retrieval cues that need reencoding into verbal memory if they are not to trigger flashbacks.

As survivors recover, trauma reminders they come across will have the potential to trigger both new verbal memories in the VAM system and the older image-based memories created at the time of the trauma. These two types of memory will compete to determine which is retrieved and whether or not the body's alarm systems will be reactivated. To begin with, the older memories may enjoy a retrieval advantage as they have already been spontaneously retrieved many times in the weeks and months following the trauma. The capacity to prevent the amygdala from initiating alarm reactions should be improved by incorporating into the new verbal memories features which will make them more likely to be retrieved than the old sensory and perceptual trauma memories. Theoretically, such an advantage might be gained from making the new memories highly distinctive.

It has long been known that the encoding of unusual or distinctive features makes retrieval more likely if some of those features are available when the time comes to recall what has been learned. For example, in trying to learn a word paired with train (such as train–cloud) it is probably easier to remember cloud if you form a bizarre image of a train flying through the air above the clouds. In other words, the memory has become highly discriminable (Eysenck, 1979; Lockhart, Craik, & Jacoby, 1976). More recent evidence goes further in showing that the encoding of unique features with the target memory improves retrieval even when these features are not available at recall. Even general reminders or cues can access these distinctive encodings (Hunt & McDaniel, 1993; Hunt & Smith, 1996). Extrapolating to a trauma context, this would suggest that the more distinctive a new memory, the more likely any trauma reminder would be to access it.

Interestingly, there are a number of therapeutic procedures that may be effective in incorporating distinctive attributes into verbal representations of trauma. Eye movement desensitization and reprocessing (EMDR) is a treatment for PTSD that has been reported to yield similar benefits to behavior therapy but in a significantly shorter time or with significantly less homework for the patient (Van Etten & Taylor, 1998). The core of the method involves three simultaneous elements: visualizing the worst moments of the trauma, holding in mind a current negative thought concerning the event, and following with their eyes the therapist's fingers as they are moved back and forth in front of the patient's face. This last element may be replaced by looking alternately at lights flashing on the left and right or attending to the therapist tapping alternately on each of the patient's hands (Shapiro, 1995). Patients attempt to distance themselves from the traumatic images, allow new thoughts, images, and associations to come to mind, and report on their mental content and level of distress at regular intervals. There is also provision for some cognitive intervention, although not in as structured a way as in cognitive therapy.

The real-time stimulus provided by the therapist's actions, which impinge directly on the person's senses as they are attending to the traumatic image, might have the effect of encoding a very distinctive set of features with the new verbal memory of the trauma. After all, it will almost certainly be the first time the person has ever tried to think about something important while following someone else's hand moving backwards and forwards just in front of their eyes. Trauma reminders would then tend to lead to the rapid reinstatement of this memory, created in a safe context, in preference to older image-based memories, thereby producing a reduction in fear.

Other forms of therapy involving the reconstruction of traumatic events in the imagination have also obtained encouraging results (Hackmann, 1998; Layden, Newman, Freeman, & Morse, 1993; Smucker, Dancu, Foa, & Niederee, 1995). For example, survivors sexually abused as children may replay traumatic moments and imagine their adult self intervening to comfort the child and prevent the occurrence of harmful and frightening acts. Most kinds of trauma-related images can similarly be manipulated in the imagination to produce a different or more reassuring outcome. Once again, these techniques reportedly bring about a relatively rapid reduction in anxiety, without requiring a repetitive and lengthy reworking of the trauma narrative. What is striking is that the new images are not more "realistic" or "believable" in the sense of being consistent with the facts. To the contrary, they are often physically impossible and at all times known to be wholly false. However, in encoding highly distinctive and sometimes bizarre attributes paired with the original trauma images, imaginal reconstruction is consistent with the principle of trying to confer a retrieval advantage onto consciously accessible memories in a separate verbal system.

Ehlers and Clark (2000) recently proposed another method for enhancing the effectiveness of cognitive restructuring which involved incorporating the more adaptive cognitions into a reliving of the traumatic event. This has been related to the proposal that there are separate memory systems by Grey, Young, and Holmes (2002) who suggested that trying to verbally restructure people's beliefs as part of standard cognitive therapy may fail to access important image-based memories. As a result the person might end up agreeing with the therapist's logic but failing to feel any different. Their intellectual beliefs or "cold" cognitions might have changed, but not their emotional beliefs or "hot" cognitions. Like Ehlers and Clark, Grey et al. proposed that cognitive restructuring should first be carried out in the normal way but then repeated within the context of a reliving session in which strong feelings and vivid images that are not verbally accessible are activated. They give a number of interesting case examples illustrating this method and its potential advantages over standard cognitive therapy.

CONCLUSIONS

Neuropsychological studies of PTSD are suggestive of a functional separation between verbal and nonverbal processing, with deficits in verbal memory and left-hemisphere hypoactivation contrasting with intact or enhanced visuospatial functioning and advantages on right-hemisphere tasks. Although this picture appears to fit well with the symptoms exhibited by PTSD patients, and with the creation of intrusive memories in nonclinical participants, it will be important to establish whether this pattern is specific to PTSD or simply replicates general findings with withdrawal or aversive states (Davidson, Jackson, & Kalin, 2000). Whatever turns out to be the case, it is likely that these findings will prove to have a general relevance for the analysis of therapeutic tasks and the design of interventions.

At present it is unclear whether the neuropsychological deficits should be regarded as causally implicated in producing or contributing to PTSD symptoms, or as secondary effects of neurobiological alterations and/or effortful attempts to manage adverse life changes or distressing intrusive and arousal symptoms. Whatever their causal status, however, they are likely to be significant in reducing the resources available to PTSD patients to cope with the demands of everyday life and, more specifically, of psychological therapy. Given the initial evidence of the link between these deficits and therapy outcome, there is a clear implication that these difficulties need to be taken into consideration, for example by reducing wherever possible demands on memory and demands for sustained mental processing.

Cognitive science has yielded a number of other important insights about the memory systems that are likely to be relevant to the processing of traumatic events. Whereas some of these are specifically relevant to fear (for example, the role of the prefrontal cortex in inhibiting learned associations), others are more general (the distinction between fast and slow memory systems). Although studies of the neurophysiology and neuroanatomy of fear have been enormously helpful in clarifying some aspects of treatment, it is important to remember that PTSD is a disorder that involves a wide range of emotions and engages in a fundamental way with the sense of self. These clinical insights are likely to be valuable in informing neuropsychological and neuroimaging studies, and helping the field to resolve current inconsistencies in findings concerning key structures such as the amygdala, hippocampus, and prefrontal cortex.

REFERENCES

Alderson, A. L., & Novack, T. A. (2002). Neurophysiological and clinical aspects of glucocorticoids and memory: A review. *Journal of Clinical and Experimental Neurophysiology, 24*, 335–355.

Andrews, B., Brewin, C. R., Rose, S., & Kirk, M. (2000). Predicting PTSD symptoms in victims of violent crime: The role of shame, anger, and childhood abuse. *Journal of Abnormal Psychology, 109*, 69–73.

Bouton, M. E., & Swartzentruber, D. (1991). Sources of relapse after extinction in Pavlovian and instrumental learning. *Clinical Psychology Review, 11*, 123–140.

Brewin, C. R. (2001). A cognitive neuroscience account of posttraumatic stress disorder and its treatment. *Behaviour Research and Therapy, 39*, 373–393.

Brewin, C. R. (2003). *Posttraumatic stress disorder: Malady or myth?* New Haven: Yale University Press.

Brewin, C. R., & Beaton, A. (2002). Thought suppression, intelligence, and working memory capacity. *Behaviour Research and Therapy, 40*, 923–930.

Brewin, C. R., Dalgleish, T., & Joseph, S. (1996). A dual representation theory of post-traumatic stress disorder. *Psychological Review, 103*, 670–686.

Brewin, C. R., & Lennard, H. (1999). Effects of mode of writing on emotional narratives. *Journal of Traumatic Stress, 12*, 355–361.

Brewin, C. R., & Smart, L. (2005). Working memory capacity and suppression of obsessional thoughts. *Journal of Behavior Therapy and Experimental Psychiatry, 36*, 61–68.

Chemtob, C. H., & Hamada, R. H. (1984). *Toward a neuropsychological model of posttraumatic stress disorder.* Paper presented at the American Psychiatric Association Region 7 Conference, Maui, HI.

Chemtob, C. H., & Taylor, K. B. (2003). Mixed lateral preference and parental left-handedness: Possible markers of risk for PTSD. *Journal of Nervous and Mental Disease, 191*, 332–338.

Conway, M. A., & Pleydell-Pearce, C. W. (2000). The construction of autobiographical memories in the self-memory system. *Psychological Review, 107*, 261–288.

Davidson, R. J., Jackson, D. C., & Kalin, N. H. (2000). Emotion, plasticity, context, and regulation: Perspectives from affective neuroscience. *Psychological Bulletin, 126,* 890–909.

Debiec, J., LeDoux, J. E., & Nader, K. (2002). Cellular and systems reconsolidation in the hippocampus. *Neuron, 36,* 527–538.

Ehlers, A., & Clark, D. M. (2000). A cognitive model of posttraumatic stress disorder. *Behaviour Research and Therapy, 38,* 319–345.

Ehlers A., Clark, D. M., Hackmann, A., McManus, F., Fennell, M., Herbert, C., & Mayou, R. (2003). A randomized controlled trial of cognitive therapy, a self-help booklet, and repeated assessments as early interventions for posttraumatic stress disorder. *Archives of General Psychiatry, 60,* 1024–1032.

Elzinga, B. M., & Bremner, J. D. (2002). Are the neural substrates of memory the final common pathway in posttraumatic stress disorder (PTSD)? *Journal of Affective Disorders, 70,* 1–17.

Evans, J. St. B. T. (2003). In two minds: Dual-process accounts of reasoning. *Trends in Cognitive Sciences, 7,* 454–459.

Eysenck, M. W. (1979). Depth, elaboration, and distinctiveness. In L. S. Cermak & F. I. M. Craik (Eds.), *Levels of processing in human memory* (pp. 89–118). Hillsdale, NJ: Erlbaum.

Fischer, A., Sananbenesi, F., Schrick, C., Spiess, J., & Radulovic, J. (2004). Distinct roles of hippocampal de novo protein synthesis and actin rearrangement in extinction of contextual fear. *Journal of Neuroscience, 24,* 1962–1966.

Foa, E. B., Dancu, C. V., Hembree, E. A., Jaycox, L. H., Meadows, E. A., & Street, G. P. (1999). A comparison of exposure therapy, stress inoculation training, and their combination for reducing posttraumatic stress disorder in female assault victims. *Journal of Consulting and Clinical Psychology, 67,* 194–200.

Foa, E. B., & McNally, R. J. (1996). Mechanisms of change in exposure therapy. In R. M. Rapee (Ed.), *Current controversies in the anxiety disorders* (pp. 329–343). New York: Guilford Press.

Foa, E. B., & Rothbaum, B. O. (1998). *Treating the trauma of rape: Cognitive-behavioral therapy for PTSD.* New York: Guilford Press.

Gray, J. R. (2001). Emotional modulation of cognitive control: Approach–withdrawal states double-dissociate spatial from verbal two-back task performance. *Journal of Experimental Psychology: General, 130,* 436–452.

Grey, N., Holmes, E., & Brewin, C. R. (2001). Peritraumatic emotional "hotspots" in traumatic memory: A case series of patients with posttraumatic stress disorder. *Behavioural and Cognitive Psychotherapy, 29,* 367–372.

Grey, N., Young, K., & Holmes, E. (2002). Hot spots in emotional memory and the treatment of posttraumatic stress disorder. *Behavioural and Cognitive Psychotherapy, 30,* 37–56.

Hackmann, A. (1998). Working with images in clinical psychology. In A. S. Bellack & M. Hersen (Eds.), *Comprehensive clinical psychology* (Vol. 6, pp. 301–318). New York: Elsevier.

Herman, J. L. (1992). *Trauma and recovery.* London: Pandora Books.

Holmes, E. A., Brewin, C. R., & Hennessy, R. G. (2004). Trauma films, information processing, and intrusive memory development. *Journal of Experimental Psychology: General, 133,* 3–22.

Horowitz, M. J. (1976). *Stress response syndromes.* New York: Aronson.

Hunt, R. R., & McDaniel, M. A. (1993). The enigma of organization and distinctiveness. *Journal of Memory and Language, 32,* 421–445.

Hunt, R. R., & Smith, R. E. (1996). Accessing the particular from the general: The power of distinctiveness in the context of organization. *Memory and Cognition, 24,* 217–225.

Jacobs, W. J., & Nadel, L. (1985). Stress induced recovery of fears and phobias. *Psychological Review, 92,* 512–531.

Klein, K., & Boals, A. (2001a). The relationship of life event stress and working memory capacity. *Applied Cognitive Psychology, 15,* 565–579.

Klein, K., & Boals, A. (2001b). Expressive writing can increase working memory capacity. *Journal of Experimental Psychology: General, 130,* 520–533.

Lattal, K. M., & Abel, T. (2004). Behavioral impairments caused by injections of the protein synthesis inhibitor anisomycin after contextual retrieval reverse with time. *Proceedings of the National Academy of Sciences, 101,* 4667–4672.

Layden, M. A., Newman, C. F., Freeman, A., & Morse, S. B. (1993). *Cognitive therapy of borderline personality disorder.* Boston: Allyn & Bacon.

LeDoux, J. E. (1998). *The emotional brain.* London: Weidenfeld & Nicolson.

Lee, J. L. C., Everitt, B. J., & Thomas, K. L. (2004). Independent cellular processes for hippocampal memory consolidation and reconsolidation. *Science, 304,* 839–843.

Lockhart, R. S., Craik, F. I. M., & Jacoby, L. L. (1976). Depth of processing, recognition and recall. In J. Brown (Ed.), *Recall and recognition* (pp. 75–102). New York: Wiley.

Maren, S., Ferrario, C. R., Corcoran, K. A., Desmond, T. J., & Frey, K. A. (2003). Protein synthesis in the amygdala, but not the auditory thalamus, is required for consolidation of Pavlovian fear conditioning in rats. *European Journal of Neuroscience, 18,* 3080–3088.

Marks, I., Lovell, K., Noshirvani, H., & Livanou, M. (1998). Treatment of posttraumatic stress disorder by exposure and/or cognitive restructuring—A controlled study. *Archives of General Psychiatry, 55,* 317–325.

McClelland, J. L., McNaughton, B. L., & O'Reilly, R. C. (1995). Why there are complementary learning systems in the hippocampus and neocortex: Insights from the successes and failures of connectionist models of learning and memory. *Psychological Review, 102,* 419–457.

McCloskey, M., & Cohen, N. J. (1989). Catastrophic interference in connectionist networks: The sequential learning problem. In G. H. Bower (Ed.), *The psychology of learning and motivation* (Vol. 24, pp. 109–165). New York: Academic Press.

Milekic, M. H., & Alberini, C. M. (2002). Temporally graded requirement for protein synthesis following memory reactivation. *Neuron, 36,* 521–525.

Nader, K. (2003). Memory traces unbound. *Trends in Neurosciences, 26,* 65–72.

Rachman, S. (1989). The return of fear: Review and prospect. *Clinical Psychology Review, 9,* 147–168.

Rauch, S. L., Shin, L. M., Whalen, P. J., & Pitman, R. K. (1998). Neuroimaging and the neuroanatomy of PTSD. *CNS Spectrums, 3*(Suppl. 2), 30–41.

Resick, P. A., Nishith, P., Weaver, T. L., Astin, M. C., & Feuer, C. A. (2002). A comparison of cognitive-processing therapy with prolonged exposure and a waiting condition for the treatment of chronic posttraumatic stress disorder in female rape victims. *Journal of Consulting and Clinical Psychology, 70,* 867–879.

Resick, P. A., & Schnicke, M. K. (1993). *Cognitive processing therapy for rape victims.* Newbury Park, CA: Sage.

Reynolds, M., & Brewin, C. R. (1999). Intrusive memories in depression and posttraumatic stress disorder. *Behaviour Research and Therapy, 37,* 201–215.

Richards, D., & Lovell, K. (1999). Behavioural and cognitive-behavioural interventions in the treatment of PTSD. In W. Yule (Ed.), *Post-traumatic stress disorders: Concepts and therapy* (pp. 239–266). Chichester, UK: Wiley.

Santini, E., Ge, H., Ren, K. Q., de Ortiz, S. P., & Quirk, G. J. (2004). Consolidation of fear extinction requires protein synthesis in the medial prefrontal cortex. *Journal of Neuroscience, 24,* 5704–5710.

Sapolsky, R. M. (2003). Stress and plasticity in the limbic system. *Neurochemical Research, 28,* 1735–1742.

Schafe, G. E., & LeDoux, J. E. (2000). Memory consolidation of auditory Pavlovian fear conditioning requires protein synthesis and protein kinase A in the amygdala. *Journal of Neuroscience, 20,* RC96(1–5).

Shapiro, F. (1995). *Eye movement desensitization and reprocessing: Basic principles, protocols, and procedures.* New York: Guilford Press.

Sloman, S. A. (1996). The empirical case for two systems of reasoning. *Psychological Bulletin, 119,* 3–22.

Smucker, M. R., Dancu, C., Foa, E. B., & Niederee, J. L. (1995). Imagery rescripting: A new treatment for survivors of childhood sexual abuse suffering from posttraumatic stress. *Journal of Cognitive Psychotherapy, 9,* 3–17.

Spivak, B., Segal, M., Mester, R., & Weizman, A. (1998). Lateral preference in posttraumatic stress disorder. *Psychological Medicine, 28,* 229–232.

Tarrier, N., Pilgrim, H., Sommerfield, C., Faragher, B., Reynolds, M., Graham, E., & Barrowclough, C. (1999). A randomized trial of cognitive therapy and imaginal exposure in the treatment of chronic posttraumatic stress disorder. *Journal of Consulting and Clinical Psychology, 67,* 13–18.

van der Kolk, B. A., McFarlane, A. C., & van der Hart, O. (1996). A general approach to the treatment of posttraumatic stress disorder. In B. A. van der Kolk, A. C. McFarlane, & L. Weisaeth (Eds.), *Traumatic stress: The effects of overwhelming experience on mind, body, and society* (pp. 417–440). New York: Guilford Press.

Van Etten, M. L., & Taylor, S. (1998). Comparative efficacy of treatments for posttraumatic stress disorder: A meta-analysis. *Clinical Psychology and Psychotherapy, 5,* 126–144.

Vasterling, J. J., Brailey, K., Constans, J. I., & Sutker, P. B. (1998). Attention and memory dysfunction in posttraumatic stress disorder. *Neuropsychology, 12,* 125–133.

Wild, J., Baxendale, S., Scragg, P., & Gur, R. C. (2002). *Verbal memory predicts outcome in posttraumatic stress disorder.* Manuscript submitted for publication.

CHAPTER 13

Pharmacological Approaches to Cognitive Deficits Associated with PTSD

MATTHEW J. FRIEDMAN

There are a number of cognitive deficits that appear to be associated with posttraumatic stress disorder (PTSD). Among adults, the focus has primarily been on memory function and information processing based in part on reports of reduced hippocampal volume among PTSD patients (Bremner, Randall, et al., 1997; Bremner, Vythilingam, et al., 2003). Among children, there has been concern that trauma/PTSD-related deficits in intelligence may be related, developmentally, to reduced intracranial and corpus callosum volumes (De Bellis et al., 2002).

The presumed circuitry underlying such abnormalities focuses on excessive activation of the amygdala by stimuli perceived to be threatening. Such activation produces outputs to a number of brain areas that mediate memory consolidation of emotional events and spatial learning (hippocampus), memory of emotional events and choice behaviors (orbitofrontal cortex), autonomic and fear reactions (locus coeruleus, thalamus, and hypothalamus), and instrumental approach or avoidance behavior (dorsal and ventral striatum) (Davis & Whalen, 2001). In PTSD, the normal checks and balances on amygdala activation have been impaired so that the restraining influence of the medial prefrontal cortex (PFC), especially the anterior cingulate gyrus and orbitofrontal cortex, are severely disrupted (Charney, 2004; Vermetten & Bremner, 2002). Disinhibition of the amygdala produces a vicious spiral of recurrent fear conditioning in which ambiguous stimuli are more likely to be appraised as threatening; mechanisms for extinguishing such responses are nullified; and key limbic nuclei are sensitized thereby lowering the threshold for fearful reactivity (Charney, Deutch, Krystal, Southwick, & Davis, 1993, 2004; Friedman, 1994; Southwick, Rasmusson, Barron, & Arnsten, Chapter 2, this volume).

The pharmacological challenge, therefore, is to identify where and how to intervene in order to rein in the amygdala and the cortical and subcortical effects it has set in motion. Although many neurobiological systems are altered among individuals with PTSD, we must first consider the adrenergic, hypothalamic–pituitary–adrenal (HPA), and glutamatergic systems because they appear to be most important with regard to cognitive deficits. Serotonergic and dopaminergic mechanisms will also be discussed.

A thorough review of PTSD-related neurochemical alterations associated with cognitive abnormalities is beyond the scope of this chapter and can be found elsewhere (Charney, 2004; Southwick et al., Chapter 2, this volume; Vermetten & Bremner, 2002). A brief summary of major findings is shown in Table 13.1.

This chapter is concerned with pharmacological interventions to reverse such alterations. It should be stated at the outset, that, with a few exceptions, I can offer little more than theoretically driven speculations rather than a review of empirical findings. This is because most research with pharmacological agents has focused on reduction of PTSD symptoms rather than amelioration of cognitive impairment. Furthermore, the lion's share of such investigations concern serotonergic agents rather than other classes of medications. Table 13.1 summarizes all the findings that will be reviewed. It specifies the mechanism of action for each pharmacological agent as well as the cognitive and clinical effects for each medication under consideration.

THE ADRENERGIC SYSTEM AND ANTIADRENERGIC AGENTS

Norepinephrine

Animal research indicates that central noradrenergic neurons play an important role in determining alertness, vigilence, orienting to novel stimuli and selective attention. All three principle adrenergic receptor systems are involved in the fear conditioning circuitry described previously. (A more thorough review is provided by Southwick, Rasmusson, Barron, & Arnsten, Chapter 2, this volume). *Beta-adrenergic receptors* mediate the enhancement of emotional memory by the amygdala (Cahill & McGaugh, 1996). Such enhancement may be related to the intrusive recollections, dissociative flashbacks and psychological/physiological reactivity provoked by exposure to traumatic stimuli that are usually seen among individuals

TABLE 13.1. Pharmacological Actions Affecting Cognition in PTSD

Pharmacological category	Specific medication	Mechanism of action	Effect on stress/fear response	Effects on cognition	Clinical findings
Adrenergic system	Propranolol	Beta-receptor antagonist.	All antiadrenergic agents: • Reduce amygdala activation. • Enhance PFC function. • Inhibit locus coeruleus activation.	All antiadrenergic agents: • Reduce consolidation of emotional memories. • Enhance working memory. • Reduce dissociative symptoms.	• All reduce PTSD symptoms (mostly reexperiencing and hyperarousal). • Propranolol reduces stress-related enhancement of emotional memories. • Prazosin reduces nightmares. • Clonidine/guanfacine enhance PFC working memory function and reduce dissociation.
	Prazosin	Alpha$_1$-receptor antagonist.			
	Clonidine/ guanfacine	Alpha$_2$-receptor antagonist.			
	Theoretical	NPY enhancer.	• Antagonizes both adrenergic and CRF activation of fear/stress response. • Suppresses adrenergic and HPA responses to stress.	• Untested. • Theoretically, should enhance cognition and working memory. • Theoretically, should reduce consolidation of emotional memories and dissociation.	• Hypothetical medication.
HPA system	Antalarmin[a]	CRF antagonist.	• Suppresses adrenergic and HPA responses to stress. • Reduces CRF release. • Reduces locus coeruleus activation. • Reduces ACTH secretion with secondary glucocorticoid elevation.	• Reduces stress-induced fearful behavior. • Should enhance cognition and working memory. • Should reduce consolidation of fearful memories and dissociation.	• Safe CRF antagonists, suitable for clinical studies, are not available.

	Hydrocortisone, other glucocorticiods.	Rectify hypocortisolism and downregulate GC receptors.	Untested.	Although HPA activation appears to be associated with PTSD, findings regarding cortisol levels and GC supersensitivity are inconsistent, therefore scenarios with medications that both increase and decrease glucocorticoid levels and GC receptor activation are presented.
	Ketoconazole	Blocks cortisol synthesis.	Reduces increased HPA activation thereby reducing potentiation of excessive adrenergic activity.	
	Mifepristone (RU-486)	GC receptor antagonist.	Reduces cortisol's neurotoxic enhancement of glutamate and calcium influx into neurons.	
Glumatergic system	Cycloserine	Partial NMDA receptor agonist.	Enhances learning, extinction, memory function, and neurogenesis.	Improvement in Wisconsin Card Sort perseverative error scores and near significant improvement in delayed recall on Auditory Verbal Learning Test.	RCT on augmentation treatment showed cognitive benefits as well as reduction in PTSD severity and general anxiety.
GABAergic agents	Benzodiazepines	$GABA_A$ receptor agonist.	Suppress stress-induced amygdala activation by inhibition of NMDA receptors.	Untested. (predict enhanced cognition by antagonizing amygdala activation if sedation and cognitive blunting can be prevented).	Clinical trials indicate no specific efficacy against core PTSD symptoms.
	Baclofen	$GABA_B$ receptor agonist.	Unclear. Might reduce stress-induced adrenergic/HPA activation. Has been effective clinically in mood and anxiety disorders.	Untested.	One small open trial showing improvement in overall PTSD symptom severity.
Anticonvulsants/ antikindling agents	Carbamazepine	AMPA antagonist. Elevates GABA. Blocks sodium channels.	Blocks sensitization/ kindling. Suppresses adrenergic arousal.	Untested.	Open trials show reduced PTSD severity, arousal, impulse control, aggression and violent behavior.

(continued)

TABLE 13.1. Pharmacological Actions Affecting Cognition in PTSD

Pharmacological category	Specific medication	Mechanism of action	Effect on stress/fear response	Effects on cognition	Clinical findings
	Valproate	• Increases brain GABA levels. • Enhances GABA receptor sensitivity.	• Blocks sensitization/kindling. • May suppress NMDA receptors.	• Untested.	• Open trials and case reports indicate clinical efficacy in PTSD.
	Lamotrigine	• Inhibits glutamate release. • Blocks voltage-dependent sodium and calcium channels.	• Blocks sensitization/kindling. • Blocks NMDA activation of amygdala.	• Inhibits dissociatve symptoms caused by ketamine and phencyclidine.	• Small, randomized trial suggests favorable effect in PTSD.
	Topirimate	• Suppresses glutamate function. • Enhances GABA activity.	• Blocks sensitization/kindling. • Blocks NMDA amygdala activation.	• Untested.	• Open trial showed suppression of PTSD reexperiencing and dissociative symptoms.
	Gabapentin	• Increases GABA turnover.	• Blocks sensitization/kindling.	• Untested.	• Case reports and chart reviews suggest effectiveness in PTSD.
	Tiagabine	• Increases GABA levels by inhibiting glial uptake.	• Blocks sensitization/kindling.	• Untested.	• Positive case reports.
	Vigabatrin	• Increases GABA by inhibiting GABA transaminase.	• Blocks sensitization/kindling. • Blocks startle response.	• Untested.	• Case reports showing reduction of insomnia, anxiety, and startle response in PTSD patients.
Selective serotonin reuptake inhibitors (SSRIs)	Paroxetine	• SSRI.	• 5-HT$_{1A}$ neurons potentiate GABA antagonism of amygdala NMDA activity. • Promotes neurogenesis in hippocampus.	• Increased hippocampal volume after 9–12 months of treatment associated with cognitive improvement in: logical, figural, verbal, and visual memory.	• FDA approval for PTSD based on three randomized clinical trials. • Broad spectrum of action against all three PTSD symptom clusters.

	Sertraline	SSRI.	• See paroxetine.	• FDA approval for PTSD based on two randomized clinical trials. • Broad spectrum of action.
	Fluoxetine	SSRI.	• See paroxetine.	• Successful randomized clinical trials in PTSD.
	Fluvoxamine	SSRI.	• See paroxetine.	• Successful open-label trials.
	Citalopram	SSRI.	• See paroxetine.	• Successful open-label trial.
Other serotonergic antidepressants	Nefazodone[b] Trazodone	SSRI plus post-synaptic 5-HT$_2$ blockade.	• In addition to potentiation of 5-HT$_{1A}$ action, blockade of 5-HT$_2$ receptors is anxiolytic. • Promotes neurogenesis.	• Untested.	• Randomized and open-label trials suggest nefazodone is as effective as sertraline. • Trazodone has limited efficacy. • Nefazodone is no longer available in the USA because of liver toxicity.
Tricyclic antidepressants (TCAs)	Imipramine Amitriptyline Desipramine	Blocks presynaptic reuptake of norepinephrine and serotonin.	• Enhance serotonergic actions at 5HT1A receptors. • Reduce adrenergic actions by downregulation of postsynaptic beta receptors. • Promote neurogenesis.	• Untested.	• Successful randomized trials for PTSD patients with imipramine and amitriptyline but not desipramine.
Monoamine oxidase inhibitors (MAOIs)	Phenelzine	Blocks enzymatic (MAO) degradation of norepinephrine, serotonin (and dopamine).	• Enhances serotonergic action at 5-HT$_{1A}$ receptors. • Downregulates postsynaptic beta receptors (and reduces locus coeruleus activity). • Promotes neurogenesis.	• Untested.	• Mixed results with phenelzine. A positive randomized trial, an inconclusive cross-over trial and mixed findings in open-label trials. • One positive open-label trial with moclobemide.
	Moclobemide	Selective MAO-A inhibitor.			

(continued)

TABLE 13.1. Pharmacological Actions Affecting Cognition in PTSD

Pharmacological category	Specific medication	Mechanism of action	Effect on stress/fear response	Effects on cognition	Clinical findings
Other antidepressants	Mirtazepine	Blocks postsynaptic 5-HT$_2$ and 5-HT$_3$ receptors.	• Anxiolytic 5-HT$_2$/5-HT$_3$ blockade. • Reduces adrenergic activity.	• Untested.	• Mirtazepine reduced PTSD symptom severity in one randomized and one open-label trial as well as in case reports. • Favorable open trials with venlafaxine and bupropion.
	Venlafaxine	Agonist action at presynaptic adrenergic alpha$_2$ receptors. Blocks presynaptic reuptake of both serotonin and norepinephrine.	• All three antidepressants promote neurogenesis. • Potentiates 5-HT and reduces adrenergic activity.		
	Bupropion	Blocks presynaptic reuptake of norepinephrine and dopamine.	• Reduces adrenergic and dopaminergic activity.		
Atypical antipsychotic agents	Risperidone Quetiapine Olanzapine	Dopamine (D$_2$) and serotonin (5-HT$_2$) blockade.	• Promotes enhanced PFC restraint of amygdala, reduces hyperarousal/ hypervigilence and blocks anxiogenic 5-HT$_2$ receptor actions.	• Untested (predict enhancement of PFC working memory and reduction in consolidation of emotional memories).	• *Risperidone* Augmentation reduced PTSD symptom severity, dissociative flashbacks and aggressive behavior—one RCT, one open trial and several case reports. • *Quetiapine* Augmentation was beneficial in reducing PTSD severity in SSRI non responders—one open trial, a retrospective chart review and case reports. • *Olanzapine* Augmentation reduced PTSD severity in SSRI non responders.

Note. ACTH, corticotropin; AMPA, alpha-amino-3-hydroxy-5-methyl-4-isoxyazoleproprionic acid; CRF, corticotropin-releasing factor; FDA, Food and Drug Administration; GABA, gamma-aminobutyric acid; GC, glucocorticoid; 5-HT, serotonin; MAO, monoamine oxidase; NMDA, N-methyl-D-aspartate; NPY, neuropeptide Y; PFC, prefrontal cortex; RCT, randomized clinical trial; SSRI, selective serotonin reuptake inhibitor; TCA, tricyclic antidepressant.

[a]Experimental medication.

[b]Withdrawn from U.S. market because of liver toxicity.

with PTSD. *Alpha$_1$-adrenergic receptors* also promote this process by facilitating the impact of beta-adrenergic enhancement of memory. This postsynaptic noradrenergic input to both beta and alpha$_1$ receptors promotes activation of the amygdala. Because the amygdala's projections to the locus coeruleus generate additional adrenergic input, it can be seen how this process can escalate and result in an upward spiral of adrenergic stimulation.

Alpha$_2$-adrenergic receptors, which provide presynaptic inhibition of amygdala catecholamine release, suppress fear conditioning and reduce consolidation of emotional memories (Davies et al., 2004). They may also play a role in dissociation since the alpha$_2$ antagonist, yohimbine (which disinhibits adrenergic activity), provoked dissociative flashbacks among Vietnam veterans with PTSD (Southwick et al., 1997, 1999). Thus, from the perspective of the amygdala, alone, agents that antagonize alpha$_1$- and beta-adrenergic receptors or enhance alpha$_2$-adrenergic activity might be expected to improve cognitive function.

Unlike the amygdala, which thrives in a climate of elevated adrenergic stimulation, the opposite is true for the PFC. High levels of catecholamines impair PFC function. In addition to modulating amygdala activity, the PFC mediates working memory. Thus, increasing adrenergic stimulation not only reduces the PFC's capacity to inhibit amygdala hyperactivity, but also impairs its cognitive role in working memory and maintenance of attention (Arnsten, 2000). Both alpha$_1$ and beta-receptor activation appear responsible for nullifying PFC activity during uncontrollable stress and these effects can be prevented with alpha$_1$-adrenergic antagonists such as prazosin (Arnsten & Jentsch, 1997) as well as with the beta-adrenergic antagonist, propranolol (Li & Mei, 1994).

To summarize, the therapeutic goal of targeting the adrenergic system is to inhibit excessive alpha$_1$ and beta-receptor activation and to augment the inhibitory influence of alpha$_2$-adrenergic receptors. The result of such treatment would be expected to reduce amygdala activation, enhance PFC function, and inhibit stimulation of the locus coeruleus and its secondary activation of other cortical and subcortical structures. Cognitive benefits should include reduced consolidation of fearful memories, enhancement of PFC working memory capability, and prevention of fragmented information processing, manifested as dissociative symptoms.

There are little empirical data to guide us. Cahill and McGaugh, (1996) have shown that the beta-adrenergic antagonist *propranolol* reduced enhancement of emotional memories among human volunteers. In small studies with clinical populations, propranolol has had beneficial effects on PTSD symptoms (including intrusive recollections and reactivity to traumatic stimuli) (Famularo, Kinscherff, & Fenton, 1988; Kolb, Burris, & Griffiths, 1984; Pitman et al., 2002; Taylor & Cahill, 2002; Vaiva et al., 2003). It should be noted that these were all small studies and that formal tests of cognitive function were not performed in any of these investigations.

Recent research with the alpha$_1$ antagonist, *prazosin*, has indicated that PTSD nightmares and other symptoms are reduced by treatment (Peskind, Bonner, Hoff, & Raskind, 2003; Raskind, Peskind, Kanter, Petrie, Radont, Thompson, et al., 2003). Since prazosin would be expected to improve PFC and reduce amygdala activation, it is expected that this agent would also improve cognition among PTSD patients.

Alpha$_2$-adrenergic agonists such as *clonidine* and *guanfacine* would also be expected to improve PFC cognitive function in addition to directly reducing amygdala activity. Animal research has shown that alpha$_2$ agonists enhance PFC working memory function (Franowicz et al., 2002; Mao, Arnsten, & Li, 1999). Again, however, the sparse, but generally favorable, clinical literature on the clinical efficacy of these agents in PTSD (Kinzie & Friedman, 2004; Kolb et al., 1984) has not included formal assessment of cognitive function.

Neuropeptide Y

Neuropeptide Y (NPY) is an amino acid neurotransmitter, colocalized in noradrenergic neurons, that inhibits the release of both norepinephrine and corticotropin-releasing factor (CRF, see later in the chapter). By virtue of its endogenous antiadrenergic actions, NPY would be expected to produce the antistress/anxiolytic benefits postulated above for antiadrenergic agents and, thereby improve cognitive function. Indirect evidence for this assertion has been obtained in studies of military personnel exposed to extreme stress in which there was an inverse relationship between NPY release and stress-induced performance decrements due to dissociation (Morgan et al., 2000, 2001). Clinically, it has been shown that, in comparison with healthy controls, PTSD patients exhibit both reduced baseline NPY levels and a blunted release of NPY in response to yohimbine stimulation (Rasmusson et al., 2000). Based on such findings, I have previously suggested that medications that enhance NPY function might ameliorate acute stress reactions, PTSD, and other stress-induced problems (Friedman, 2002). No pharmacological agents of this nature are currently available.

CORTICOTROPIN-RELEASING FACTOR AND THE HYPOTHALAMIC-PITUITARY-ADRENAL SYSTEM

Corticotropin-Releasing Factor

Corticotropin-releasing factor (CRF) has a dual role in the human stress response. As a neurotransmitter it promotes release of norepinephrine from the locus coeruleus, thereby enhancing amygdala and reducing PFC activity as described previously. As a hypothalamic hormone, activated by stressful stimuli and threat appraisal, it releases corticotropin (ACTH) from the pituitary gland which then promotes release of cortisol and other glucocorticoids from the adrenal cortex. Vietnam veterans with PTSD have been shown to have elevated resting levels of cerebrospinal fluid CRF (Baker et al., 1999; Bremner, Licinio, et al., 1997) and enhanced hypothalamic release of CRF (Yehuda, 2002). Specified research on cognitive deficits associated with CRF concentration has not been carried out. Preclinical studies with the CRF receptor antagonist, antalarmin, have demonstrated reductions in cerebrospinal fluid CRF, reduced stress-induced fearful behavior, and suppression of both adrenergic and HPA responses to stress (Habib et al., 2000). Given its key role in mobilizing the human stress response as well as its increased expression among PTSD patients, there is good reason to predict that CRF antagonists might have beneficial clinical effects on PTSD-related symptoms and cognitive deficits. Although CRF antagonists are currently utilized in animal research and under development by pharmaceutical companies, none are available for clinical use.

Glucocorticoids

Glucocorticoids, such as cortisol, appear to impair PFC functions (such as working memory and amygdala restraint) by enhancing catecholamine levels during activation of the stress response (Arnsten, 2000; Roozendaal, McReynolds, & McGaugh, 2004). Although excessive HPA system activity does appear to be associated with trauma exposure and PTSD, it is controversial how this may be manifested. On the one hand, it may be expressed by elevated cortisol levels, as has been found in some PTSD patients and in children exposed to sexual trauma. On the other hand, it may be expressed by reduced cortisol levels associated with supersensitivity of glucocorticoid receptors (De Bellis et al., 1994; Friedman et al., 2001; Heim, Newport, Bonsall, Miller, & Nemeroff, 2001; Lemieux & Coe, 1995; Rasmusson & Friedman, 2002; Rasmusson et al., 2001; Yehuda, 2002; Yehuda, Boisoneau, Lowy, & Giller, 1995).

From a cognitive perspective, it has been proposed that abnormal HPA activity may have neurotoxic effects through activation of excitatory amino acids resulting in calcium influx into susceptible neurons (McEwen et al., 1992; Sapolsky, 2000). From a PTSD perspective, the theory that acute (or chronic) cortisol elevation and/or glucocorticoid receptor supersensitivity is neurotoxic has been invoked to explain reduced corpus callosum and intracranial volumes observed among traumatized children (De Bellis et al., 2002) and reduced hippocampal volumes among adults with PTSD (Bremner, Randall, et al., 1997; Bremner et al., 2003; Yehuda, 1999). In the only study that systematically explored the association between reduced hippocampal volume and cognitive impairment among PTSD patients, Vermetten and associates (Vermetten, Vythilingam, Southwick, Charney, & Bremner, 2003) observed decrements in verbal declarative memory that improved after an increase in hippocampal volume following antidepressant treatment (see later in the chapter). Since decrements in corpus callosum, hippocampus, or overall intracranial volume would be expected to have serious adverse effects on many key cognitive operations, it is important to explore the glucocorticoid neurotoxic hypothesis with the following caveat: it remains an open question whether such structural abnormalities precede the onset of PTSD or whether such reductions in brain nuclei develop after the occurrence of PTSD. Twin studies with war-zone-exposed Vietnam veterans and their nontraumatized monozygotic brothers indicate that both sets of twins have reduced hippocampal volume (Gilbertson et al., 2002). In addition, ongoing prospective studies with traumatized Israelis who developed PTSD have, as yet, failed to detect decrements in hippocampal volume associated with PTSD onset (Bonne et al., 2001). Taken together, those two studies suggest that reduced volumes of brain structures constitute a risk factor for PTSD but do not represent a serious consequence of this disorder.

Such considerations notwithstanding, it is useful to consider pharmacological strategies that might either prevent or ameliorate PTSD-related neurotoxic effects mediated by excessive HPA activity. With regard to early intervention, potential treatments might include CRF antagonists or NPY enhancers, which would reduce the intensity of the acute stress response (Friedman, 2002). If the problem is excessive cortisol levels, a medication that inhibits cortisol synthesis (such as ketoconazole) or that blocks glucocorticoid receptors (such as mifepristone, RU-486) might be considered. If the problem is reduced cortisol and supersensitive glucocorticoid receptors, the opposite approach might be indicated in which glucocorticoids would be administered to downregulate supersensitive glucocorticoid receptors. Indeed, it has been shown that acute *hydrocortisone* treatment for septic shock effectively prevents the later development of PTSD (Schelling et al., 2001).

We will return to prevention of neurotoxicity later in this discussion when we consider glutamate antagonists, such as lamotrigine, which by inhibiting the release of excitatory amino acids, protect neurons by preventing toxic calcium influx. We will also consider treatments that promote neurogenesis and that have been shown to increase hippocampal volume in PTSD patients when we consider selective serotonin reuptake inhibitors (SSRIs) and other antidepressant medications.

THE GLUTAMATE AND GAMMA-AMINOBUTYRIC ACID SYSTEMS AND ANTICONVULSANT MEDICATIONS

Glutamate is the major excitatory, while gamma-aminobutyric acid (GABA) is the primary inhibitory neurotransmitter in the brain. Monoamines (such as norepinephrine, serotonin, and dopamine) have received the most attention in the past because effective clinical agents (such as antidepressants and antipsychotic medications) are known to alter monoaminergic function. An important shift in focus has began to occur because our growing understanding of glutamatergic and GABAergic mechanisms indicates their crucial function in mediating most cognitive operations, their importance in the human stress response, and their probable role in the pathophysiology of PTSD. Anticonvulsant agents, also known as mood stabilizers, exert their primary actions on glutamate and/or GABA activity. Such actions also have potential importance in ameliorating cognitive deficits associated with PTSD.

Glutamate

There are two families of glutamate receptors: inotropic, which exert their actions through neuronal receptor ion channels, and metabotropic, which act by coupling with receptor-bound G proteins. There are three types of inotropic glutamate receptors named after the agonists to which they are differentially sensitive: N-methyl-D-aspartate (NMDA), alpha-amino-3-hydroxy-5-methyl-4-isoxyazolepropionic acid (AMPA), and kainate. We focus on inotropic receptors in the following discussion. There are also three types of metabotropic receptors (M Glu I, II, and III), which act on intracellular messenger systems. Metabotropic receptors, through modulation of glutamate, GABA, and serotonin appear to mediate anxiolytic and antipsychotic actions (Zarate, Quirox, Payne, & Manji, 2002).

During the fear response NMDA receptors in the amygdala activate the fear circuit described previously. NMDA antagonists such as certain anticonvulsants inhibit such actions (Berlant, 2003; Davis & Whalen, 2001; Paul, Nowak, Layer, Popik, & Skolnick, 1994). In addition to enhancing the startle response and anxious behavior, AMPA receptors mediate long-term potentiation, sensitization, and kindling of brain neurons, which is an important neurobiological model of PTSD (Post, Weiss, & Smith, 1995; Post, Weiss, Li, Leverich, & Pert, 1999; Walker & Davis, 2002). Kainate receptors appear to promote fear and anxiety through actions in the periaqueductal gray and frontal cortex where they promote reduction of benzodiazepine (e.g., GABAergic) sites.

NMDA receptors are of great importance in cognition. They are crucial for all forms of learning, including fear conditioning (Bardgett et al., 2003; Liang, Hon, & Davis, 1994; Nakazawa et al., 2002) and extinction (Davis, 2002; Falls, Miserendino, & Davis, 1992; van der Meulen, Bilbija, Joosten, de Bruin, & Feenstra, 2003). They also play a major role in neurogenesis, the production of new neurons (Gould, McEwen, Tanapat, Galea, & Fuchs, 1997; Nacher, Alonso-Llosa, Rosell, & McEwen, 2003; Okuyama, Takagi, Kawai, Miyake-Takagi, & Takeo, 2004). AMPA receptors may also promote neurogenesis through activation of brain-derived neurotropic factor (BDNF) (Mackowiak, O'Neill, Hicks, Bleakman, & Skolnick, 2002). An important model of dissociation involves the interplay of NMDA and AMPA receptors. Based on the observation that low doses of NMDA receptor antagonists such as ketamine or phencyclidine can produce alterations in thought content and processes such as paranoia, loosening of associations, tangentiality, and ideas of reference, while higher doses can produce dissociative symptoms such as slowed time perception (regarding the intensity, shape and color of objects), alterations in body perceptions, and derealization. The proposed model is that NMDA blockade intensifies glutamate stimulation of AMPA receptors (Chambers et al., 1999; Krystal, Bennett, Bremner, Southwick, & Charney, 1995). It is noteworthy that the dissociative effects of ketamine are blocked by lamotrigine, an anticonvulsant that inhibits glutamate release (Anand et al., 2000).

D-*Cycloserine* is a partial NMDA receptor agonist that has positive effects on memory deficits in animals (Monahan, Handelman, Hood, & Cordi, 1989; Thompson, Moskal, & Disterhoft, 1992), in elderly volunteers (Jones, Wesnes, & Kirby, 1991) and in Alzheimer's disease patients (Schwartz, Hashtroudi, Herting, Schwartz, & Deutsch, 1996). In a 12-week double-blind, placebo-controlled crossover design, PTSD patients currently treated with other medications were randomized to augmentation treatment with either D-cycloserine or placebo. Significant reductions in PTSD and anxiety (but not depression) symptom severity were observed. Furthermore, D-cycloserine treatment was associated with significant improvement in Wisconsin Card Sort perseverative error scores and near significant improvement in delayed recall on the Auditory Verbal Learning Test (Heresco-Levy et al., 2002).

Thus, the centrality of glutamatergic actions in cognitive deficits associated with PTSD has strong support both theoretically and from laboratory research. Such deficits include stress-induced problems with information processing, working memory, declarative memory, and dissociation.

Gamma-Aminobutyric Acid and Benzodiazepine Medication

GABA is the brain's major inhibitory neurotransmitter that suppresses stress-induced actions of the amygdala. GABA receptors within the basolateral amygdala inhibit glutamatergic excitation. Furthermore, serotonin enhances this GABAergic suppression of the amygdala (Berlant, 2003; Stutzmann & LeDoux, 1999), which is a major mechanism through which serotoninergic agents ameliorate both the acute stress response and PTSD symptomatology.

PTSD patients exhibit both reduced GABA plasma levels (Vaiva, Thomas, Ducroq, Fontaine, Boss, Devos, Rascle, et al., 2004) and reduced benzodiazepine receptor activity in the amygdala, PFC, and other brain areas (Bremner et al., 2000). Because benzodiazepine receptors are a part of the GABA$_A$ receptor complex, these findings suggest that deficiencies in GABAergic mechanisms in the amygdala, PFC, and elsewhere result in insufficient protection against the activating effects of norepinephrine and glutamate. It is possible that intrusive recollections, hyperarousal symptoms, and disinhibited social and emotional behavior observed among PTSD patients may be due to such deficient GABAergic function (Morgan, Krystal, & Southwick, 2003). It should be noted in this regard that pretreating animals later exposed to inescapable shock with benzodiazepines blocks stress-induced increases in norepinephrine in the amygdala, cortex, locus coeruleus, hypothalamus, and hippocampus (Drugan, Ryan, Minor, & Maier, 1984; Grant, Huang, & Redmond, 1980).

With regard to cognition, there is probably a therapeutic window within which enhancement of GABAergic activity will block the adverse cognitive effects of excessive norepinephrine and glutamate activity associated with acute stress, PTSD, and dissociative states. Excessive GABAergic activity, however, can impair cognitive function through dulling of the sensorium and suppression of cortical activity.

Given the above discussion, one might expect that treatment with benzodiazepines might ameliorate PTSD symptoms. Unfortunately, this has not been the case. A randomized clinical trial with *alprazolam* did not reduce core reexperiencing or avoidant/numbing symptoms, although it did lead to improvement in insomnia and generalized anxiety (Braun, Greenberg, Dasberg, & Lerer, 1990). Treatment of recently traumatized emergency room patients with *clonazepam* (Gelpin, Bonne, Peri, Brandes, & Shalev, 1996) or the hypnotic benzodiazepine, *temazepam* (Mellman, Bustamante, David, & Fins, 2002) did not prevent the later development of PTSD. Other open trials with benzodiazepines have also been unsuccessful (Friedman, Davidson, Mellman, & Southwick, 2000).

Benzodiazepines act at GABA$_A$ receptors. *Baclofen* is a medication that activates GABA$_B$ receptors. Previous studies have shown that GABA$_B$ agonists have been effective in treating mood and anxiety disorders (Breslow et al., 1989; Krupitsky et al., 1993). An open-label study with baclofen was carried out, in which 9 of 11 veterans with PTSD experienced improvement in overall PTSD symptom severity, although there was no improvement in reexperiencing symptoms (Drake et al., 2003). As usual, specific tests of cognitive function were not included in this protocol. It does appear, however, that further trials with baclofen are warranted.

Anticonvulsant/Antikindling Agents

Anticonvulsant agents have been sporadically tested in small single-site studies for almost 20 years. Only one small, randomized clinical trial has been carried out. Interest in this class of medications was initially prompted by their antikindling actions, since there has been great interest in sensitization/kindling hypotheses for a long time (Friedman, 1994; Post et al., 1995, 1999). More recently, appreciation of glutamatergic and GABAergic actions of anticonvulsants as well as detection of abnormalities in these two systems among PTSD patients has raised the level of interest in this class of medications. Finally, the development of several new anticonvulsant/mood stabilizers in recent years has motivated the pharmaceutical industry to support clinical trials utilizing these agents with PTSD patients.

What follows is a brief description of each anticonvulsant tested with PTSD patients, its mechanism of action, and the result of clinical trials. At the outset, it is important to recognize that all anticonvulsants may produce neurological symptoms and cognitive impairment as a side effect. Such side effects may include impaired concentration, memory problems, sedation, and confusion. Therefore, when treating PTSD, one must always weigh the relative risk of such side effects against the benefit of PTSD symptom reduction and improved cognition.

Carbamazepine

Carbamazepine is an antikindling agent thought to act by blocking sodium channels. Its antikindling effect suggests action at AMPA receptors. Chronic carbamazepine treatment has also been shown to elevate GABA concentrations in certain brain regions. There is also evidence that it antagonizes noradrenergic arousal (Berlant, 2003; Iancu, Rosen, & Moshe, 2002). Three open-label studies with veterans and adolescents observed improvement in PTSD symptom severity, impulse control, anger, and violent behavior (Lipper et al., 1986; Looff, Grimley, Kuller, Martin, & Shonfield, 1995; Wolfe, Alavi, & Mosnaim, 1988). A large retrospective study with military personnel indicated the effectiveness of carbamazepine in PTSD (Viola et al., 1997). Case reports with carbamazepine (Steward & Bartucci, 1986) and its close relative, oxcarbamazepine (Berigan, 2002a) have also been positive.

Valproate

Valproate is an antikindling agent that increases brain GABA levels, enhances GABA receptor sensitivity, and may suppress NMDA receptors (Berlant, 2003; Iancu et al., 2002). Four open-label trials and two case reports indicate the effectiveness of valproate for PTSD (Berigan & Holzgang, 1995; Clark, Canive, Calais, Qualls, & Tuason, 1999; Fesler, 1991; Goldberg, Cloitre, Whiteside, & Han, 2003; Petty et al., 2002; Szymanski & Olympia, 1991).

Lamotrigine

Lamotrigine inhibits glutamate release, blocks voltage-dependent sodium channels, antagonizes calcium channels, may block serotonin ($5\text{-}HT_2$) receptors, and may potentiate dopaminergic transmission (Goa, Ross, & Chrisp, 1993; Xie & Hagan, 1998). The only study on lamotrigine in PTSD is the only randomized clinical trial with any anticonvulsant. This was a 10-week trial in which 10 patients were randomized to lamotrigine and 5 to placebo monotherapy. Although the investigators reported amelioration of PTSD in 50% (5/10) of lamotrigine patients in contrast to 25% (1/4) placebo patients (Hertzberg et al., 1999), their interpretation has been challenged (Berlant, 2003) based on a reanalysis of these data. Given the low statistical power due to the small sample size, further studies with lamotrigine are certainly warranted, given its unique pharmacological profile.

Topirimate

Topirimate is an extremely interesting anticonvulsant that suppresses glutamate function while enhancing GABAergic activity (Chengappa, John, & Parepally, 2002). It has antikindling actions as well, probably through AMPA blockade (Zullino, Krenz, & Besson, 2003). From a theoretical perspective, it seems like an excellent medication for PTSD patients. From a clinical perspective, it is one of the few psychotropic medications available that promotes weight loss rather than weight gain (Van Ameringen, Mancini, Pipe, Campbell, & Oakman, 2002). An open-label trial with 35 PTSD patients focused exclusively on reexperiencing symptoms such as nightmares, intrusive recollections, and flashbacks. Overall, 71% patients had complete remission of those symptoms and 21% reported a partial response (Berlant & van Kammen, 2002). Further trials are warranted in which the full spectrum of PTSD symptoms as well as cognitive function are monitored.

Gabapentin

Gabapentin appears to increase GABA turnover in certain brain regions (Berlant, 2003). Evidence regarding its efficacy in PTSD is sparse. Three case reports describe amelioration of PTSD symptoms (Berigan, 2002b; Brannon, Labbate, & Huber, 2000; Malek-Ahmadi, 2003). The most extensive report is a retrospective chart review of 30 patients, most of whom (90%) received another medication in addition to gabapentin. Since dropout rates and adverse side effects (especially excessive daytime sedation) were significant (Hamner, Brodrick, & Labbate, 2001), further research is clearly needed.

Tiagabine

Tiagabine is an antikindling agent that inhibits glial GABA reuptake, thereby increasing GABA concentration at both GABA-A and GABA-B receptors. Three case reports describe its effectiveness in PTSD (Berigan, 2002c; Schwartz, 2002; Taylor, 2003).

Vigabatrin

Vigabatrin increases GABA levels through inhibition of GABA transaminase (Berlant, 2003). A report on five cases of PTSD treated with this agent emphasized its reduction of the startle response along with improvement in anxiety and insomnia (Macleod, 1996).

   To summarize, anticonvulsant agents have diverse actions on glutamate, GABA, and other neurotransmitters. Findings are generally favorable regarding amelioration of PTSD symptoms but all but one of these reports are either open-label trials or case reports. The single randomized trial (with lamotrigine) included only 15 patients and lacked sufficient statistical power. Cognitive performance was not assessed formally in any of these trials, so it is impossible to determine whether reduction in PTSD symptoms was reliably associated with improved information processing or memory function. Finally, these are not benign medications and their clinical utilizations may produce adverse side effects regarding cognitive operations.

THE SEROTONIN SYSTEM AND ANTIDEPRESSANT MEDICATIONS

The Serotonin System

The serotonergic system has important interactions with the adrenergic, HPA, glutamate, GABA, and dopamine systems. Most serotonin neurons have their origin in two midbrain loci, the dorsal and median raphe nuclei, respectively, which have extensive connections with key limbic structures mediating stressful or threatening stimuli. Excessive stress, HPA activity, or PTSD produces downregulation of anxiolytic, 5-HT_{1A} and upregulation of anxiogenic, 5-HT_{2A} receptors.

   There also appear to be synergistic interactions between 5-HT_{1A} and GABA receptors with regard to acute stress and PTSD. It is thought that stimulation of 5-HT_{1A} receptors in the amygdala potentiates GABA neurons which, in turn, antagonize the excitatory glutamate neurotransmission that mediates stress-related amygdala activation (Charney, 2004; Vermetten & Bremner, 2002). This model suggests three potential amygdala-based target sites for pharmacological intervention: antagonism of glutamate, potentiation of GABA, and enhancement of serotonin neurotransmission.

As with NMDA receptors, serotonin 5-HT_{1A} receptors also promote neurogenesis in the hippocampus. It has been shown that selective serotonin reuptake inhibitors (SSRIs), as well as all clinically effective antidepressants promote neurogenesis through activation of BDNF and cyclic adenosine monophosphate (cAMP) (Duman, Nakagawa, & Malberg, 2001). This obviously has important implications for cognitive function, as discussed previously with regard to the reduced hippocampal volume of brain structures observed among PTSD patients.

Clinical studies have long indicated that many symptoms observed among PTSD patients are associated with serotonin deficiency such as impulsivity, suicidal behavior, rage, aggression, depression, panic, obsessional thoughts, and chemical dependency (Friedman, 1990). Furthermore, since the serotoninergic agonist M-chorophenylpiperazine (mCPP) can provoke panic reactions and dissociative flashbacks in PTSD but not control subjects (Southwick et al., 1997), there is reason to presume that serotonin 5-HT-2 antagonists might be clinically useful in this regard.

Selective Serotonin Reuptake Inhibitors

SSRIs are the treatment of choice for PTSD patients as attested by three independent clinical practice guidelines (American Psychiatric Association, in press; Friedman et al., 2000; VA/DoD, 2004). The only two medications to receive approval as indicated treatments for PTSD by the U.S. Food and Drug Administration are the SSRIs, sertraline and paroxetine. Multisite randomized clinical trials with *sertraline* (Brady et al., 2000; Davidson, Rothbaum, van der Kolk, Sikes, & Farfel, 2001) and *paroxetine* (Marshall, Beebe, Oldham, & Zaninelli, 2001; Tucker et al., 2001) demonstrated that both agents significantly reduced PTSD symptoms in contrast to placebo. It was also shown that if sertraline treatment was extended from 12 to 36 weeks that 55% of nonresponding patients would convert to medication responders (Lonborg et al., 2001). Finally, discontinuation of SSRI treatment is associated with clinical relapse and a return of PTSD symptoms (Davidson, Pearlstein, et al., 2001; Martenyi, Brown, Zhang, Koke, & Prakash, 2002; Rapaport, Endicott, & Clary, 2002). Randomized clinical trials with *fluoxetine* (Martenyi, Brown, Zhang, Prakash, & Koke, 2002; van der Kolk et al., 1994) and open-label studies with *fluvoxamine* (De Boer, Op den Velde, Falger, Hovens, De Groen, & Van Duijn, 1992; Escalona, Canive, Calais, & Davidson, 2002; Marmar, Schoenfeld, Weiss, Metzler, Zatzick, Wu, et al., 1996) and *citalopram* (Seedat, Lockhat, Kaminer, Zungu-Dirwayi, & Stein, 2001) indicate that these SSRIs are also effective agents. As with other medications discussed previously, most research has focused on reduction of PTSD symptoms with one notable exception (see later discussion). Since SSRIs have a broad spectrum of action and are effective for PTSD reexperiencing, avoidance/numbing, and hyper-arousal symptoms, they have a general positive impact on cognition by improving concentration and attenuating the distraction of intrusive recol-lections. Furthermore, within the amygdala, inhibition of glutamatergic ex-citation through serotonergic potentiation of GABAergic activity would be expected to have the beneficial cognitive effects produced by any interven-tion that reduces stress-induced amygdala activation.

A very exciting recent study with the SSRI paroxetine addresses two important questions regarding cognitive deficits among PTSD patients: de-clarative memory and hippocampal volume. Vermetten and associates (2003) assessed declarative memory and hippocampal volume among 20 PTSD patients who completed 9–12 months of treatment with paroxetine. These investigators observed a significant improvement in Wechsler Mem-ory Scale—Revised performance after treatment in the following domains: logical memory (delayed recall and percent retention) and figural memory (immediate recall). Significant improvement was also observed with the Se-lective Reminding Test in verbal memory (total recall, long-term storage, long-term retrieval, continuous long-term retrieval, and delayed recall) as well as in visual memory (total recall, long-term storage, long-term re-trieval, and continuous long-term retrieval). Most remarkably, these inves-tigators also observed a 4.6% increase in mean hippocampal volume as measured by magnetic resonance imaging (MRI).

Other Serotonergic Antidepressants

Nefazadone and *trazodone* are two antidepressants that enhance seroton-ergic activity through a dual mechanism that combines an SSRI action with postsynaptic, 5-HT$_2$ blockade. As with most other medications reviewed, there are no published studies in which cognitive function was monitored in conjunction with treatment. Trials with nefazadone have been much more promising, including a randomized trial in which treatment with nefazadone was as effective as sertraline (Saygin, Sungur, Sabol, & Cetin-kaya, 2002). Similar positive results have been obtained in open-label nefazadone trials (Davis, Nugent, Murray, Kramer, & Petty, 2000; Hertz-berg, Feldman, Beckham, Moore, & Davidson, 1998; Hidalgo et al., 1999). Despite these promising results, nefazadone has been recently withdrawn from the American market because of liver toxicity. The reason for includ-ing nefazadone in this review is to demonstrate the utility of non-SSRI med-ications that enhance serotonergic actions among PTSD patients.

Trazodone has limited efficacy in monotherapy for PTSD. Due to its sedating effects and serotoninergic action, it is often used in conjunction with SSRIs to counter medication-induced insomnia (Friedman et al., 2000).

OTHER ANTIDEPRESSANTS

Although SSRIs are the current first-line medications for PTSD, it is useful to consider other effective antidepressants whose action is not restricted to the serotonergic system. These include tricyclic antidepressants (TCAs), monoamine oxidase inhibitors (MAOIs), and newer agents such as mirtazapine, venlafaxine, and bupropion.

Tricyclic Antidepressants

These medications block presynaptic reuptake of both serotonin and norepinephrine. Some TCAs exert their actions primarily on serotonin reuptake (e.g., amitriptyline), others primarily on norepinephrine reuptake (e.g., desipramine), and some on both neurotransmitter systems (e.g., imipramine). From the previous discussion, it is clear why serotonin enhancement might be beneficial for PTSD patients. Blockade of adrenergic reuptake (which is also effective for panic disorder) probably exerts its therapeutic action either through enhancement of (presynaptic inhibitory) alpha$_2$ receptors and/or through downregulation of postsynaptic beta receptors. In either case, the end result is a reduction in adrenergic activity in the amygdala, PFC, and locus coeruleus. Randomized clinical trials with *imipramine* (Kosten, Frank, Dan, McDougle, & Giller, 1991) and *amitriptyline* (Davidson et al., 1990) but not *desipramine* (Reist et al., 1989) have demonstrated symptom reduction in PTSD patients.

One consequence of the effectiveness and benign side effect profiles of SSRIs and newer antidepressants has been a loss of investigator interest in older but still effective agents such as TCAs and MAOIs. A remarkable exception to this is a prospective study comparing imipramine with the hypnotic, chloral hydrate, among pediatric burn patients in which imipramine treatment was effective in treating young burn victims with acute stress disorder (Robert, Blakeney, Villarreal, Rosenberg, & Meyer, 1999).

Monoamine Oxidase Inhibitors

MAOIs block the intraneuronal metabolic breakdown of serotonin, norepinephrine, dopamine, and other monoamines. By preventing enzymatic destruction of these neurotransmitters, more is available for presynaptic release. Thus, their therapeutic action may result from downregulation of postsynaptic receptors and, possibly, by downregulating adrenergic activity in the locus coeruleus (Davidson, Walker, & Kilts, 1987). A randomized clinical trial with the MAOI, *phenelzine*, with Vietnam combat veterans was extremely successful in reducing reexperiencing and arousal PTSD symptoms (Kosten et al, 1991). Results have been mixed in open-label trials

(Davidson et al., 1987; Lerer, Ebstein, Shestatzky, Shemesh, & Greenberg, 1987; Milanes, Mack, Dennison, & Slater, 1984), and a small, methodologically flawed 5-week crossover study had negative results (Shestatzky, Greenberg, & Lerer, 1988). Finally, an open trial with the reversible MAO-A inhibitor, moclobemide (Neal, Shapland, & Fox, 1997) reported improvement in all three PTSD symptom clusters. Again, no formal testing of cognitive function was carried out in any of these investigations.

Newer Antidepressants

Mirtazepine

Mirtazepine has both serotonergic actions (blockade of postsynaptic 5-HT$_2$ and 5-HT$_3$ receptors) as well as action at presynaptic alpha$_2$-adrenergic receptors. In one randomized trial (versus placebo) (Davidson et al., 2003) and one open-label 8-week trial in Korea (Bahk et al., 2002), mirtazepine effectively reduced PTSD symptom severity. An interesting case report describes the usefulness of mirtazepine for traumatic nightmares (or for postawaking memory of such nightmares) among 300 refuges who had previously failed to benefit in this regard from other medications (Lewis, 2002).

Venlafaxine

Venlafaxine blocks presynaptic reuptake of norepinephrine and serotonin. It also has a much less potent effect on blocking dopamine reuptake. Although there have been promising reports, it has not been tested adequately as a treatment for PTSD (Hamner & Frueh, 1998).

Bupropion

Bupropion blocks presynaptic reuptake of norepinephrine and dopamine, but not serotonin. Anecdotal evidence and open trials suggests that it may be effective in PTSD (Canive, Clark, Calais, Qualls, & Tuason, 1998).

THE DOPAMINERGIC SYSTEM AND ANTIPSYCHOTIC MEDICATIONS

Dopamine

During uncontrollable stress, amygdala activation produces PFC dopamine release (Charney, 2004). There is evidence that dopamine D$_1$ receptor agonists can produce stress-induced PFC impairments in working memory (Zahrt, Taylor, Mathew, & Arnsten, 1997) and that both D$_1$ and D$_2$ receptor antagonists can prevent such cognitive deficits (Arnsten, 2000; Druzin, Kurzina, Malinina, & Kozlov, 2000).

Excessive dopamine release may have a role in PTSD hyperarousal, hypervigilence, and possibly in provoking the brief paranoid/psychotic states sometimes observed among PTSD patients. It is surprising how little PTSD research has focused on dopamine in comparison with neurotransmitters discussed previously. Elevated urinary and plasma dopamine concentrations have been found among PTSD subjects (Hamner & Diamond, 1993; Lemieux & Coe, 1995; Yehuda et al., 1994).

There is one report that the D2A1 dopamine receptor allele increases the risk for PTSD (Comings, Muhleman, & Gysin, 1996). It is interesting, in this regard, that PTSD patients with the D2A1 allele show more improvement in social functioning (but not depression or anxiety) following paroxetine treatment, in contrast to the PTSD patients who do not posses the D2A1 allele. Thus, the bad news is that this allele may increase risk of developing PTSD, but among those affected with this disorder, the D2A1 allele may be prognostic for better responsivity to SSRI treatment in social function, but not clinical symptoms.

Atypical Antipsychotic Medications

There is a small but growing literature on favorable results with atypical antipsychotic agents. This contrasts with a general consensus that conventional antipsychotic agents (e.g., chlorpromazine or haloperidol) have no place in PTSD treatment because of a very unfavorable risk–benefit ratio due to questionable clinical usefulness plus serious side effects, especially tardive dysknesia (Friedman et al., 2000). One the other hand, atypical antipsychotics have two actions, D_2 receptor blockade (which they share with conventional antipsychotics) and a unique $5\text{-}HT_2$ receptor antagonism. As a result, they not only have a much more benign side effect profile (e.g., rare extrapyramial complications), but also unique therapeutic actions, such as efficacy against negative symptoms of schizophrenia. In PTSD treatment, atypicals have usually been utilized as adjunctive agents for refractory patients who have failed to respond to SSRIs or other antidepressants. Although there is little empirical evidence to guide general practice, these medications are usually prescribed to ameliorate dissociation, hypervigilance/paranoia, psychosis, hyperarousal, irritability, and aggression. There have not been any systematic attempts to asses enhancement of cognition among PTSD patients treated with atypical antipsychotics. As with the vast majority of medications discussed in this review, the focus has been on symptom reduction with the implication that amelioration of intrusive recollections, dissociative, psychogenic amnesia, and global cognitive problems indicates the potential utility of those medications for improving more specific cognitive operations.

There are published reports on three antipsychotic medications: risperidone, quetiapine and olanzapine. Results from a randomized trial (Hamner, Faldowski, et al., 2003), an open-label trial (Monnelly, Ciraulo, Knapp, & Keane, 2003), and several case reports with *risperidone* as adjunctive therapy suggest that it reduces overall PTSD symptom severity in addition to reducing dissociative flashbacks and aggressive behavior. Similar findings have been obtained with *quetiapine* as an adjunctive agent in which an open-label trial (Hamner, Deitsch, Brodrick, Ulmer, & Lorberbaum, 2003), a retrospective client review (Sokolski, Densen, Lee, & Reist, 2003), and several case reports indicate beneficial effects in reducing PTSD symptoms among refractory patients who had failed to respond to SSRIs and other medications. Finally, a randomized trial with *olanzapine* (Stein, Kline, & Matloff, 2002) also indicated its effectiveness as an adjunctive agent in reducing PTSD symptoms among chronic patients who had failed to respond to other agents.

To summarize, what little research has been conducted on dopamine mechanisms in PTSD patients suggests that dopamine blockade might be a beneficial approach. Small open-label and randomized trials with atypical antipsychotics as adjunctive agents for nonrespondant chronic PTSD patients have been encouraging. Little more than PTSD symptom severity has been monitored in these trials but there are indications that successful treatment enhances PFC function in general and improves cognition with respect to working memory, information processing, dissociation, hypervigilance/paranoia, and psychotic symptoms.

SUMMARY

It is clear that PTSD is associated with impairments in cognitive function. Our growing understanding of the underlying pathophysiology of this disorder has gradually narrowed this focus to alterations in information processing, working memory, declarative memory, dissociation, and related symptoms. Neuropharmacological mechanisms associated with altered amygdala, hippocampal, and prefrontal cortex function include abnormal adrenergic, HPA, glutamatergic, GABAergic, serotonergic, and dopaminergic function. There are, potentially, a number of pharmacological interventions that might improve PTSD-related cognitive disruption while ameliorating clinical symptoms. With the exception of one study regarding the SSRI, paroxetine (Vermetten et al., 2003), this possibility has not been addressed systematically in clinical research. Hopefully, this important area will begin to receive the attention it deserves.

REFERENCES

American Psychiatric Association (in press). Practice guideline for the treatment of patients with acute stress disorder and posttraumatic stress disorder. *American Journal of Psychiatry.*

Anand, A., Charney, D. S., Oren, D. A., Berman, R. M., Hu, X. S., Capiello, A., & Krystal, J. H. (2000). Attenuation of the neuropsychiatric effects of ketamine with lamotrigine: Support for hyperglutamatergic effects of N-methyl-D-aspartate receptor antagonists. *Archives of General Psychiatry, 57,* 270–276.

Arnsten, A. F. T. (2000). Stress impairs PFC function in rats and monkeys: Role of dopamine D1 and norepinephrine alpha-1 receptor mechanisms. *Progress in Brain Research, 126,* 183–192.

Arnsten, A. F. T., & Jentsch, J. D. (1997). The alpha-1 adrenergic agonist, cirazoline, impairs spatial working memory performance in aged monkeys. *Pharmacology, Biochemistry, and Behavior, 58,* 55–59.

Bahk, W. -M., Pae, C. -U., Tsoh, J., Chae, J. -H., Jun, T. -Y., Chul-Lee, & Kim, K. -S. (2002). Effects of mirtazepine in patients with post-traumatic stress disorder in Korea: A pilot study. *Human Psychopharmacology, 17,* 341–344.

Baker, D. G., West, S. A., Nicholson, W. E., Ekhator, N. N., Kasckow, J. W., Hill, K. K., Bruce, A. B., Orth, D. N., & Gerociati, T. D. (1999). Serial CSF corticotropin-releasing hormone levels and adrenocortical activity in combat veterans with posttraumatic stress disorder. *American Journal of Psychiatry, 156,* 585–588.

Bardgett, M. E., Boeckman, R., Krochmal, D., Fernando, H., Ahrens, P. & Csernansky, J. G. (2003). NMDA receptor blockade and hippocampal neuronal loss impair fear conditioning and position habit reversal in C 57Bl/6 mice. *Brain Research Bulletin, 60,* 131–142.

Berigan, T. (2002a). Oxcarbazepine treatment of posttraumatic stress disorder. *Canadian Journal of Psychiatry, 10,* 973–974.

Berigan, T. (2002b). Gabapentin and PTSD (letter). *Journal of Clinical Psychiatry, 63,* 744.

Berigan, T. (2002c). Treatment of posttraumatic stress disorder with tiagabine. *Canadian Journal of Psychiatry, 8,* 788.

Berigan, T. R., & Holzgang, A. (1995). Valproate as an alternative in post-traumatic stress disorder: A case report. *Military Medicine, 6,* 318.

Berlant, J. L. (2003). Antiepileptic treatment of posttraumatic stress disorder. *Primary Psychiatry, 10,* 41–49.

Berlant, J. L., & van Kammen, D. P. (2002). Open-label topiramate as primary or adjunctive therapy in chronic civilian post-traumatic stress disorder: A preliminary report. *Journal of Clinical Psychiatry, 63,* 15–20.

Bonne, O., Brandes, D., Gilboa, A., Gomori, J. M., Shenton, M. E., Pitman, R. K., & Shalev, A. Y. (2001). Longitudinal MRI study of hippocampal volume in trauma survivors with PTSD. *American Journal of Psychiatry, 158,* 1248–1251.

Brady, K., Pearlstein, T., Asnis, G.M., Baker, D., Rothbaum, B., Sikes, C. R., & Farfel, G. M. (2000). Efficacy and safety of sertraline treatment of posttraumatic stress disorder. *Journal of the American Medical Association, 283,* 1837–1844.

Brannon, N., Labbate, L., & Huber, M. (2000). Gabapentin treatment for post-traumatic stress disorder. *Canadian Journal of Psychiatry, 45*, 84.

Braun, P., Greenberg, D., Dasberg, H., & Lerer, B. (1990). Core symptoms of posttraumatic stress disorder unimproved by alprazolam treatment. *Journal of Clinical Psychiatry, 51*, 236–238.

Bremner, J. D., Innis, R. B., Southwick, S. M., Staib, L., Zoghbi, S., & Charney, D. S. (2000). Decreased benzodiazepine receptor binding in prefrontal cortex in combat related posttraumatic stress disorder. *American Journal of Psychiatry, 157*, 1120–1126.

Bremner, J. D., Licinio, J., Darnell, A., Krystal, J. H., Owens, M. J., Southwick, S. M., Nemeroff, C. B., & Charney, D. S. (1997). Elevated CSF corticotropin-releasing factor concentrations in posttraumatic stress disorder. *American Journal of Psychiatry, 154*, 624–629.

Bremner, J. D., Randall, P. K., Vermetten, E., Staib, L. H., Bronen, R. A., Mazure, C., Capelli, S., McCarthy, G., Innis, R. B., & Charney, D. S. (1997). Magnetic resonance imaging-based measurement of hippocampal volume in posttraumatic stress disorder related to childhood physical and sexual abuse: A preliminary report. *Biological Psychiatry, 41*, 23–32.

Bremner, J. D., Vythilingam, M., Vermetten, E., Southwick, S. M., McGlashan, T., Nazeer, A., Khan, S., Vaccarino, L. V., Soufer, R., Garg, P. K., Ng, C. K., Staib, L. H., Duncan, J. S., & Charney, D. S. (2003). MRI and PET study of deficits in hippocampal structure and function in women with childhood sexual abuse and posttraumatic stress disorder. *American Journal of Psychiatry, 160*, 924–932.

Breslow, M. F., Fankhauser, M. P., Potter, R. L., Meredith, K. E., Misiaszek, J., & Hope, D. G., Jr. (1989). Role of γ-aminobutyric acid in antipanic drug efficacy. *American Journal of Psychiatry, 146*, 353–356.

Cahill, L., & McGaugh, J. L. (1996). Modulation of memory storage. *Current Opinion in Neurobiology, 6*, 237–242.

Canive, J. M., Clark, R. D., Calais, L. A., Qualls, C., & Tuason, V. B. (1998). Bupropion treatment in veterans with posttraumatic stress disorder: An open study. *Journal of Clinical Psychopharmacology, 18*, 379–383.

Chambers, R. A., Bremner, J. D., Moghaddam, B., Southwick, S., Charney, D. S., & Krystal, J.H. (1999). Glutamate and PTSD: Toward a psychobiology of dissociation. *Seminars in Clinical Neuropsychiatry, 4*, 274–281.

Charney, D. S. (2004). Psychobiological mechanisms of resilience and vulnerability: Implications for the successful adaptation to extreme stress. *American Journal of Psychiatry, 161*, 195–216.

Charney, D. S., Deutch, A. Y., Krystal, J. H., Southwick, S. M., & Davis, M. (1993). Psychobiologic mechanisms of posttraumatic stress disorder. *Archives of General Psychiatry, 50*, 295–305.

Chengappa, K. N. R., John, V., & Parepally, H. (2002). The use of topiramate in psychiatric disorders. *Primary Psychiatry, 9*, 43–49.

Clark, R. D., Canive, J. M., Calais, L. A., Qualls, C. R., & Tuason, V. B. (1999). Divalproex in posttraumatic stress disorder: An open-label clinical trial. *Journal of Traumatic Stress, 12*, 395–401.

Comings, D. E., Muhleman, D., & Gysin, R. (1996). Dopamine D_2 receptor (DRD2) gene and susceptibility to posttraumatic stress disorder: A study and replication. *Biological Psychiatry, 40,* 368–372.

Davidson, J., Kudler, H., Smith, R., Mahorney, S. L., Lipper, S., Hammett, E. B., Saunders, W. B., & Cavenar, J. (1990). Treatment of post-traumatic stress disorder with amitriptyline and placebo. *Archives of General Psychiatry, 47,* 259–266.

Davidson, J. R. T., Pearlstein, T., Londborg, P., Brady, K. T., Rothbaum, B., Bell., J., Maddock, R., Hegel, M. T., & Farfel, G. (2001). Efficacy of sertraline in preventing relapse of posttraumatic stress disorder: Results of a 28-week double-blind, placebo-controlled study. *American Journal of Psychiatry, 158,* 1974–1981.

Davidson, J. R. T., Rothbaum, B. O., van der Kolk, B.A., Sikes, C. R., & Farfel, G. M. (2001). Multicenter, double-blind comparison of sertraline and placebo in the treatment of posttraumatic stress disorder. *Archives of General Psychiatry, 58,* 485–492.

Davidson, J., Walker, J. U., & Kilts, C. (1987). A pilot study of phenelzine in posttraumatic stress disorder. *British Journal of Psychiatry, 150,* 252–255.

Davidson, J. R. T., Weisler, R. H., Butterfield, M. I., Casat, C. D., Connor, K. M., Barnett, S., & van Meter, S. (2003) Mirtazapine vs. placebo in posttraumatic stress disorder: A pilot trial. *Biological Psychiatry, 53,* 188–191.

Davies, M. F., Tsui, J., Flannery, J. A., Li, X. C., DeLorey, T. M., & Hoffman, B. B. (2004). Activation of alpha2 adrenergic receptors suppresses fear conditioning: Expression of c-Fos and phosphorylated CREB in mouse amygdala. *Neuropsychopharmacology, 29,* 229–239.

Davis, M. (2002). Role of NMDA receptors and MAP kinase in the amygdala in extinction of fear: Clinical implications for exposure therapy. *European Journal of Neuroscience, 16,* 395–398.

Davis, L. L., Nugent, A. L., Murray, J., Kramer, G. L., & Petty, F. (2000). Nefazodone treatment for chronic posttraumatic stress disorder: An open trial. *Journal of Clinical Psychopharmacology, 20,* 159–164.

Davis, M., & Whalen, P. J. (2001). The amygdala: Vigilance and emotion. *Molecular Psychiatry, 1,* 13–34.

De Bellis, M. D., Chrousos, G. P., Dorn, L. D., Burke, L., Helmers, K., Kling, M. A., Trickett, P. K., & Putnam, F. W. (1994). Hypothalamic–pituitary–adrenal axis dysregulation in sexually abused girls. *Journal of Clinical Endocrinology and Metabolism, 78,* 249–255.

De Bellis, M. D., Keshaven, M. S., Shiflett, H., Iyengar, S., Beers, S. R., Hall, J., & Moritz, G. (2002). Brain structure in pediatric maltreatment-related posttraumatic stress disorder: A sociodemographically matched study. *Biological Psychiatry, 52,* 1066–1078.

De Boer, M., Op den Velde, W., Falger, P. J., Hovens, J. E., De Groen, J. H., & Van Duijn, H. (1992). Fluvoxamine treatment for chronic PTSD: A pilot study. *Psychotherapy and Psychosomatics, 57,* 158–163.

Drake, R. G., Davis, L. L., Cates, M. E., Jewell, M. E., Ambrose, S. M., & Lowe, J. S. (2003). Baclofen treatment for chronic posttraumatic stress disorder. *Annals of Pharmacotherapy, 37,* 1177–1181.

Drugan, R. C., Ryan, S. M., Minor, T. R., & Maier, S. F. (1984). Librium prevents the analgesia and shuttlebox escape deficit typically observed following inescapable shock. *Pharmacology, Biochemistry, and Behavior, 21*, 749–754.

Druzin, M. Y., Kurzina, N. P., Malinina, E. P., & Kozlov, A. P. (2000). The effects of local application of D_2 selective dopaminergic drugs into the medial prefrontal cortex of rats in a delayed spatial choice task. *Behavioural Brain Research, 109*, 99–111.

Duman, R. S., Nakagawa, S., & Malberg, J. (2001). Regulation of adult neurogenesis by antidepressant treatment. *Neuropsychopharmacology, 25*, 836–844.

Escalona, R., Canive, J. M., Calais, L. A., & Davidson, J. R. (2002). Fluvoxamine treatment in veterans with combat-related post-traumatic stress disorder. *Depression and Anxiety, 15*, 29–33.

Falls, W. A., Miserendino, M. J., & Davis, M. (1992). Extinction of fear-potentiated startle: Blockage by infusion of an NMDA antagonist into the amygdala. *Journal of Neuroscience, 12*, 854–863.

Famularo, R., Kinscherff, R., & Fenton, T. (1988). Propranolol treatment for childhood posttraumatic stress disorder, acute type. *American Journal of Diseases of Children, 142*, 1244–1247.

Fesler, F. A. (1991). Valproate in combat-related posttraumatic stress disorder. *Journal of Clinical Psychiatry, 52*, 361–364.

Franowicz, J. S., Kessler, L., Dailey-Borja, C. M., Kobilka, B. K., Limbird, L. E., & Arnsten, A. F. T. (2002). Mutation of the alpha2A-adrenoceptor impairs working memory performance and annuls cognitive enhancement by guanfacine. *Journal of Neuroscience, 22*, 8771–8777.

Friedman, M. J. (1990). Interrelationships between biological mechanisms and pharmacotherapy of posttraumatic stress disorder. In M. E. Wolfe & A. D. Mosnaim (Eds.), *Posttraumatic stress disorder: Etiology, phenomenology, and treatment* (1st ed., pp. 204–225). Washington, DC: American Psychiatric Press.

Friedman, M. J. (1994). Neurobiological sensitization models of post-traumatic stress disorder: Their possible relevance to multiple chemical sensitivity syndrome. *Toxicology and Industrial Health, 10*, 449–462.

Friedman, M. J. (2002). Future pharmacotherapy for PTSD: Prevention and treatment. *Psychiatry Clinics of North America, 25*, 1–15.

Friedman, M. J., Davidson, J. R. T., Mellman, T. A., & Southwick, S. M. (2000). Guidelines for pharmacotherapy and position paper on practice guidelines. In E. B. Foa, T. M. Keane, & M. J. Friedman (Eds.), *Effective treatments for PTSD: Practice guidelines from the International Society for Traumatic Stress Studies* (pp. 84–105). New York: Guilford Press.

Friedman, M. J., McDonagh-Coyle, A. S., Jalowiec, J. E., Wang, S., Fournier, D. A., & McHugo, G. J. (2001). *Neurohormonal findings during treatment of women with PTSD due to childhood sexual abuse.* Symposium presented at the annual meeting of the International Society for Traumatic Stress Studies, New Orleans, LA.

Gelpin, E., Bonne, O., Peri, T., Brandes, D., & Shalev, A. Y. (1996). Treatment of recent trauma survivors with benzodiazepines: A prospective study. *Journal of Clinical Psychiatry, 57*, 390–394.

Gilbertson, M. W., Shenton, M. E., Ciszewski, A., Kasai, K., Lasko, N. B., Orr, S. P., &

Pitman, R. K. (2002). Smaller hippocampal volume predicts pathologic vulnerability to psychological trauma. *Nature Neuroscience, 5,* 1242–1247.

Goa, K. L., Ross, S. P., & Chrisp, P. (1993). Lamotrigine: A review of pharmacological properties and clinical efficacy in epilepsy. *Drugs, 46,* 152–176.

Goldberg, J. F., Cloitre, M., Whiteside, J. E., & Han, H. (2003). An open-label pilot study of divalproex sodium for posttraumatic stress disorder related to childhood abuse. *Current Therapeutic Research, 64,* 45–54.

Gould, E., McEwen, B. S., Tanapat, P., Galea, L. A. M., & Fuchs, E. (1997). Neurogenesis in the dentate gyrus of the adult tree shrew is regulated by psychosocial stress and NMDA receptor activation. *Journal of Neuroscience, 17,* 2492–2498.

Grant, S. J., Huang, Y. H., & Redmond, D. E. (1980). Benzodiazepines attenuate single unit activity in the locus coeruleus. *Life Sciences, 27,* 2231.

Habib, K. E., Weld, K. P., Rice, K. C., Pushkas, J., Champoux, M., Listwak, S., Webster, E. L., Atkinson, A. J., Schulkin, J., Contoreggi, C., Chrousos, G. P., McCann, S. M., Suomi, S. J., Higley, J. D., & Gold, P. W. (2000). Oral administration of a corticotropin-releasing hormone receptor antagonist significantly attenuates behavioral, neuroendocrine, and autonomic responses to stress in primates. *Proceedings of the National Academy of Sciences of the United States of America, 97,* 6079–6084.

Hamner, M. B., Brodrick, P. S., & Labbate, L. A. (2001). Gabapentin in PTSD: A retrospective, clinical series of adjunctive therapy. *Annals of Clinical Psychiatry, 3,* 141–146.

Hamner, M. B., Deitsch, S. E., Brodrick, P. S., Ulmer, H. G., & Lorberbaum, J. P. (2003). Quetiapine treatment in patients with posttraumatic stress disorder: An open trial of adjunctive therapy. *Journal of Clinical Psychopharmacology, 23*(1), 15–20.

Hamner, M. B., & Diamond, B. I. (1993). Elevated plasma dopamine in posttraumatic stress disorder: A preliminary report. *Biological Psychiatry, 33,* 304–306.

Hamner, M. B., Faldowski, R. A., Ulmer, H. G., Frueh, B. C., Huber, M. G., & Arana, G. W. (2003). Adjunctive risperidone treatment in post-traumatic stress disorder: A preliminary controlled trial of effects on comorbid psychotic symptoms. *International Clinical Psychopharmacology, 18,* 1–8.

Hamner, M. B., & Frueh, B. C. (1998). Response to venlafaxine in a previously antidepressant treatment-resistant combat veterans with post-traumatic stress disorder. *International Journal of Clinical Psychopharmacology, 13,* 233–234.

Heim, C., Newport, J. D., Bonsall, R., Miller, A. H., & Nemeroff, C. B. (2001). Altered pituitary–adrenal axis responses to provocative challenge tests in adult survivors of childhood abuse. *American Journal of Psychiatry, 158,* 575–581.

Heresco-Levy, U., Kremer, I., Javitt, D. C., Goichman, R., Reshef, A., Blanaru, M., & Cohen, T. (2002). Pilot-controlled trial of D-cycloserine for the treatment of post-traumatic stress disorder. *International Journal of Neuropsychopharmacology, 5,* 301–307.

Hertzberg, M. A., Butterfield, M. I., Feldman, M. E., Beckham, J. C., Sutherland, S. M., Connor, K. M., & Davidson, J. R. (1999). A preliminary study of lamotrigine for the treatment of posttraumatic stress disorder. *Biological Psychiatry, 45,* 1226–1229.

320   CLINICAL APPLICATIONS

Hertzberg, M. A., Feldman, M. E., Beckham, J. C., Moore, S. D., & Davidson, J. R. (2002). Three- to four-year follow-up to an open trial of nefazodone for combat-related posttraumatic stress disorder. *Annals of Clinical Psychiatry, 14,* 215–221.

Hidalgo, R., Hertzberg, M. A., Mellman, T., Petty, F., Tucker, P., Weisler, R., Zisook, S., Chen, S., Churchill, E., & Davidson, J. (1999). Nefazodone in posttraumatic stress disorder: Results from six open-label trials. *International Clinical Psychopharmacology, 14,* 61–68.

Iancu, I., Rosen, Y., & Moshe, K. (2002). Antiepileptic drugs in posttraumatic stress disorder. *Clinical Neuropharmacology, 25,* 225–229.

Jones, R. W., Wesnes, K. A., & Kirby, J. (1991). Effects of NMDA modulation in scopolamine dementia. *Annals of the New York Academy of Science, 640,* 241–244.

Kinzie, J. D., & Friedman, M. J. (2004). Psychopharmacology for refugee and asylum seeker patients. In J. P. Wilson & B. Drozdek (Eds.), *Broken spirits: The treatment of asylum seekers and refugees with PTSD.* New York: Brunner-Routledge Press.

Kolb, L. C., Burris, B. C., & Griffiths, S. (1984). Propranolol and clonidine in the treatment of the chronic post-traumatic stress disorders of war. In B. A. van der Kolk (Ed.), *Post-traumatic stress disorder: Psychological and biological sequelae* (pp. 97–107). Washington, DC: American Psychiatric Press.

Kosten, T. R., Frank, J. B., Dan, E., McDougle, C. J., & Giller, E. L. (1991). Pharmacotherapy for post-traumatic stress disorder using phenelzine or imipramine. *Journal of Nervous and Mental Disease, 179,* 366–370.

Krupitsky, E. M., Burakov, A. M., Ivanov, G. F., Krandashova, G. F., Lapin, I. P., Grinenko, A. J., & Borodkin, Y. S. (1993). Baclofen administration for the treatment of affective disorders in alcoholic patients. *Drug and Alcohol Dependence, 33,* 157–163.

Krystal, J., Bennett, A. L., Bremner, J. D., Southwick, S. M., & Charney, D. S. (1995). Toward a cognitive neuroscience of dissociation and altered memory functions in post-traumatic stress disorder. In M. J. Friedman, D. S. Charney, & A. Y. Deutch (Eds.), *Neurobiological and clinical consequences of stress: From normal adaptation to post-traumatic stress disorder* (pp. 239–269). Philadelphia: Lippincott-Raven.

Lemieux, A. M., & Coe, C. L. (1995). Abuse-related posttraumatic stress disorder: Evidence for chronic neuroendocrine activation in women. *Psychosomatic Medicine, 57,* 105–115.

Lerer, B., Ebstein, R. P., Shestatsky, M., Shemesh, Z., & Greenberg, D. (1987). Cyclic AMP signal transduction in posttraumatic stress disorder. *American Journal of Psychiatry, 144,* 1324–1327.

Lewis, J. D. (2002). Mirtazepine for PTSD nightmares (letter). *American Journal of Psychiatry, 159,* 1948–1949.

Li, B.-M., & Mei, Z.-T. (1994). Delayed response deficit induced by local injection of the alpha-2 adrenergic antagonist yohimbine into the dorsolateral prefrontal cortex in young adult monkeys. *Behavioral and Neural Biology, 62,* 134–139.

Liang, K. C., Hon, W., & Davis, M. (1994). Pre- and posttraining infusion of N-methyl-D-aspartate receptor antagonists into the amygdala impair memory in an inhibitory avoidance task. *Behavioral Neuroscience, 108,* 241–253.

Lipper, S., Davidson, J. R. T., Grady, T. A., Edinger, J. D., Hammett, E. B., Mahorney, S. L., & Cavenar, J. O., Jr. (1986). Preliminary study of carbamazepine in posttraumatic stress disorder. *Psychosomatics, 27*, 849–854.

Lonborg, P. D., Hegel, M. T., Goldstein, S., Goldstein, D., Himmelhoch, J. M., Maddock, R., Patterson, W. M., Rausch, J., & Farfel, G. M. (2001). Sertraline treatment of posttraumatic stress disorder: Results of weeks of open-label continuation treatment. *Journal of Clinical Psychiatry, 62*, 325–331.

Looff, D., Grimley, P., Kuller, F., Martin, A., & Shonfield, L. (1995). Carbamazepine for PTSD. *Journal of the American Academy of Child Adolescent Psychiatry, 6*, 703–704.

Mackowiak, M., O'Neill, M. J., Hicks, C. A., Bleakman, D., & Skolnick, P. (2002). An AMPA receptor potentiator modulates hippocampal expression of BDNF: An in vivo study. *Neuropharmacology, 43*, 1–10.

Macleod, A.D. (1996). Vigabatrin and posttraumatic stress disorder. *Journal of Clinical Psychopharmacology, 2*, 190–191.

Malek-Ahmadi, P. (2003). Gabapentin and posttraumatic stress disorder. *Annals of Pharmacotherapy, 37*, 664–666.

Mao, Z.-M., Arnsten, A. F. T., & Li, B.-M. (1999). Local infusion of alpha-1 adrenergic agonist into the prefrontal cortex impairs spatial working memory performance in monkeys. *Biological Psychiatry, 46*, 1259–1265.

Marmar, C. R., Schoenfeld, F., Weiss, D. S., Metzler, T., Zatzick, D., Wu, R., Smiga, S., Tecott, L., & Neylan, T. (1996). Open trial of fluvoxamine treatment for combat-related posttraumatic stress disorder. *Journal of Clinical Psychiatry, 57*, 66–70.

Marshall, R. D., Beebe, K. L., Oldham, M., & Zaninelli, R. (2001). Efficacy and safety of paroxetine treatment for chronic PTSD: A fixed-dose-placebo-controlled study. *American Journal of Psychiatry, 158*, 1982–1988.

Martenyi, F., Brown, E. B., Zhang, H., Koke, S. C., & Prakash, A. (2002). Fluoxetine v. placebo in prevention of relapse in post-traumatic stress disorder. *British Journal of Psychiatry, 181*, 315–320.

Martenyi, F., Brown, E. B., Zhang, H., Prakash, A., & Koke, S. C. (2002). Fluoxetine versus placebo in posttraumatic stress disorder. *Journal of Clinical Psychiatry, 63*, 199–206.

McEwen, B. S., Angulo, J., Cameron, H., Chao, H. M., Daniels, D., Gannon, M. N., Gould, E., Mendelson, S., Sakai, R., Spencer, R., et al. (1992). Paradoxical effects of adrenal steroids on the brain: Protection versus degeneration. *Biological Psychiatry, 31*, 177–199.

Mellman, T. A., Bustamante, V., David, D., & Fins, A. I. (2002). Hypnotic medication in the aftermath of trauma (letter). *Journal of Clinical Psychiatry, 63*, 1183–1184.

Milanes, F. J., Mack, C. N., Dennison, J., & Slater, V. L. (1984). Phenelzine treatment of post-Vietnam stress syndrome. *VA Practitioner*, 40–49.

Monahan, J. B., Handelman, G. E., Hood, W. F., & Cordi, A. A. (1989). DCS, a positive modulator of N-methyl-D-aspartate receptor, enhances performance of learning tasks in rats. *Pharmacology, Biochemistry and Behavior, 34*, 649–653.

Monnelly, E. P., Ciraulo, D. A., Knapp, C., & Keane, T. (2003). Low dose risperidone as adjunctive therapy for irritable aggression in posttraumatic stress disorder. *Journal of Clinical Psychopharmacology, 23*, 193–196.

Morgan, C. A., III, Krystal, J. H., & Southwick, S. M. (2003). Toward early pharmacologic post-traumatic stress intervention. *Biological Psychiatry, 53,* 834–843.

Morgan, C. A., III, Wang, S., Mason, J., Southwick, S. M., Fox, P., Hazlett, G., Charney, D. S., & Greenfield, G. (2000). Hormone profiles in humans experiencing military survival training. *Biological Psychiatry, 47,* 891–901.

Morgan, C. A., III, Wang, S., Rasmusson, A., Hazlett, G., Anderson, G., & Charney, D. S. (2001). Relationship among cortisol, catecholamines, neuropeptide-Y and human performance during exposure to uncontrollable stress. *Psychosomatic Medicine, 63,* 412–422.

Nacher, J., Alonso-Llosa, G., Rosell, D. R., & McEwen, B. S. (2003). NMDA receptor antagonist treatment increases the production of new neurons in the aged rat hippocampus. *Neurobiology of Aging, 24,* 273–284.

Nakazawa, K., Quirk, M. C., Chitwood, R. A., Watanabe, M., Yeckel, M. F., Sun, L. D., Kato, A., Carr, C. A., Johnston, D., Wilson, M. A., & Tonegawa, S. (2002). Requirement for hippocampal CA3 NMDA receptors in associative memory recall. *Science, 297,* 211–218.

Neal, L. A., Shapland, W., & Fox, C. (1997). An open trial of moclobemide in the treatment of post-traumatic stress disorder. *International Journal of Clinical Psychopharmacology, 12,* 231–232.

Okuyama, N., Takagi, N., Kawai, T., Miyake-Takagi, K., & Takeo, S. (2004). Phosphorylation of extracellular-regulating kinase in NMDA receptor antagonist-induced newly generated neurons in the adult rate dentate gyrus. *Journal of Neurochemistry, 88,* 717–724.

Paul, I. A., Nowak, G., Layer, R. T., Popik, P., & Skolnick, P. (1994). Adaptation of the N-methyl-D-aspartate receptor complex following chronic antidepressant treatments. *Journal of Pharmacology and Experimental Therapeutics, 1,* 95–102.

Peskind, E. R., Bonner, L. T., Hoff, D. J., & Raskind, M. A. (2003). Prazosin reduces trauma-related nightmares in older men with chronic posttraumatic stress disorder. *Journal of Geriatric Psychiatry and Neurology, 16*(3), 165–171.

Petty, F., Davis, L. L., Nugent, A. L., Kramer, G. L., Tetent, A., Schmitt, A., & Stone, R. C. (2002). Valproate therapy for chronic, combat-induced posttraumatic stress disorder. *Journal of Clinical Psychopharmacology, 1,* 100–101.

Pitman, R. K., Sanders, K. M., Zusman, R. M., Healy, A. R., Cheema, F., Lasko, N. B., Cahill, L., & Orr, S. P. (2002). Pilot study of secondary prevention of posttraumatic stress disorder with propranolol. *Biological Psychiatry, 51,* 189–192.

Post, R. M., Weiss, S. R. B., Li, H., Leverich, G. S., & Pert, A. (1999). Sensitization components of posttraumatic stress disorder; implications for therapeutics. *Seminars in Clinical Neuropsychiatry, 4,* 282–294.

Post, R. M., Weiss, S. R. B., & Smith, M. A. (1995). Sensitization and kindling: Implications for the evolving neural substrate of PTSD. In M. J. Friedman, D. S. Charney, & A.Y. Deutch (Eds.), *Neurobiological and clinical consequences of stress: From normal adaptation to post-traumatic stress disorder* (pp. 135–147). Philadelphia: Lippincott-Raven.

Rapaport, M. H., Endicott, J., & Clary, C. M. (2002). Posttraumatic stress disorder and Quality of life: Results across 64 weeks of sertraline treatment. *Journal of Clinical Psychiatry, 63,* 59–65.

Raskind, M. A., Peskind, E. R., Kanter, E. D., Petrie, E. C., Radont, A., Thompson, C.,

Dobie, D.J ., Hoff, D., Rein, R. J., Straits-Troster, K., Thomas, R., & McFall, M. M. (2003). Prazosin reduces nightmares and other PTSD symptoms in combat veterans: A placebo-controlled study. *American Journal of Psychiatry, 160*, 371–373.

Rasmusson, A. M., & Friedman, M. J. (2002). The neurobiology of PTSD in women. In R. Kimerling, P. Ouimette, & J. Wolfe (Eds.), *Gender and PTSD* (pp. 43–75). New York: Guilford Press.

Rasmusson, A. M., Hauger, R. L., Morgan, C. A., III, Bremner, J. D., Southwick, S. M., & Charney, D. S. (2000). Low baseline and yohimbine stimulated plasma neuropeptide Y (NPY) levels in combat-related PTSD. *Biological Psychiatry, 47*, 526–539.

Rasmusson, A. M., Lipschitz, D. S., Wang, S., Hu, S., Vojvoda, D., Bremner, J. D., Southwick, S. M., & Charney, D. S. (2001). Increased pituitary and adrenal reactivity in premenopausal women with PTSD. *Biological Psychiatry, 50*, 965–977.

Reist, C., Kauffman, C.D., Haier, R.J., Sangdahl, C., DeMet, E.M., Chicz-DeMet, A., & Nelson, J.N. (1989). A controlled trial of desipramine in 18 men with posttraumatic stress disorder. *American Journal of Psychiatry, 146*, 513–516.

Robert, R., Blakeney, P. E., Villarreal, C., Rosenberg, L., & Meyer, W. J., III (1999). Imipramine treatment in pediatric burn patients with symptoms of acute stress disorder: a pilot study. *Journal of the American Academy of Child and Adolescent Psychiatry, 38*, 873–882.

Roozendaal, B., McReynolds, J. R., & McGaugh, J. L. (2004). The basolateral amygdala interacts with the medial prefrontal cortex in regulating glucocorticoid effects on working memory impairment. *Journal of Neuroscience, 24*, 1385–1392.

Sapolsky, R. M. (2000). Glucocorticoids and hippocampal atrophy in neuropsychiatric disorders. *Archives of General Psychiatry, 57*, 925–935.

Saygin, M. Z., Sungur, M. Z., Sabol, E. U., & Cetinkaya, P. (2002). Nefazadone versus sertraline in treatment of posttraumatic stress disorder. *Bulletin of Clinical Psychopharmacology, 12*, 1–5.

Schelling, G., Briegel, J., Roozendaal, B., Stoll, C., Rothenhäusler, H. B., & Kapfhammer, H. P. (2001). The effect of stress doses of hydrocortisone during septic shock on posttraumatic stress disorder in survivors. *Biological Psychiatry, 50*, 978–985.

Schwartz, B. L., Hashtroudi, S., Herting, R. L., Schwartz, P., & Deutsch, S. I. (1996). D-cycloserine enhances implicit memory in Alzheimer patients. *Neurology, 46*, 420–424.

Schwartz, T. L. (2002). The use of tiagabine augmentation for treatment-resistant anxiety disorders: A case series. *Psychopharmacology Bulletin, 2*, 53–57.

Seedat, S., Lockhat, R., Kaminer, D., Zungu-Dirwayi, N., & Stein, D. J. (2001). An open trial of citalopram in adolescents with post-traumatic stress disorder. *International Clinical Psychopharmacology, 16*, 21–25.

Shestatzky, M., Greenberg, D., & Lerer, B. (1988). A controlled trial of phenelzine in posttraumatic stress disorder. *Psychiatry Research, 24*, 149–155.

Sokolski, K. N., Densen, T. F., Lee, R. T., & Reist, C. (2003). Quetiapine for treatment of refractory symptoms of combat-related post-traumatic stress disorder. *Military Medicine, 168*, 486–489.

Southwick, S. M., Krystal, J. H., Bremner, J. D., Morgan, C. A., Nicolaou, A. L., Nagy, L. M., Johnson, D. R., Heninger, G. R., & Charney, D. S. (1997). Noradrenergic and serotonergic function in posttraumatic stress disorder. *Archives of General Psychiatry, 54,* 749–758.

Southwick, S. M., Paige, S. R., Morgan, C. A., Bremner, J. D., Krystal, J. H., & Charney, D. S. (1999). Adrenergic and serotonergic abnormalities in PTSD: Catecholamines and serotonin. *Seminars in Clinical Neuropsychiatry, 4,* 242–248.

Stein, M. B., Kline, N. A., & Matloff, J. L. (2002). Adjunctive olanzapine for SSRI-resistant combat-related PTSD: A double-blind, placebo-controlled study. *American Journal of Psychiatry, 159,* 1777–1779.

Steward, J. T., & Bartucci, R. J. (1986). Posttraumatic stress disorder and partial complex seizures. *American Journal of Psychiatry, 1,* 113–114.

Stutzmann, G. E., & LeDoux, J. E. (1999). GABAergic antagonists block the inhibitory effects of serotonin in the lateral amygdala: A mechanism for modulation of sensory inputs related to fear conditioning. *Journal of Neuroscience, 11,* RC8.

Szymanski, H. V., & Olympia, J. (1991). Divalproex in post-traumatic stress disorder. *American Journal of Psychiatry, 8,* 1086–1087.

Taylor, F. B. (2003). Tiagabine for posttraumatic stress disorder: A case series of 7 women. *Journal of Clinical Psychiatry, 64,* 1421–1425.

Taylor, F. B., & Cahill, L. (2002). Propranolol for reemergent posttraumatic stress disorder following an event of retraumatization: A case study. *Journal of Trauma Stress, 15,* 433–437.

Thompson, L. T., Moskal, J. R., & Disterhoft, J. F. (1992). Hippocampus-dependent learning facilitated by a monoclonal antibody or D-cycloserine. *Nature, 356,* 638–641.

Tucker, P., Zaninelli, R., Yehuda, R., Ruggiero, L., Dillingham, K., & Pitts, C. D. (2001). Paroxetine in the treatment of chronic posttraumatic stress disorder: results of a placebo-controlled, flexible-dosage trial. *Journal of Clinical Psychiatry, 62,* 860–868.

VA/DoD Clinical Practice Guideline Working Group (2004). *Management of posttraumatic Stress.* Found at: *http://www.oqp.med.va.gov/cpg/PTS/PTS_base.htm*

Vaiva, G., Thomas, P. Ducroq, F., Fontaine, M., Boss, V., Devos, P., et al. (2004). Low posttrauma GABA levels as a predictive factor in the development of acute posttraumatic stress disorder. *Biological Psychiatry, 55,* 250–254.

Vaiva, G., Ducrocq, F., Jezequel, K., Averland, B., Lestavel, P., Brunet, A., & Marmar, C. R. (2003). Immediate treatment with propranolol decreases posttraumatic stress disorder two months after trauma. *Biological Psychiatry, 54,* 947–949.

van Ameringen, M., Mancini, C., Pipe, B., Campbell, M., & Oakman, J. (2002). Topiramate treatment for SSRI-induced weight gain in anxiety disorders. *Journal of Clinical Psychiatry, 63,* 981–984.

van der Kolk, B. A., Dreyfuss, D., Michaels, M., Shera, D., Berkowitz, R., Fisler, R., & Saxe, G. (1994). Fluoxetine versus placebo in posttraumatic stress disorder. *Journal of Clinical Psychiatry, 55,* 517–522.

van der Meulen, J. A., Bilbija, L., Joosten, R. N., de Bruin, J. P., & Feenstra, M. G.

(2003). The NMDA-receptor antagonist MK-801 selectively disrupts reversal learning in rats. *Neuroreport, 14,* 2225–2228.

Vermetten, E., & Bremner, J. D. (2002). Circuits and systems in stress. II. Applications to neurobiology and treatment in posttraumatic stress disorder. *Depression and Anxiety, 16,* 14–38.

Vermetten, E., Vythilingam, M., Southwick, S. M., Charney, D. S., & Bremner, J. D. (2003). Long-term treatment with paroxetine increases verbal declarative memory and hippocampal volume in posttraumatic stress disorder. *Biological Psychiatry, 54,* 693–702.

Viola, J., Ditzler, T., Batzer, W., Harazin, J., Adams, D., Lettich, L., & Berigan, T. (1997). Pharmacological management of posttraumatic stress disorder: Clinical summary of a five-year retrospective study, 1990–1995. *Military Medicine, 162,* 616–619.

Walker, D. L., & Davis, M. (2002). The role of amygdala glutamate receptors in fear learning, fear-potentiated startle, and extinction. *Pharmacology, Biochemistry, and Behavior, 3,* 379–392.

Wolfe, M. E., Alavi, A., & Mosnaim, A. D. (1988). Posttraumatic stress disorder in Vietnam veterans: Clinical and EEG findings; possible therapeutic effects of carbamazepine. *Biological Psychiatry, 23,* 642–644.

Xie, X., & Hagan, R. M. (1998). Cellular and molecular actions of lamotrigine: Possible mechanisms of efficacy in bipolar disorder. *Neuropsychobiology, 38,* 119–130.

Yehuda, R. (1999). Linking the neuroendocrinology of post-traumatic stress disorder with recent neuroanatomic findings. *Seminars in Clinical Neuropsychiatry, 4,* 256–265.

Yehuda, R. (2002). Current status of cortisol findings in post-traumatic stress disorder. *Psychiatry Clinics of North America, 2,* 341–368.

Yehuda, R., Boisoneau, D., Lowy, M. T., & Giller, E. L. (1995). Dose-response changes in plasma cortisol and lymphocyte glucocorticoid receptors following dexamethasone administration in combat veterans with and without posttraumatic stress disorder. *Archives of General Psychiatry, 52,* 583–593.

Yehuda, R., Giller, E. L., Southwick, S. M., Kahana, B., Boisoneau, D., Ma, X., & Mason, J. W. (1994). Relationship between catecholamine excretion and PTSD symptoms in Vietnam combat veterans and holocaust survivors. In M. M. Murburg (Ed.), *Catecholamine function in post-traumatic stress disorder: Emerging concepts* (pp. 203–220). Washington, DC: American Psychiatric Press.

Zahrt, J., Taylor, T. R., Mathew, R.G., & Arnsten, A. F. T. (1997). Supranormal stimulation of dopamine D1 receptors in the rodent prefrontal cortex impairs spatial working memory performance. *Journal of Neuroscience, 17,* 8525–8535.

Zarate, C. A., Quirox, J., Payne, J., & Manji, H. K. (2002). Modulators of the glutamatergic system: Implications for the development of improved therapeutics in mood disorders. *Psychopharmacology Bulletin, 4,* 35–83.

Zullino, D. F., Krenz, S., & Besson, J. (2003). AMPA blockade may be the mechanism underlying the efficacy of topiramate in PTSD. *Journal of Clinical Psychiatry, 4,* 219–220.

Index